FLEXIBLE INDIA

FLEXIBLE INDIA

YOGA'S CULTURAL

and

POLITICAL TENSIONS

SHAMEEM BLACK

Columbia University Press
New York

Columbia University Press
Publishers Since 1893
New York   Chichester, West Sussex
cup.columbia.edu

Library of Congress Cataloging-in-Publication Data
Names: Black, Shameem, 1976– author.
Title: Flexible India : Yoga's cultural and political tensions / Shameem Black.
Description: New York : Columbia University Press, [2024] |
Includes bibliographical references and index.
Identifiers: LCCN 2023024093 (print) | LCCN 2023024094 (ebook) |
ISBN 9780231206020 (hardback) | ISBN 9780231206037 (trade paperback) |
ISBN 9780231556286 (ebook)
Subjects: LCSH: Yoga—Social aspects. | Yoga—India.
Classification: LCC BL1238.52 .B58 2024 (print) | LCC BL1238.52 (ebook) |
DDC 181/.45—dc23/eng/20230914
LC record available at https://lccn.loc.gov/2023024093
LC ebook record available at https://lccn.loc.gov/2023024094

Printed in the United States of America

Cover design: Milenda Nan Ok Lee
Cover photo: Mo Eid / Pexels

FOR ANDY, SANYA, AND
JASPER, WITH LOVE

CONTENTS

ACKNOWLEDGMENTS

This book was written on unceded Ngunnawal and Ngambri land. I would like to begin by offering respect to the traditional custodians and their enduring traditions of sharing knowledge, and express my thanks that I can think and write on this country.

This manuscript started as work in motion. I first began to reflect on the possibilities of yoga's imaginative power as I pushed my children to sleep in their pram. Many of these ideas later took shape in the car on Canberra's roads. Years on, my children now outrace me down mountains. Though I may never clear the jumps on Mount Stromlo, finishing this book feels like a big leap.

In that time I have acquired many debts. When I joined the School of Culture, History and Language in the College of Asia and the Pacific at the Australian National University, I gained a wonderful community of colleagues who have broadened my thinking far beyond my comfort zone of traditional literary studies. I thank Andrew MacIntyre, Jacqueline Lo, Brij Lal, Ken George, and Simon Haberle for making this work possible. The College of Asia and the Pacific gave concrete assistance for fieldwork, symposia, and public events through research grants in the Asia-Pacific Innovation Program. I would like to thank Suzy Andrew, Dipika Nand, Joanna Cousins, Kirsten Farrell, and Gouri Banerji for their expertise and warmth. Collaborating with these professional staff in our school has allowed me to appreciate how much academic research relies on the work they do.

The ANU has been home to many inspiring scholars in South Asian studies who have shared their expertise and leads with me, including Assa Doron, Kirin Narayan, Ken George, McComas Taylor, Peter Friedlander, Meera Ashar, Stephanie Majcher, Chris Diamond, Aditya Balasubramanian, Dipesh Chakrabarty, Kuntala Lahiri-Dutt, Chaitanya Sambrani, Barbara Nelson, John Powers, Felix Pal, Annie McCarthy, Tanya Jakimow, and Anuradha Sajjanhar. I was fortunate to have the chance to convene a symposium on yoga with Patrick McCartney. I thank the ANU's South Asia Research Institute (SARI) for its role in encouraging exchanges of ideas, the Global Organisation of People of Indian Origin for collaborating on events for the International Day of Yoga, and YellowEdge consulting for the opportunity to share a vision of India through the lens of yoga to public servants. My undergraduate students and PhD candidates in South Asian studies have offered enthusiastic and insightful perspectives, as well as many great yoga stories.

Beyond the ANU's borders, many wonderful colleagues in South Asian studies have strengthened this work. I thank Joseph Alter and Andrea Jain for sharing their work on yoga with Australian audiences. I am grateful to the University of Michigan, SOAS University of London, the Australia India Institute, Jagiellonian University Institute for the Study of Religions, the Modern Yoga Research Group, Nanyang Technological University, the Jaipur Literature Festival, the Consul General of India in Melbourne, and the journals *South Asia*, *Race and Yoga*, *Australian Feminist Studies*, *Contemporary South Asia*, *The Asian American Literary Review*, and *Textual Practice* for opportunities to present and publish my research. I am grateful to all the academics involved, especially Kama Maclean, Suzanne Newcombe, Karen O'Brien-Kop, Craig Jeffrey, Matylda Ciolkosz, Balbinder Singh Bhogal, Theo Wildcroft, James Mallinson, Jatin Dua, Matthew Hull, Clemente Beghi, Wernmei Yong Ade, Jennifer Musial, Richard Robinson, and Barry Sheils.

I am deeply grateful to colleagues who have offered insights from the diverse fields of gender and cultural studies, anthropology, and literary studies. In my program in Gender, Media and Cultural Studies, I have benefited over the years from the conviviality and intellectual spark of my colleagues Hyaeweol Choi, Ariel Heryanto, Margaret Jolly, Peter Jackson, Katerina Teaiwa, Nayahamui Rooney, Ari Heinrich, Ross Tapsell, Janit Feangfu, Jen Mason, Roald Maliangkaij, and Ying Xin Show. I give warm thanks to Rosanne Kennedy, Lia Kent, Matt Tomlinson, Tanya Agathocleous, Debjani Ganguly, Maryam Wasif Khan, Trang Ta, Leslie Barnes, Shengyu Fan, Hannah McCann, and Monique Rooney, among others, for commenting on my work; engaging in discussions over conference panels, coffee shop tables, and Zoom; and giving me the benefit of their considerable expertise and kindness. Special thanks to Carol Hayes, who did not live to see this book in print, but whose inimitable voice of encouragement I still hear in the corridors.

This book reflects a broader desire to link academic thinking to creative work. As my program in Gender, Media and Cultural Studies has developed in this direction, I thank my school for letting me buy all those beautiful art materials. They are changing the way we as academics, PhD candidates, and students think by inviting us to use our hands as well as our heads. Parts of this book originated in writing workshops run with Kirin Narayan and Katerina Teaiwa, two colleagues who have created opportunities for creative and engaged research for Asian and Pacific studies and provided me with continual inspiration and support. Warm thanks to Kirin for reading parts of this manuscript, offering insights into how to weave critique with creativity, and hosting so many delicious lunches. I thank my academic collaborators Natasha Fijn and Shimona Kealy, along with our project manager, Sumithri Venketasubramanian and events manager Lea Collins, for bringing to life our School Flagship project *Cultural Creativity and Research in Asia and the Pacific*. I am grateful to the participants in my 2022 workshop "CUT: Deconstructing the Yoga Pant," and to Ginger Gorman at *BroadAgenda* for inviting me to reflect on this workshop for the University of Canberra's 50/50 by 2030 Foundation. Cutting up those pants and watching them transform into fresh, surprising shapes serves as a keen reminder of what yoga's flexible forms can offer.

Part of chapter 1 first appeared as "Yogic Style in Motion: Experiments in Power and Knowledge," *Textual Practice* 36, no. 4 (2022): 605–25.

Chapter 1 also draws on contextualizing material first presented in "State Spectacles of Yoga: Invisible India and India Everywhere," *South Asia: Journal of South Asian Studies* 46, no. 1 (2023): 1-17. Part of chapter 4 first appeared as "The Yoga Mysteries," *The Asian American Literary Review* 10, no. 1 (Spring/Summer 2019): 153–64. Parts of chapters 5 and 6 first appeared as "Flexible Indian Labor: Yoga, Information Technology Migration, and U.S. Technoculture," *Race and Yoga* 1, no. 1 (2016): 23–41. I am grateful to these journals for the ability to incorporate revised forms of my work in this book. I warmly thank the anonymous peer reviewers for Columbia University Press, whose insights and acumen have strengthened this work, Philip Leventhal for his sustained expertise and support as an editor, and Leslie Kriesel for outstanding copyediting and production editing. All errors are mine alone.

Thank you to all from beyond the borders of the university who have taught me in the course of writing this book. I owe a debt of gratitude to Alan Goode and the teachers at Yoga Mandir in Canberra for teaching me yoga and for collaborating with me on self-reflective yoga in the Australian university space. I am grateful to the advanced yoga practitioners who generously spoke with me in India and Singapore. This study would not have been possible without my parents and extended family in the United States and my family in India, Singapore, and the United Kingdom, who have shared with me their experiences, histories, and networks in the world of yoga. Although we are many miles apart, writing this has helped me feel closer to all of them.

Although this project has taken me into my family's past, I also see it as a passport to the future. This book is dedicated to my partner, Andy, without whose love, editorial eye, and endless school pickups I couldn't have written it, and to our children, Sanya and Jasper, on their own unique journeys within a flexible India.

NOTE ON TRANSLITERATION

I have aimed to balance precision and accessibility when I represent Sanskrit words in the Roman alphabet. As much as possible, I have been guided by the International Alphabet of Sanskrit Transliteration to represent the full range of Sanskrit sounds. However, for some commonly used words, diacritics can add more mystery than clarity. For these words I have retained familiar English spellings.

FLEXIBLE INDIA

PROLOGUE

The Bracelet

When I was ten, I bought a silver bracelet in Bombay. We often went to the silver markets with my aunt, who knew all the vendors of beautiful things in the city. In the crowded markets I stayed close to my mother. The air would have been warm, the skies would have glowed through the haze, the glass counters in the markets would have been smudged by the restless rubbing of hands. Around the corner there would have been fresh pomegranates squeezed into shakes so thick and rich and tangy I taste them thirty years on. The exchange would have been confusing. It would have necessitated the regal head sweeping of my aunt, whose long black hair, tossed just the right way, would indicate to the merchant what price we were willing to pay.

Endlessly flexible, soft-spoken, and luminous, the beauty of silver captured me right from the beginning. I loved the way silver took on the shape of one's imagination. I loved its balance of gleam and tarnish, lunar sheen, and generosity to geometric pattern and organic folly. I loved its quiet elegance, so distinct from the brazenness of the more expensive and voluble gold.

The metal of the bracelet was forged in intricate layers, seemingly infinite bands of tiny *v*'s framing a raised set of images. At the two ends were faces with bulbous cheeks and towering headdresses enclosing a script I could not read. But as soon as I saw the bracelet held written words, I knew it was mine. It was distant kin to the novels and poems that defined my world. It was silver language.

When I got back to my aunt's flat, I asked for help in reading the bracelet. My cousins looked at it. My aunt and uncle and mother looked at it. Among them, they could read Hindi, Marathi, Gujarati, Cantonese, and English. It wasn't any of those languages.

Over the years, the silver bracelet traveled with me. The raised script remained bright, while the silver surrounding it grew darker with each succeeding year. It enclosed my wrist at elegant dinner parties in India and at American school dances in crepe-papered lunchrooms. I wore it in polished marble halls when I was an undergraduate and when I walked those same halls in my first academic job. On the days when I couldn't recognize any dishes in an Indian restaurant or keep straight the order of Indian festivals, the bracelet kept me connected.

I wore it when I began to practice yoga in the basement of a university gym in Northern California. It flowed with me to studios where English on the walls mimicked the calligraphic curves of Devanagari script, form-fitting tops I couldn't afford sat alongside carafes of free organic tea, and I learned to let my voice loose into the rising notes of "Om" before and after a class.

Wearing silver always felt right. It went with jeans, it went with silk. It traveled well. When I moved to Australia, I left most of my jewelery in my mother's keeping, but I took the bracelet.

Three decades after the silver bracelet came into my hands, I wore it to lunch with a few colleagues from the fourth floor of the Baldessin building. The fourth floor was home to people who chanted in Sanskrit, sang in the Himalayas, read nineteenth-century Gujarati novels, and painted watercolors of Varanasi. We sat down together at a round table in the Street Theatre café. "Perhaps someone at this table can solve my thirty-year mystery," I said, handing them the bracelet. "What does this say?"

"It's Tibetan," one said immediately. Two colleagues peered over it together, working it out. They handed it to a third around the circle.

"It's your mantra," he said. "See, in Tibetan script, here is the *Om*." My flexible silver bracelet, bringing me full circle into this book.

1

SETTING UP

Yoga's Flexible Forms

I n 1984, in a Bombay living room, my uncle stands on his head. It's supposed to be good for his blood pressure. It's thirty years before a newly elected prime minister will declare a national ministry for yoga, create a United Nations day for the practice, and eventually preside over the largest yoga class in the world.

As India rises unevenly in economic clout and global standing, yoga is its cipher. When I was an eight-year-old with big glasses, I only saw my uncle's dark curls balanced beside the colonial cabinet that housed his Johnnie Walker. In this account of yoga's imaginative life in twenty-first-century English, I peer beyond the visible contours of postural practice to show how creative visions of yoga in popular fiction, digital media, public spectacle, and soft power strategies legitimate competing meanings of Indianness today. These visions, created by Indians, the Indian diaspora, and Westerners not of Indian descent, take shape in the controversial border zone of English that connects elements of India to public spheres beyond the nation's borders. Yoga offers a lens through which to understand key tensions in twenty-first-century ideas of India and Indianness, especially in light of national aspirations, capitalist expansions, global mobilities, political violations, and quests for cultural recognition. Challenging popular perceptions that yoga is primarily about spiritual growth or physical well-being, this book reframes yoga as a deeply political exercise in how to imagine the world.

David Gordon White declares that "'yoga' has a wider range of meanings than nearly any other word in the Sanskrit lexicon."[1] Like a palimpsest, the story of yoga is the tale of meanings inscribed upon meanings. Although it may be tempting to limit the iconic sign of modern yoga to a person in expensive engineered fabric stretching and sweating through a ninety-minute class, the fiction, media, art, and political spectacle that I bring to light portray a much more complex picture. In this book, I use the word "yoga" to signal a constellation of practices, traceable in some way to genealogies from the Indian subcontinent, that seek transformative person making through the disciplining of body, mind, or energy.[2] In creative works of the twenty-first century, yoga can appear as postural practice, breath control, mental discipline, religious devotion, philosophical perception, martial training, social service, and political critique (among other items). Complex histories echo through this sign, refracting the ideals and anxieties of social life in motion.

Yoga has been interpreted historically in many ways. The word once meant the yoke that harnesses bullocks to the plow, and this metaphor for connection continues to loom large in twenty-first-century accounts.[3] Through diverse philosophical, religious, and ascetic traditions, the language of yoga has offered tools to refine perceptions of the world and achieve liberation from nets of illusion.[4] In devotional practices, yoga can be described as a way to unite with the divine.[5] Yoga has provided a path for the pursuit of supernatural power and political strength, often through bodily austerity and religious ritual.[6]

At the turn of the millennium, the concept of yoga in English is informed not only by these enduring histories but also by the major transformations of Indian colonial modernity. In the late nineteenth and early twentieth centuries, as scholars have shown, yoga was imagined in new ways. Cosmopolitan physical culture, anticolonial activism, religious militancy, spiritual entrepreneurship, health and fitness norms, beauty ideals, capitalist imperatives, and social justice pursuits have all invoked the language of yoga to engage with emerging needs and goals.[7] As scholars have shown, many elements that have contributed to the making of modern yoga come from well beyond the South Asian region.[8] The changes wrought in this period, amplified by the intensive takeup of yoga in the twentieth and twenty-first centuries, have shaped how yoga is portrayed in a mobile English. Without judging representations of yoga as authentic or inauthentic, this book aims to evaluate the political and social significance of twenty-first-century creative work that appears under yoga's sign.

Who is such yoga for? Diverse representations from this century show both change and continuity in the history of the practice. Early textual sources from India envision the yogi as a sage from a mystical tradition who inhabits the margins of mainstream life.[9] From that imagined starting point, where the idealized yogi is male, ascetic, and detached from society, yoga has become a practice suited in at least in some respects to distinctly different conditions. Through capitalist consumerism, spiritual entrepreneurship, mass media, and public health programs, yoga in India and internationally has expanded its reach. Once a practice largely for men without household responsibilities, it has grown popular with women facing unending demands on their paid and unpaid labor.[10] Yet, at the same time, the practice has often continued to serve patriarchal hierarchies and prescriptive ideas of gender.[11] While elite controls over yogic teachings have yielded to broader access for more people, powerful mechanisms—such as the pricing strategies of the market or social perceptions about which castes, classes, bodies, or races truly belong—have continued to govern how yoga has spread.[12] The nuances of these demographic changes have played out around the world in relation to local intersecting hierarchies that include caste, religion, gender, race, ethnicity, class, and ability. Exploring the tensions between expanded access and resilient hierarchy, this book unfolds an account of how yoga's imaginative power can be used to support competing ends.

Is yoga primarily a tool for liberation or an instrument of oppression? Entering an important debate within the study of yoga, I suggest that the world of imagination offers evidence for both. I will explore how yoga can be imagined as free and freeing, yet costly and constraining at the same time. Like Farah Godrej, whose work explores how racial capitalism and state violence can find both ally and adversary in the practice of yoga,[13] I linger on the tension between these different possibilities. Mapping how cultural visions of yoga help to reconfigure hegemonies within ideas of India, and how they work to question social hierarchies, is a key purpose of this book.

One strand of *Flexible India* critiques how yoga is often imagined in flexible ways to mask or perpetuate inequalities. Advocates of a right-wing Hindu nationalism, committed to seeing India as a sanctified Hindu land rather than as a liberal secular state, have sometimes imagined yoga as a path to restoring an ideal that relies on hierarchies and exclusions, especially of caste, gender, and religion. Banking on globalized discourses that portray yoga as a practice of peaceful cosmopolitanism, healthy living, and progressive politics, such advocates can recruit unsuspecting allies across the world to enshrine yoga more deeply within ideals that reinforce ideologies of inequality. Although the history of yoga is significant to a wide range of people, including those oppressed for their caste or gender,[14] many globally circulating images of yoga purposefully or inadvertently bolster the claims to legitimacy of hegemonic social systems. Visions of the practice thus sometimes create points of agreement between secular liberalism and Hindu nationalism, often seen as adversaries. Although many cultural practices in twenty-first-century India are seen to exemplify "culture wars" between liberal and conservative agendas, *Flexible India* argues that images of yoga in English can offer a "culture peace," or a set of unwitting allies and concealed contradictions, that mask such tensions in India and beyond. This allows states, corporations, and people to think of themselves as welcoming and tolerant, even if they continue to support practices that render minority or subjugated populations increasingly vulnerable.

Elements of this study will thus confirm the power of yoga to delude, seduce, and subjugate. As Andrea R. Jain argues in *Peace Love Yoga* (2020), yoga is frequently harnessed for "gestural subversions" that critique capitalist or political inequalities at a surface level but remain aloof from deeper change.[15] Gestural subversion can be found within the landscape of yoga in English-language creative work. So too can points where yoga is used to render individuals complicit in their own exploitation, a yogic imaginative capacity articulated by Lee Siegel in *Trance-Migrations* (2014) as the power to hypnotize.[16] Waving a peacock feather, the yogi as storyteller invents fictional worlds designed to reveal deeper reality to the listener. But to be hypnotized, as *Trance-Migrations* reveals, can involve surrender to capitalist extraction, sexual violation, and imperial power. As a metaphor for Gramscian hegemony, yogic hypnosis is so disturbing because the hypnotist continually insists that he (and it usually is a he) cannot make the hypnotized do anything they do not really desire. Such nets of coercion continue to shadow the narrative landscape I explore.

In looking to the world of artistic imagination, I also reveal how yoga can be called upon to offer critically reflective tools that expose hierarchical structures of power. Although imaginative work cannot be expected to usher in political or economic transformation on its own, it can shift perceptions by making normalized or invisible structures of power more seeable. This capacity has made it useful for a wide range of practitioners.[17] To enhance yoga's resources for political critique, I remix the traveling yogic concept of *svādhyāya*, a Sanskrit word that traditionally means studying texts in isolation. Rethought through twentieth-century contexts of practice, *svādhyāya* has come to carry the new responsibility of "studying oneself," as a tool to promote critical reflection. This remixed *svādhyāya* offers a lens through which to explore written and visual creative work from India, its diaspora, and the West, where yoga is used for self-studies that expose the illusions used to justify hierarchies of power. By building interpretative tools and amplifying imaginative voices, yoga can offer political critique on changing ideas of Indianness. A remixed *svādhyāya* can also provide a potential yogic counter-optic for the commodified or hypnotized subject, exposing how the pernicious and liberatory elements of the practice can be deeply entangled. This vision offers a twenty-first-century reinterpretation of a long-standing aspiration for yoga: to see the contours of a previously invisible world.

WHY ENGLISH?

The sojourns of yoga through novels, poems, videos, tourist campaigns, political speeches, court cases, and many other cultural texts bring to light fierce quests for power over visions of India. When the villain is an old Indian guru who kills with a fake Sanskrit text, a female tantric who murders through mantras, or an assassin who deploys banned chemical weapons, we witness new stories of Indianness trying to be born. From such imaginary deaths arise new, and often surprising, cultural life.

Flexible India argues that imaginative visions of yoga in English project new powers onto the practice that rewrite what it means to be Indian in a twenty-first-century world. By tracking yoga's sojourns in the English language, I seek to bring fresh insight from fictional stories, visual culture, and political spectacle to the current boom in scholarship on yoga, which has grown into a sizable field since Mircea Eliade's *Yoga: Immortality and Freedom* (1954).[18] Both extending and undoing my past research as a scholar of postcolonial literature in English, this book brings approaches from literary and cultural studies to illuminate written and visual creative work. Building on the work of anthropologists, historians, and religious studies scholars who have explored yoga's modern historical transformations in response to competing social demands,[19] I bring together creative voices of the Indian state, Indian writers, the Indian diaspora, and Westerners without ethnic or national ties to India. Their visions of yoga in the twenty-first century allow contradictory ideas of Indianness to flourish.

The full story of yoga is told across many languages.[20] In the South Asian context, yoga is deeply informed by Sanskrit, Tamil, Tibetan, Persian, and many other textual genealogies. In this century, yoga has been linked to the heightened political prominence of Hindi, even as imaginative work from other Indian languages reminds us how ideas of yoga have long shaped ways of knowing in different regional approaches.[21] Internationally, yoga can be found in a wealth of popular culture, where works as diverse as French novels, Chinese tourism videos, and Korean horror films all turn to the practice to respond to key changes of the new millennium. Each linguistic tradition brings new depth and possibility for the practice. The meanings of yoga that are articulated through multiple South Asian and non-South Asian languages, which lie beyond the scope of this book, may well bring to light social, political, and philosophical valences that are distinctly different from the ones I explore. These possibilities offer exciting future directions for comparative multilingual scholarship.

Within this broader linguistic landscape, yoga in English represents a significant and distinctive phenomenon. English served as an influential language through which yoga was remediated and reproduced in the twentieth century in India. "Modern, transnational yoga was and is a predominantly anglophone phenomenon," argues Mark Singleton in *Yoga Body* (2010).[22] English was used to promote dialogue among north Indians, south Indians, and Westerners in influential ashrams, was deployed to articulate visions of yoga beyond India's borders in twentieth-century print culture, and came to constitute part of a larger discourse of Indian religious cosmopolitanism that Srinivas Aravamudan calls "Guru English."[23] Picking up where Aravamudan leaves off, I explore the changing valence of this tradition as it is shaped by twenty-first-century anxieties. While yoga has afforded some opportunities for Indians to expand their authority in a transnational frame, it has also become a new space where Aravamudan's gurus *lose* their English to new publics. This contest over authority is part of what makes yoga in English worth watching.

Yoga in English is especially significant because this phenomenon draws attention to India's ongoing engagements with colonialism and capitalism. These forces have developed English into an Indian language with its own distinctive history, often in relation to other Indian languages.[24] The history of that English has long been shaped by ongoing debates about its own Indianness, so much so that anxiety has come to govern the particular way that the language belongs to India. In this context, yoga and English occupy contradictory, yet twinned symbolic roles that embed questions of Indianness in both content and form. Yoga is often portrayed as ancient, indigenous, and spiritual, while English is often assumed to be hypermodern, imported, and technocratic. Imaginative discourses of yoga seek to resolve the anxieties of Indianness created by and through English while capitalizing on the benefits that have flowed to and from the language. Interweaving close readings of literary studies with remixed concepts from yogic traditions, social and economic histories, and autoethnographic reflections, I seek to show how yoga and English engage questions of Indianness in multiple and entangled ways. These readings challenge the assumption that "yoga" is authentically Indian while "English" remains forever foreign. Instead, their dialectical engagement envisions multiple flexible Indias where colonial and capitalist logics cannot be wished away, but must be negotiated time and again.

Over the past decade, my research has uncovered dozens of creative texts in English that envision something they all call "yoga" alive in diverse social worlds. These works of imagination resurrect spiritual seekers in the icy Himalayas, mock the spandex societies of Los Angeles, and track assassins in mystical lands. Yoga has journeyed into the heart of genres as different as urban fantasies, realist novels, spiritual quests, social satires, life writings, murder mysteries, legal judgments, confessional poetry, chick lit, soft porn, tourist advertisements, and mockumentary dramas. I analyze creative works from India, the United States, Canada, the United Kingdom, Singapore, and New Zealand, drawing on in-country fieldwork and primary research conducted over eight years. India and the United States offer the largest bodies of primary evidence, so I consider them in the most depth.

As I mapped repeated themes across authors, nations, and genres, an insistent set of preoccupations began to take shape in handwritten notes that encircled my office walls. Expanding Hindu nationalism, multicultural social negotiations, global capitalist labor politics, and social justice aspirations all organically rose to prominence. In selecting which texts to linger on, I have chosen ones that illustrate these key themes in detail, reveal connections across creative texts from different parts of the world, and present a diverse ecology of literary and visual form. Complementing sociology, communications, and media studies, where scholars have analyzed the codes and patterns that shape representations of yoga in periodical culture, social media, and pop culture,[25] I bring a literary scholar's interpretative lens and a commitment to close readings to explore these creative works.

Found in the marketing blazes of mainstream presses and in the shadowy worlds of self-publishing, some works may be household names, while for others, I may well be their only close reader. Over the years, academic colleagues as well as acerbic uncles have wondered aloud why I have chosen to write about curious novels or obscure poems. These niche works are valuable, I suggest, for two reasons. First, works that fly below the radar of establishment gatekeepers provide a particularly vivid window into uncensored cultural logics. The very rawness of these writings exposes vivid power dynamics that are often muffled within, but vital to, more mainstream articulations. Second, other works go unnoticed by mainstream readers because they challenge dominant groups to reconsider their points of privilege. These texts may not have many readers, but they should. Writing about them is one way to share these critical perspectives with a broader audience. In calling attention to this diverse range of imaginative practice, I show how yoga in English is used to legitimate unseen norms of possibility for new flexible Indias across borders.

This book begins with a close look at English cultural production in India and expands to investigate visions of yoga in spaces where English connects India to other parts of the world. Although this landscape by no means captures the totality of such images, I aim to showcase dynamic and dominant spaces where changing concepts of India are taking shape. Inspired by what Tessa Morris-Suzuki calls "liquid area studies," my approach takes imaginative visions as both "flows" and "vortices" that challenge conventional divides among area, ethnic, and diaspora studies.[26] Visions of yoga flow across borders through traveling texts. Even and especially in periods where the mobility of people has been blocked, the mobility of words and images through English has shaped social meanings for the practice. At the same time, visions of yoga form vortices that compress diverse voices in English from India, its diaspora, and the West, joining the political implications of individual cultural practice with the cultural politics of states.

HOW YOGA SHAPES IDEAS OF INDIA

Flexible India explores how yoga is used to imagine India at a moment of political and cultural rise. Its first major concern is the theoretical question of what constitutes "India" and "Indianness" at particular historical junctures. Ideas of India, under any circumstances, are diverse and contested, often mixing plurality and expansiveness with exclusion and othering.[27] But yoga adds a new complication. Unlike in well-studied culture industries such as Bollywood, where Indian casts and production teams predominate, people of all different nationalities, ethnicities, and backgrounds practice yoga. Yoga thus raises intriguing theoretical questions about where its Indianness might lie, especially as people around the world pursue its techniques under deracinated health and wellness regimes. Political spectacle and imaginative storytelling produce and legitimate flexible ideas of Indian identity within such expansion.

While the story of yoga has unfolded over many centuries, the twenty-first century has seen it ascend to new heights. Yoga has caught the eye of public health officials seeking to combat disease, corporations hoping to capitalize on a sizable industry, and government officials aiming to capture its benefits for national gain. This landscape encompasses rising Indian ambitions for greater international influence, anxieties brought by economic liberalization, globalized political violence, and quests for cultural recognition within and beyond national borders. Yoga has loomed even larger as India has confronted the ravages of a worldwide pandemic.

I explore how and why such a cultural practice may work to address specific national contradictions in a world of economic and social transformation. Mapping the explosion of state support for yoga in Narendra Modi's first term as India's prime minister (2014–2019), *Flexible India* reads this newfound state enthusiasm against a transnational world of energetic popular culture. Exploring how yoga has assumed new power in Modi's India as a globally acceptable way to promote projects that appeal to the Hindu right, I build on interdisciplinary work on the reach of expanding Hindutva, or the idea of India as a nation with a fundamentally Hindu essence.[28] Bringing to light new empirical bodies of Indian and Western creative work, I illuminate the expanding cultural logics that connect these worlds. Western popular fiction and media can be recruited as an unexpected ally for Hindu nationalism beyond India's borders. Visions of yoga are thus used to shape an image of a new flexible India for the twenty-first century.

The second major concern of this study is investigating ideas of Indianness in the context of racial and gendered politics beyond the nation's borders. I focus on the United States, where a large yoga industry, coupled with a long history of migration from India and a complex history of racial inequality, bring these ideas into stark relief. U.S. representations of yoga and Indianness are informed by broader anxieties over race, gender, identity, and status, which have made questions of cultural recognition urgent preoccupations. In the first decades of the new millennium, an enthusiasm for the rise of Indian culture has sometimes emerged at the expense of actual Indians. Demographic data on yoga practice in the United States suggests that yoga is often taught within "an industry run by and for White women."[29] The rhetoric of cultural appropriation calls attention to this dissonance: cultural practices can be celebrated to such an extent that people from those practices' homelands are erased from the picture, while benefit flows are redirected toward more dominant social groups. As Amanda Lucia has shown, yoga can be used to produce "white utopias" that perpetuate landscapes of inequality.[30] Practitioners who embrace yoga without considering these dynamics may cultivate flexible personhoods that implicate them within political projects they may not consciously want to support.

Here I offer a fresh perspective on how to think about cultural recognition within a complex U.S. racial landscape. Broader attempts to decenter Western narratives of whiteness inform debates about the Indianness of yoga. In some cases, Hindu nationalist yoga advocates present themselves as marginalized, thus aligning themselves with the social justice claims of other U.S. minorities, while simultaneously promoting majoritarian views that reaffirm Hindu-centric and upper-caste definitions of ideal Indianness. At other points, Indian (and more broadly, South Asian) diasporic yoga advocates take more critical positions, challenging the hegemonies associated with whiteness and with Hindu nationalism. By looking at this diversity of voices, I contribute to broader conversations about how ideas of Indianness can be used to negotiate questions of recognition.

These questions emerge within a time of significant pressure on the U.S. yoga industry to acknowledge its implications within intersectional racial politics. As Stephanie Evans's *Black Women's Yoga History* (2021) and Cara Hagan's *Practicing Yoga as Resistance* (2021) show, yoga has long offered value to U.S. communities of color in navigating the perils of life within landscapes of racial inequality. Yet these histories often remain invisible within mainstream accounts, even as diverse practitioners of color, including African American, Native American, Latinx, and other U.S. racialized minority groups, seek to understand the social significance of their practice.[31] Works of the imagination can bring to light the lived complexity of yoga and the ambivalent meaning that the signifier "India" plays in this U.S. conversation.

The third thematic concern of this book links racial and gendered politics to economic structures by investigating yoga in the context of global capitalism, transnational labor, and the cultural logics of neoliberalism. As Andrea Jain, Sarah Sharma, and Laurah Klepinger have revealed, the increased global popularity of yoga is deeply indebted to capitalist exchanges, neoliberal paradigms, and structures of labor inequality in which individuals are expected to seek freedom and flourishing through the market.[32] Building on these accounts, I show how imaginative visions of yoga may create "a capitalist provision that provisions capitalism."[33] These visions reveal how practices of incorporation can help to make capitalism intimate, embodied, and resilient.

Yoga, I argue, can be imagined as a set of practices that promote capitalist projects of self-making through the illusion of being outside capitalist values of exchange. In different landscapes, these illusions have taken different shapes. In India, access to yoga has often been made most affordable through the devotional regimes of spiritual empires, where mass yoga camps offer alternatives to expensive studio models that remain out of reach for many. Attendees pay for admission by opening themselves to the spiritual and political claims of the yoga providers. These beliefs can also shape them as proto-consumers of spiritual wellness products and practices in the context of caste, gender, religious, and ethnic hierarchies. In Western and other Asian contexts, where market mechanisms have loomed large, access to yoga has been shaped not only by the price of a class but also by unstated social norms about what kind of body belongs in such a space. These differing sites of incorporation (and exclusion) offer insights into how capitalism shapes regimes of personhood. Precisely because yoga in both postural and devotional inflections offers a self-help tool for navigating the precarious nature of modern life, exposing its economic reliance on uneven and unpredictable labor structures hints at the need to confront these contradictions. Stories and spectacles help to establish where and how yoga recruits new bodies to neoliberal ideas of labor under capitalism, and where and how it promotes alternative ways of thinking and feeling, helping us gain a clearer sense of how visions of yoga both reinforce capitalist logics and introduce notes of self-reflective critical dissonance.

The fourth concern, which draws most directly on my past work in literary theory, involves cross-cultural representation. For cultural, ethnic, and diaspora studies, this book offers a renewed assessment of what Satya Mohanty has called "discursive domination," or representation that constrains others considered to be socially different from an assumed norm.[34] I examine where discursive domination still flourishes, and where cultural practices like yoga may offer a promising approach for projects of cross-cultural recognition. Precisely because many yoga philosophies promote visions of ultimate values, a rising number of practitioners concerned with social justice have inquired how the practice might engage with difference without embracing inevitably partial universals or insisting upon insurmountable signs of perpetual otherness.

As I show across multiple chapters, yoga continues to be imagined through structures of discursive domination that should trouble us. In some cases, imaginative representations of yoga from outside India's borders attest to the durable dynamics of Said's Orientalism, in which India becomes knowable as an ancient source of spiritual exoticism. In other cases, the idea of India is rendered completely irrelevant as the flow of yoga's benefits is channeled toward Western practitioners. And in yet other cases, Indian image producers have offered self-Orientalized visions that serve the needs of particular groups within the broader landscape of global capitalism. In multiple cases, it can be argued that complex ideas of India are flattened into predictable commodities.

Yet these durable logics are not without challenge. In the most theoretically intriguing set of creative texts, cultural representations of yoga inquire how multicultural practitioners can productively engage with ideas of India beyond a dynamic of domination. Looking at their experiments as a form of remixed *svādhyāya*, or critical self-reflection, I investigate how yogic storytellers seek to create new voices capable of a different approach. The most promising efforts at cross-cultural representation invite us to think directly about the problem. Drawing on the theories of representation I advanced in *Fiction Across Borders* (2010), I argue that borders are most effectively crossed when stories give substantial attention to their own positions of privilege and make sacrifices to reduce inequalities. Without subscribing to philosophically and historically untenable ideas of uncontaminated cultural practice, the new voices I examine encourage their audiences to consider the potential dissonance between the hypervaluation of a cultural product and the undervaluation of people from that culture. Thus these works forward a productive yoga-inspired way to cross-cultural representation. When harnessed for such self-study, visions of yoga can potentially inspire resistance to injustice, exploitation, and hierarchy.

Finally, the fifth dimension of this study, which for me has been its most transformative, is the layering of different voices. At various points, personal essays frame key ideas from a more intimate point of view. Drawing on experiences that have shaped me as a scholar, I see in yoga a metaphor for the flexibility in identity and practice often demanded of India's diaspora. In personal spaces defined by borders, gaps, silences, and fault lines, the common English translation of yoga as a "join" or "yoke" takes on new resonance. Clarity of broader perception emerges through careful study of the self as it positions itself in new and challenging poses. I use writing to conduct a self-study that aims to yield greater clarity about the surrounding world. This aspiration leads me to yoke life writing to scholarly analysis. The most hopeful finding of this book is that yoga works best for social justice and democratic connection when it is understood in a self-reflective way. As part of a broader yoga community of scholar-practitioners, I seek to let a life of practice inform my writing.[35]

This method finds strength from traditions that challenge impersonal scholarly voice, especially within feminist and ethnic studies. Like Nancy

Miller, Saidiya Hartman, Ann Cvetkovich, and Carrie Preston (to name only a few), I turn to life writing as a theoretical mode that may say what critical analysis alone cannot.[36] This approach joins the work of writers in South Asian studies, such as Sara Suleri, Amitava Kumar, Kirin Narayan, and Lee Siegel, who for decades have enlarged the literary styles—and thus the ways of knowing—found in academic writing.[37] Weaving ethnography, close reading, life writing, history, and fiction, they animate the power of imagination within analytical work.

Flexible India builds in particular on the writings of Narayan and Siegel, who are both, in very different ways, drawn to yoga. From Narayan I find inspiration in the power of family story. In *My Family and Other Saints* (2007), Narayan invites us to ask how spiritual quests shape and reshape what a family can be across national and cultural divides. This book is informed by my experiences as a member of a Shia Muslim family once based in Gujarat and reshaped by colonial and postcolonial circuitry connecting India, Hong Kong, the United States, and Australia. Like Narayan, I grew up "hahlf and haylf" in a multiracial family, insider and outsider to many worlds at once, and the questions set in motion by those experiences propel this book.[38] From Siegel's writing, I draw on the power that speculation can proffer. As academics we live into our subjects, even to the point where we might seem in their thrall. I have drawn comfort from predecessors like Siegel who ask what can be gained by making ourselves vulnerable, allowing ourselves to be hypnotized by our subjects even as we seek to expose their illusions.[39] Yoga has put me in unusual positions from which I seek to learn.

FLEXIBILITIES IN MOTION

Through the intensified spread of postural practice in the 1990s, yoga has come to conjure the ideal of flexibility. Yet this ideal goes beyond supple anatomy. As the primary metaphor for this study, flexibility can be understood as a project of resilience, sustaining and sometimes revitalizing particular power relations in times of stress and change. We can think of it as the quest to extend in different directions, to adjust to changing conditions, to meet the expectations of competing demands, and to bend without breaking. Such flexibility may be physical, spiritual, social, and/or political, often at the same time. In working with this metaphor, I draw strength from conceptual frameworks that have sought to understand how the emergence of flexibilities may also testify to rigid boundaries. This dialectic is a key part of this book.

As a way of thinking about identity and belonging in the context of political border making, the flexibility promised through yoga can be considered in light of Catherine Malabou's philosophical concept of plasticity. Through Hegel, Malabou approaches plasticity as "a capacity to receive form and a capacity to produce form."[40] She argues that "the process of plasticity is dialectical because the operations which constitute it, the seizure of form and the annihilation of all form, emergence and explosion, are contradictory."[41] The flexibility of yoga is most overtly imagined in ways that call attention to receiving form: a person becoming, literally or metaphorically, more capable of taking on new shapes. Through yoga, diverse groups of people can be asked to adjust their senses of self, nation, community, or value to suit the needs of changing political structures, whose contours form the metaphorical molds into which individuals are expected to flow. That can both conceal and expose plasticity's dialectical investment in the powers producing (or annihilating) such forms. In this way, the flexibilities sought through visions of yoga are not only exemplars of adaptive change but also integral to understanding the survival of invisible structural rigidities.

These rigidities emerge in key political spaces that judge and define belonging. The flexibilities projected onto yoga, and the India it can signify, thus invite us to consider the ongoing resonance of Aihwa Ong's "flexible citizenship," a critical vocabulary for emergent global mobilities in the 1990s, defined as "the cultural logics of capitalist accumulation, travel, and displacement that induce subjects to respond fluidly and opportunistically to changing political-economic conditions."[42] In Ong's work, the word "flexible" challenges the authority of the nation-state. Whereas once states authorized a fixed set of rights, the turn of the millennium shed light on "the assemblage"—a lively mix of state and nonstate actors, such as refugee camps, cyberspaces, and cit-ies—as places for political claims.[43] The potential fragility of the state under these conditions could be understood as part of Zygmunt Bau-man's concept of "liquid modernity," or a moment of transition in which modern sovereign institutions had become weak.[44] State author-ity could be challenged by the flexibilities of the neoliberal market.

Yet as Ong also argued, flexibility soon became a tool for states to define new power for themselves. In the first decades of the twenty-first century, such flexibilities yielded what Ravinder Kaur has articulated in *Brand New Nation* (2020) as the new enclosing of nations. In this process, the global flows of capital investment do not break down the nation; instead, they contain it. Like my silver bracelet, these flows appear to bend to the contours of the emerging postcolonial nation while they also encircle that national identity into a fixed form. The nation becomes what Kaur calls "an income-generating asset: a new imaginary of the national territory as an infrastructure-ready enclo-sure for capital investment, its cultural identity distilled into a com-petitive global brand and its inhabitants—designated as demographic dividend—income-generating human capital that can be plowed back to generate more economic growth."[45] The widespread practice of nation branding in the early 2000s, a time of high economic optimism for countries like India, treated the nation as a capitalist product that must be differentiated from others through clear imaginative bound-aries. In this sense, the flexibilities that once might have challenged the state now lie at the heart of state policy, direction, and identity. The metaphor of flexibility thus links mobility with fixity.

Flexibility further sheds light on the paradoxes shaping India's dias-pora, often considered the largest diaspora in the world. Although—or because—in the early twenty-first century many people experienced more voluntary mobility than at any other time in the modern era, nations like India simultaneously expanded and constrained ideas of national belonging. Whereas the state of India in the early twentieth century showed limited desire to claim a connection to its overseas population, the 1990s inaugurated a process of selective recognition that created strategic flexibilities in the concept of citizenship. These twenty-first-century overseas citizenship regimes, designed to enclose and manage India's diaspora, reveal how the creation of such flexibilities can reflect the hardening of national borders.[46] Within emerging enclosures, certain kinds of subjects could be hailed as belonging to India: those with capital and those with documentation (such as proof of domiciles, passports, and birth certificates) could become legible and desirable to the state. Other subjects were excluded. Even before India's Citizenship Amendment Act of 2019, widely seen as a discriminatory anti-Muslim approach to citizenship, schemes available to India's diaspora created very particular forms of recognition, often defining India against Pakistan and Bangladesh, excluding applicants whose Indian parent had passed away, or relying on documentation that was particularly difficult for women to procure. Such forms of flexible belonging to India, therefore, were also part of a broader project of enclosing and recognizing an idealized but incomplete diaspora.

In seeking to explore changing ideas of India and Indians in the world, I build upon Purnima Mankekar's concept of "unsettlement." Mankekar's work articulates how the idea of India emerges through regimes of affect and temporality within transnational public cultures. She argues that in these public cultures, the idea of India is profoundly "unsettled"—a term that beautifully captures the way national and diasporic perspectives mutually alter each other. "Unsettlement," Mankekar argues, "occurs on two registers here: at the level of subject formation, as when subjects are formed through unsettlement; and as a framework for thinking about the relationship between media, public culture, and culture/cultural change."[47] It signals a dense affective experience felt by many Indians both in India and in the diaspora. It also offers "an analytic toward a feminist project of denaturalizing and unpacking the totalizing claims of nationhood."[48] Such a project inspires and sustains *Flexible India*.

If "unsettlement" captures the dissonances within competing ideas of India, "flexibility" points to the creative work that conceals these contradictions and thus renders them more resilient. Flexibility as an imaginative formation is useful to the state, which has deployed the practice to build alliances with and demand recognition from communities that hold competing political beliefs. A portable practice like yoga exemplifies an ideal of flexibility that can complement or compensate for some of the twenty-first-century limitations that have constrained belonging and mobility in an Indian context. Yoga has often been able to travel in ways that people from India, or of Indian descent, have not. It has thus rendered certain ideas of India mobile while concealing the material exclusions shaping Indian bodies. In this sense, yoga can offer a metaphor for the twinned rise of seeming opposites that have shaped the early decades of the millennium and peaked with the global pandemic: world networks coupled with national enclosures, seemingly endless image circulation paired with hardened political boundaries, and tolerant universalism hand in hand with fundamentalist ideologies.

The flexibility projected through and onto yoga is sometimes envisioned as a specifically Indian cultural contribution that resonates with its Hindi and Punjabi sister art *jugaad*. Amit Rai defines the twenty-first-century colloquialism *jugaad* as a "makeshift way of getting around obstacles."[49] Whether we understand it as workaround problem solving for the poor, frugal innovation in neoliberal business discourse, or everyday life improvisational performance culture, *jugaad* both extends and contests global capitalism. Management discourse, extolling *jugaad* as "*doing more with less*" through "flexible thinking and action,"[50] has been quick to hail it as an exemplary practice that contrasts with more formalized Western modes of innovation. Such literature praises creative workarounds as moral entrepreneurship while often obscuring attention to the underlying structural problems that prompt them. Yet, as Rai's ethnography shows, *jugaad* is far more complex. Its flexibilities can be turned to many ends, sometimes compelling businesses to respond to the needs of subaltern consumers, sometimes allowing subaltern voices to thrive despite obstacles, and sometimes creating new resilience for the tyranny of gender and caste hierarchies. Yoga also has been imagined as an ideal Indian tool to resolve problems linked to national aspirations and global capitalism, yet its flexibilities yield both utopian and dystopian possibilities. Complementing the technological space where *jugaad* reigns supreme, yoga reveals how analogue personmaking projects produce flexibilities both hegemonic and resistant.

Flexibility, as a concept applied to personhood, helps to illuminate competing demands and quests for power. Debates about culturally specific forms of Indian personhood since the mid-twentieth century have contrasted a Western image of the "individual" with an Indian experience of being "dividual," or a person called into being through transactions that expand relationships throughout the course of a lifetime.[51] Assa Doron intervenes by introducing the idea of the "nodal person" to capture changing forms of Indianness in the twenty-first century. Personhood emerges through relationships with connective objects (exemplified by the mobile phone), which allow particular people to develop forms of selfhood that are at once individualistic and nested within social obligations.[52] Focusing on visions of a cultural practice rather than of a physical object, I stretch this idea to suggest that the imaginative and performative dimensions of yoga construct flexible forms of selfhood as a response to competing ideal visions of Indianness. The metaphor of the flexible person yokes neoliberal understandings of individualized self-perfection and relational understandings of community resilience. It also reveals how a particular person may be flexibly invested in political and social goals at odds with each other. This concept of "flexible personhood" thus contributes to broader conversations in South Asian studies that explore the diverse ways personhoods dynamically engage both individual and collective dimensions.[53]

Finally, the metaphor of flexibility invites us to locate its power within what seems to be its most familiar world, yet in other ways is its most recent domain: the universe of bodily health and fitness. In the late eighteenth century, the word "flexibility" in English usually described the pliant or adaptive qualities of objects, language, or thought. Its link to human anatomy emerged first through music, indicating the movability of voice and fingers. Not until the mid-nineteenth century did the *Oxford English Dictionary* record a meaning that refers to the mobility of human limbs within physical exercise. In the 1860s, colonial publications in South Asia, such as *The Pioneer*, reflected this new attention to muscular flexibility in the context of army drills.[54] By the 1870s, lozenges were sold in India to promote "flexibility, agility, and power of the muscles"[55]—a promise that suggests how flexibility had gained new value as a physical ideal of fitness that could be pursued through the market.

The intimacy between yoga and flexibility took some time to develop, and it did so in highly gendered ways. From the 1920s on, as scholars have shown, yoga as a postural practice flourished within an emergent transnational culture of health and fitness.[56] Mark Singleton argues that Western cultures of fitness from the mid-nineteenth century onward tended to emphasize strength for male bodies and suppleness for female ones.[57] This gendered division shaped how Indian yoga was imagined within health and fitness as well. Yoga promoted for men a strong masculine body suitable for anticolonial activism. In contrast, flexibility in its own right represented a modern, health-oriented way to promote femininized virtues. European women in India, for instance, were encouraged to take up stretching in emulation of Burmese dancers, whose "trained flexibility is a grace" and "who never become fat."[58] Such promises (or coercions), over time, have insinuated themselves into the heart of yoga as a health and fitness practice, both in India and beyond. Grounded in an illusion of effortlessness, flexibility as an ideal conceals relentless gendered discipline, both bodily and social, at work.

In this book, I look upon flexibility with both yearning and fear. It is my strength. In practicing yoga, in the extension of limbs, I am opened into histories, stories, and sensations that expand the boundaries of personhood. When my shoulders pull back, my dignity rises. Yet I cannot ignore the histories through which this flexibility, so generative for me in some ways, also extends social expectations about my body, my time, and my value.

Flexibility, enshrined as a goal within the imagined worlds of health and fitness, is always about something just out of reach. Fitness culture of the twenty-first century, in India and beyond, has been propelled by capitalist structures of labor (in my university world, the chairs, desks, and screens) that lead to bodily problems that workers are expected to correct with their own time, money, and energy. This responsibility can lead to a gendered, as well as classed, "'third shift' of fitness practices" that follows a first shift of paid labor and a second shift of household work.[59] In India, analogous to global trends elsewhere, this third shift has emerged as a response to the economic liberalization of the 1990s, which helped to create an aspirational middle class for whom physical fitness exudes moral and professional value.[60] The imperative is also distinctively national. In 2019, India launched the Fit India Movement to promote an active population. Borrowing grandeur from the moral seriousness of the Quit India campaign, the Fit India movement asks citizens to make the following pledge: "I promise to myself that I will devote time for physical activity and sports every day and I will encourage my family members and neighbours to be physically fit and make India a fit nation."[61] Especially during the global pandemic, yoga was heavily promoted by the Indian government as a fitness practice that could be done under lockdown conditions. The pursuit of fitness as a dedicated activity, ennobled as the work of disciplined, moral, beautiful, and potentially wealthy people, conceals economic and political systems at work.

As a fitness practice, yoga prompts questions: Just what are we trying to be fit for? Just what are we fitting into? Just what, and who, does not fit?

REMIXING *SVĀDHYĀYA*: BUILDING THE TOOLS

The floorboards press up. Beyond the striated blackness of the backs of my eyelids, sound waves take shape in the air. Words fall down to the wood. One day, a new set of syllables flutters into ears, onto skin, into the hollow of chests extended upward. "*Svādhyāya* is self-study." Over time, this word takes different shapes. It perches on a metal chair. It lies on the floor. It entangles bent knees. Unlike most words I know, it does not write itself in clear script across my mind. It is nowhere to be found in the book of life that my brain is constantly writing and reading. It is all sound wave, all motion.

In order to challenge some of the flexible formations within which yoga is enlisted, I turn to yoga's past for inspiration. Drawing on diverse Indian texts that include philosophical writings, stone inscriptions, imperial accounts, postural manuals, and modern fiction, I describe here a twentieth-century Indian reinterpretation of the Sanskrit yogic concept of *svādhyāya*, sometimes translated into English as "self-study." Once used to describe one kind of textual encounter, the recitation of memorized texts, *svādhyāya* has developed over time to denote a different kind of textual practice: a dynamic and embodied observational inquiry that analytically connects selfhoods to structures.[62] This remixed *svādhyāya* offers a critical tool that can help to enhance yoga's imaginative resources for political critique in the twenty-first century.

Exploring the creative potential of Indian yogic histories speaks to my broader interest in contributing to projects of decolonizing knowledge. By working with ideas from South Asian genealogies, I join a widespread critique of assumptions that the West provides theoretical form while non-Western sites, such as India, simply provide empirical content. Scholars in Asia, inspired by the suggestive possibilities of Takeushi Yoshimi's 1960 lecture on "Asia as Method," have argued for decoloniality as a project that refuses the Western dominance of concepts and frames without retreating into nationalist essentialism. For Ichiyo Muto, decolonizing means "we must soberly recognize how power originating in the West is exercised globally, nationally, locally, nay in all creases of our brains and must find ways to overcome it."[63] Such an overcoming, famously articulated by Dipesh Chakrabarty as "provincializing Europe," remains an ongoing project.[64]

However, while concepts linked to the roots of precolonial societies can be celebrated in some places as means of resistance to ongoing colonial and capitalist dispossession, India presents an ambivalent story. In twenty-first-century India, concepts of civilizational deep time have been reanimated not to support Adivasi or other communities understood as indigenous[65] but to justify majoritarian agendas linked to cultural expressions of right-wing Hindu nationalism. This position, given significant shape in the early twentieth century, contends that India was once a Hindu civilization whose grandeur diminished through the Mughal and British empires. According to this line of thought, India should seek to revive its glorified Hindu past to rise on a world stage. India's politicians have therefore routinely invoked ancient texts to inform their aspirations for India's future.[66] This idealized Hindu past is frequently implicated in hierarchies of gender, caste, and religion, placing many Indians in subordinated social positions. Suhas Palshikar argues that this project of "religio-cultural homogenisation" and "the search for Hindu cultural hegemony" is growing in strength in twenty-first-century India.[67] Even movements not identified as Hindu nationalist can direct followers toward utopian visions that bolster this hegemony.[68] Yoga—a practice that can be seen to offer a pathway to such an idealized past—has gained new visibility as an emblem of India that can suit the needs of Hindu nationalism.[69]

Often linked to these elite hierarchies of gender, caste, and religion, textual elements of yoga may need their own decolonizing.[70] Sanskrit, the language most closely identified with the roots of yoga, is often extolled as a perfect language for a perfected Hindu society, yet access to Sanskrit has been historically limited for those not upper caste or male.[71] "Coming from a lower-caste background, I personally have no attachment to Sanskrit," writes Prachi Patankar. "In fact, I reject it as a language of 'divine knowledge' that was only available to brahmins. It was used as a means to keep spiritual knowledge away from the majority of the people so they would have no choice but to follow the brahmins' edicts on ritual and spiritual practice."[72] In India's northeast, where diverse indigenous and Christian communities challenge Indian state authority, Arkotong Longkumer shows how Sanskrit serves as an imperial tool for Hindu nationalists to reinscribe the region as Indic.[73] For many Indians, the sound of Sanskrit is the sound of being left out or being taken over.

Gods, imagined in particular ways, also do their part to uphold imperial ideas. Shiva, a deity associated with yoga in contexts that include twentieth-century colonial and twenty-first-century Indian government accounts,[74] has been recruited as the hero of Amish Tripathi's best-selling Shiva trilogy, which offers a worldview befitting soft Hindutva and neoliberal nationalism. These novels dramatize an ancient political utopia known as Ram Rajya, or the rule of Ram, which India's Bharatiya Janata Party (BJP), the mainstream political party associated with Hindutva, has invoked to project its political ambitions.[75] ' "[Lord Ram] created our systems, our rules, our ideologies, everything,"' declares one character in *The Immortals of Meluha* (2008), the first book in the trilogy. '"The term 'Ram Rajya' is considered the gold standard in how an empire must be administered, in order to create a perfect life for all its citizens."' Shiva is impressed: '"[Ram] must have been quite a man! For he truly created a paradise right here on earth." '[76] Far from contesting empire as an unjust form of political governance, such visions recuperate imperial ambitions for Hindutva imaginaries. Although Shiva offers some critique of the social hierarchies that underpin Ram's supposedly perfect world, the novel is frequently compatible with popular visions that glorify an idealized Hindu past.

There is a clear danger, then, in looking to India's yogic histories. Such a project may seem all too close to textual practices where exclusionary visions of nationalism justify gendered, caste-based, and religious hierarchy. Those practices participate in projects of decolonizing insofar as they seek strength in non-Western modalities, but they leave undisturbed, and sometimes even justify, other discourses of domination. I do not wish to give yoga's past, and its generative possibilities for the present, over to such ends. Yoga has been, and can be, more than a simple tool for elite power. Although decolonizing knowledge requires much more than looking to an Indian past replete with its own hierarchies and hegemonies, I suggest that a process of reflective remix may offer critical tools for yoga in the twenty-first century.

At this point, I might turn to the more hopeful legacies of the north Indian Sant, or poet-saint, movements where yoga has grown in the context of spiritual quests open to all castes, genders, and religions. Often led by those of the lowest caste, Sant traditions have provided a wellspring of inspiration for egalitarian politics in modern India. In these *bhakti* traditions anchored in devotion, influenced by Nath yogis and Sufi mystics, understandings of yoga are often focused on meditative practices.[77] Sant gurus have drawn upon Vedic teachings to articulate an egalitarian yoga of sacred light and sound, realizing a more radical potential within those teachings than the upper-caste orthodoxy they are often seen to support.[78] Spiritual liberation, in these traditions, requires social justice and rejection of discriminatory systems of caste.[79]

Such Sant beliefs have informed the spiritual life of influential Dalit political figures.[80] Although these traditions can themselves be bent to serve the interests of the powerful, their yoking of spiritual quests to social demands for equality offers powerful inspiration for yoga in the twenty-first century.

Instead I turn to a concept from within the heart of elite tradition: *svādhyāya*. Although it may seem perverse, *svādhyāya* has called to me because it exemplifies the contradictions propelling me to write this book. Like scholars of years past, I was trained within established institutions where socially dominant forms of race, class, gender, and religion took their authority for granted. Over time, I've come to question many of the things I learned, thought, and believed in those stone courtyards and walled libraries. I find redemptive the idea that concepts created to serve one set of masters can be changed, stretched, and transformed until they yield new possibility.

Svādhyāya claims a genealogy in Vedic texts dating to approximately 1000–800 B.C.E. In tracing the concept across texts that include the *Brāhmaṇas* and *Manu*, Dermot Killingley argues that *svādhyāya* signified a textual practice in which a person (assumed to be male) would recite a memorized section of the Vedas without the presence of a teacher and outside the context of a separate ritual. With time, *svādhyāya* came to constitute its own merit-making ritual that helped to transmit the Vedas orally.[81] *Svādhyāya* served as a multidimensional person-making activity, conferring "brahminhood (*brāhmaṇya*), appropriate behaviour (*pratirūpa-caryā*), fame (*yaśas*) and social status (*loka-pakti*)."[82] The practice of recitation was thus linked to a deepened understanding of revelatory knowledge, the accumulation of social capital for elite men, and the mnemonic stability of Vedic texts. The potential transformations available through this seemingly static practice emerge in Patañjali's *Yogasūtra*, estimated by Philipp Maas to have been composed and compiled between 325 and 425 C.E.[83] *Svādhyāya* reappears as one of the five observances, or *niyamas*, of yoga. As translated by James Mallinson and Mark Singleton, Patañjali's text reads, "(2.44) From recitation [arises] union with one's chosen deity."[84] Repetition—of spoken words or hierarchical social structures—appears to be key.

While one strand of *svādhyāya* concerns the divine, evidence of *svādhyāya* in medieval periods suggests that the concept could also signify social standing. In this period, *svādhyāya* came to be seen as one of the five major kinds of Vedic sacrifice.[85] Archaeological surveys, produced through the University of Mysore under M. H. Krishna in the late 1920s, document stone inscriptions with the word *svādhyāya*. In three stone inscriptions dated approximately to 1065–1085 C.E. and written in Kannada, patrons setting up sites for a deity are described as "possessed of *Yama* (restraint), *Niyama* (discipline), *Svâdhyâya* (study), *Dhyâna* (meditation), *Dhârana* (keeping the mind collected), *Mauna* (silence), *Anushthâna* (performance of duties), *Japa* (repetition of sacred formulae) and *Samâdhi* (absorption in holy thought)."[86] The repetition of these attributes across three epigraphs suggests that *svādhyāya* was associated with elite capital and religious worthiness.

Portraits of *svādhyāya* seen by cultural outsiders offer a glimpse of how the concept might operate within dynamics of cross-cultural engagement. Like many other aspects of yogic practice, *svādhyāya* was of interest to Mughal emperors as a way of understanding their Hindu subjects. In the late sixteenth century, Abu al-Fazl, Akbar's court historian, produced the Persian *Ā 'īn-i Akbarī* to cast Hindu philosophy in a favorable light for an elite Muslim audience.[87] This vision of *svādhyāya* presents a practice aimed at liberation, gesturing toward a world not fully under imperial Mughal control. Audrey Truschke argues that while British scholars tended to assimilate Indian systems of learning to their own categories, Abu al-Fazl's approach could not simply be equated with discourses of domination. "Abu al-Fazl's basic goal," Truschke argues, "revolved around integrating Sanskrit discourses within Mughal learning in order to drastically change the latter in accordance with Akbar's royal wisdom."[88] From the heart of imperial power may emerge subversive forms of cross-cultural engagement that lend historical resources for decolonizing reinterpretations of what Sanskrit concepts like *svādhyāya* can offer.

With the modern yoga renaissance of the twentieth century, the meaning of *svādhyāya* shifted from reciting memorized texts in isolation to a concept invested in new ideas of the self. One of the most influential figures to remediate *svādhyāya* in twentieth-century yogic practice was B. K. S. Iyengar, who helped to popularize yoga as a postural practice in the mid-twentieth century.[89] Inspired by neo-Vedantic ideas and devotional Srivaisnavism as well as by Theosophy and Harmonialism,[90] Iyengar helped to reshape yoga through the institutions he created; the popular writing, such as instruction manuals, that he produced; and the transnational brand he fostered.[91] *Light on Yoga* (1966), which became an enduring twentieth-century text on yoga in English, represents a cross-cultural recasting of key yogic concepts.[92] Iyengar remediates *svādhyāya* to speak to social needs within a transnational mid-twentieth-century moment.

> Sva means self and adhyāya means study or education. Education is the drawing out of the best that is within a person. Svādhyāya, therefore, is the education of the self.
>
> Svādhyāya is different from mere instruction like attending a lecture where the lecturer parades his own learning before the ignorance of his audience. When people meet for svādhyāya, the speaker and listener are of one mind and have mutual love and respect. There is no sermonising and one heart speaks to another. The ennobling thoughts that arise from svādhyāya are, so to speak, taken into one's bloodstream so that they become a part of one's life and being.
>
> The person practicising svādhyāya reads his own book of life, at the same time that he writes and revises it.[93]

In contrast to the earlier Sanskrit emphasis on a subject working in isolation, *Light on Yoga* translates the word "self" in a different way, possibly influenced by Romantic and psychoanalytical ideas of personhood with interiority. It implies new kinds of cognitive and performative activity, such as observation, analysis, and inquiry. In Iyengar's translation, the two halves of the word now bear a remixed relationship to each other. Instead of speaking aloud memorized texts, the self is recast as both subject and object of study, blending observational inquiry with the transformative powers attributed to education. Breaking the word into the English "self" and "education" resituates the Sanskrit concept into new intellectual genealogies. *Light on Yoga* takes a syncretic approach that had gained currency in India's late colonial period[94] and recalibrates yogic philosophies within texts that would make sense to readers schooled in Judeo-Christian and Western traditions.[95] Against the specter of rote learning and social reproduction of norms emerges an educative practice that (despite the masculine pronoun) appears democratic, egalitarian, and embodied.

Whereas earlier sources stress the isolated quality of *svādhyāya*, Iyengar portrays it as a social engagement: "the speaker and listener are of one mind and have mutual love and respect." The passage goes on to make *svādhyāya* foundational to political action: "According to Śri Vinobā Bhāve (the leader of the Bhoodan movement), svādhyāya is the study of one subject which is the basis or root of all other subjects or actions, upon which the others rest, but which itself does not rest upon anything."[96] Vinoba Bhave was a Gandhian political disciple whose Bhoodan movement aimed to redistribute land to low-caste villagers.[97] Though the effort was politically limited by paternalistic reliance on the noblesse oblige of elites, Iyengar suggests that the education of the self, in a remixed yogic context, might inspire a social vision with the potential to subvert the replication of Vedic-authorized hierarchies.

Finally, Iyengar introduces a new metaphor: a vision of *svādhyāya* as the iterative act of reading, writing, and revising a book of life. This direct invocation of literacy and authorship as a metaphor within yogic practice offers a new way of understanding the relationship between body and word. Challenging hierarchical understandings in which words are above or below practice, Iyengar places words *within* practice. His rhetoric mingles metaphors of embodiment with metaphors of literacy, so that thoughts enter the bloodstream while practitioners read, write, and revise their worlds and worldviews. This approach refuses to make choices between body and thought, words and practice, self and other, or personhood and politics.

What might a decolonizing imaginative approach inspired by a remixed *svādhyāya* draw from these historical genealogies, how might such an approach be experienced by writers and readers, and how might it be practiced in language? Four elements from the history I wish to stress for twenty-first-century decolonizing textual practice include *repetition*; the cycle of *reading, writing, and revising*; *embodied thinking*; and *cross-cultural engagement*.

Repetition, a key part of the history of *svādhyāya*, may allow writers to resist dominant systems of power by emphasizing process over product. In this context, practices focused on repetition bring a certain political resistance to the distinction-making process so crucial to capitalism. The origins of *svādhyāya* in the recitation of memorized texts hint at the transformative value and even liberation possible through a sustained engagement with a practice that appears to stay the same. When a body is held in the same way each time, observation can become attuned to subtle differences in outer and inner worlds. Such detailed observation can illuminate how power structures shape everyday life. As described by Candace Brunette-Debassige, who practiced yoga as a way to clarify her identity as an Indigenous woman within colonial history: "I can now observe my mind without judgment and can recognize that my mind is deeply influenced by its exposure to external messages."[98] The focused work of repeated action allows her to perceive not only sensations within her body but also structural layers of power that shape her world. These perceptions can shed light on the social meanings attributed to hierarchical categories—such as race, caste, gender, nation, or ability—that shape how diverse bodies move through the world.

As a way of engaging what Iyengar calls a "book of life," *svādhyāya* explicitly becomes open to a critical practice in which observation and study can emerge in dialogue with intersectional political concerns. Dianne Bondy describes how it allows her to revise external perceptions about racial identity into activist critique: "Because people stare at me like they have never seen a black person do yoga before, I have learned to sit in my discomfort and use the practice of self-study. Such experiences have also encouraged me to speak out about preconceived notions of what is 'different' (versus what is within 'the norm') in the yoga community. . . . Let's agree to study who we are and what we stand for."[99] Such *svādhyāya* may be considered in relation to the idea of "cognitive ecologies," or "a distributed but interconnected system or assemblage of social, material, bodily, and psychological resources and mechanisms."[100] *Svādhyāya* helps to distribute such resources. It offers sensory experience and verbal reflection felt across the whole body rather than simply experienced in the mind. In contrast to the unidirectional model of "mere instruction," Iyengar's *svādhyāya* implies a form of study that is dialogic. Presenting reading, writing, and revising as a cognitive ecology allows for a practice that is observational, creative, and constantly in motion: a worldview capable of adding layers of increasing subtlety. This attentiveness can move perception in different directions and link experiences of individual selfhood to political concerns for equality and justice.

This method challenges divisions between literacy and embodiment. As phenomenological accounts of postural yoga suggest, the practice draws attention to the "inherent relation between the body's inside and outside."[101] Bodies are not confined to conventional understandings of contained physical selves. "If I sink my weight down to the ground and begin to turn my inner gaze toward the soles of my feet, I quickly encounter the difficulty of marking the boundaries of my body," writes Oren Ergas in an investigation of how postural practice promotes philosophical inquiry. "Where do my feet end? Where does the earth begin?"[102] Divisions between bodies and writing can represent artificial constructs that rest on erasing the bodily experiences of writing and reading. The pacing, texture, and tone of words can affect breathing—elongating or quickening, deepening or speeding it. Writing is a physical and postural practice, requiring body work as varied as the skill and strength needed to carve stone inscriptions, to control a pen, or to type on a digital device. Aligned with feminist interpretations that have stressed the repressive historical forces that render writing bodies invisible,[103] this approach invites us to consider how imaginative power requires anatomical, mental, conceptual, and political states.

Finally, the embodied repetitions that can stimulate revised analytic gazes animate historical intimacies between *svādhyāya* and cross-cultural engagement. Many genealogies would stress the way *svādhyāya* is distinctly not cross-cultural. It has been used to shape strong boundaries around elite male personhood and to elevate the social standing of particular people over others. Yet *svādhyāya* might also be seen, in the work of texts as different as the early modern *Ā 'īn-i Akbarī* and Iyengar's mid-twentieth-century *Light on Yoga*, as a practice that invites diverse "others" to engage. The style implied by Iyengar's metaphor links *svādhyāya* to an observational exchange that brings some element of the "other" into the "bloodstream" of the self. Combined with a critical gaze that takes in intersecting political and social fields, this ongoing practice offers the capacity to perceive new dimensions within the politics of cross-cultural practice: to ask who benefits and who pays in such an economy of exchange.

Svādhyāya might take writers and readers into a process in which observing or engaging with the writer in a moment of practice alters the words in their journey to a page, where the roles of writer and reader are fluid rather than fixed. It might bring to light a writer's process of sharing ideas with people from different social locations or within movements for social justice, making it visible rather than hiding such cross-cultural engagements behind the scenes. It might live in attention to writing and other forms of textuality as bodily acts that reflect on political conditions governing what certain bodies are allowed or encouraged to do. In this sense, *svādhyāya* does not need to perform expected aesthetic markers of Indianness or remain focused on sacred texts to animate significant elements of Indian histories for decolonial ends. Outside the pressures to recode images of India into commodifiable nationalist and Orientalist products, it can instead offer a resource for creative reinterpretation, a living Indian remix composed of contradictory genealogies.

It is by embracing *svādhyāya*'s transformation—its history of remediation, cross-cultural dynamics, compatibility with different ideas of personhood, and contradictions—that we can best reclaim it for a decolonizing approach. This gives strength to a form of knowledge and power articulated by key Indian innovators but does not pretend to be uncontaminated by historical change or by diverse cultural forces. In this way, a remixed *svādhyāya* can yield new forms of critical self-reflection.

MAPPING THE CHAPTERS

In chapter 2, "Conducting Mass Practice," I begin by investigating the flexible Indianness that yoga's imaginative power affords the Indian state. Especially since the election of Narendra Modi in 2014, yoga has become a symbol of a new India rising in the world. Yet this equation between the practice and the nation, made so emphatically, conceals profound anxieties about the Indianness of yoga. Yoga is appealing as a national symbol because it is globally popular, but because it is globally popular, many people across the world do not think of it as particularly Indian. The state has therefore energetically worked to reclaim the "Indianness" of yoga in order to use the practice for India's political aspirations. Following the clues offered by state-authored and state-authorized texts, including tourist campaigns, media reporting, political speeches, and India's tax code, I trace how the state in the twenty-first century creates new conditions for yoga to legitimate an idealized national identity.

These conditions of flexibility conceal profound cultural tensions. India's nation-branding campaigns offer yoga as the country's gift to the world, but the appearance of cosmopolitan giving strategically asserts yoga as national property. India has embraced new technologies, such as websites, databases, and intellectual property regimes, to produce an image of yoga as authentic and traditional. Its heightened prominence in national public culture, exemplified by Modi leading Indians in practice on International Yoga Day, projects an image of peaceful power that erases Indian histories of violence. Through the culture peace of yoga, India can be all things to all people, while rarely calling anyone to account for these contradictions.

Fictional visions of yoga both amplify and erase ideas of India in the late twentieth- and early twenty-first centuries. In chapter 3, "Aligning Both Hands," I journey into visions of yoga within Indian and diasporic popular fiction in English. In many places, such fiction serves as the right-hand man (and it often is a man) of the Indian state, frequently colluding with the project to reclaim yoga for India by giving it to the world.

Novels like Mohan Ashtakala's *The Yoga Zapper* (2015) offer cultural fantasies of how yoga recruits Western (often white) bodies to validate an Indian, and especially Vedic, religious and philosophical universe. These fantasies are gendered in ways that remasculinize yoga, linking visions of an idealized Indian world to conservative gender norms. I suggest that the act of bestowing yogic authority beyond recognizably Indian bodies forwards larger aims for the nation of India. These projects envision flexible personhoods that appear cosmopolitan and inclusive, yet are also eerily compatible with domestic social hierarchies.

At the same time, competing currents within Indian popular culture reveal a different understanding of yoga tied more to Tantra, devotional practice, and the search for raw power in a neoliberal age—a vision that jars with the Vedic health and wellness image projected by the Indian state. What seem like new and unexpected portraits of yoga are often the uncanny heirs to the folkloric traditions that scholars have tracked across South Asia's many languages.[104] Drawing energy from what scholars have described as "left hand" traditions of religious practice, in which the violation of ethical codes and moral norms provokes important transformations, these darker currents indicate how older formations of the yogi as a frightening specter gain new currency. In Atul Merchant's self-published thriller *Taskari* (2014), for instance, yogic philosophies justify the use of chemical weapons against Pakistani terrorists. Attention to such diverse fiction expands and complicates our understanding of how cosmopolitan histories of yoga can be turned toward nationalist and even fundamentalist political projects. Such novels reveal cultural logics that the state publicly disavows, but which haunt the image India presents to the world.

Yet the weaving of the left hand within the right also generates possibilities for a critical practice of *svādhyāya*. While such novels show how peaceful ideals of Vedic life rely on violent practices, feminist mysteries by Shweta Taneja harness the Tantric possibilities of yoga to critique India's gender and caste-based hierarchies. The yogi as the spy or assassin takes on new life as a way to make sense of twenty-first-century challenges that include India's embrace of neoliberalism and its anxieties over national and gendered security.

Visions of yoga offer the imaginative power of a culture peace, or a set of unwitting alliances and concealed contradictions, to Western countries as well. In chapter 4, "Assuming Corpse Pose," I tell the story of how yoga's increased popularity internationally can allow countries like the United States to think of themselves as well-disposed toward India in exactly the same period when people of South Asian descent have experienced new vulnerabilities in public space. Using the United States as a case in point, I argue that yoga can be made to serve as an invisible framing device that distinguishes acceptable visions of South Asia from unacceptable ones.

The growing popularity of yoga has sometimes masked exclusion, surveillance, and even violence against communities of South Asian descent. Yoga murder mysteries, cropping up in the United States, yield insight into how India becomes a specter that must be killed off for the practice to thrive in U.S. culture. Close readings of U.S. court decisions on yoga tell an uncannily similar story. As the practice crystallizes debates over the legitimate visibility of Indianness within public schools, these legal documents frame Indianness as a potential problem. Likewise, as yoga has become a calming presence in U.S. airports, the airplane after September 11 has become decidedly less comfortable for brown-skinned travelers from the subcontinent. The imaginative flexibility accessed through yoga, I suggest, has enabled the United States to think of itself as cosmopolitan and open at precisely the historical moment in which South Asian American communities have experienced new vulnerabilities in the war on terror. The flexibilities that conceal India's contradictions, therefore, are also useful to the U.S. state.

In chapter 5, "Bending Over Backward," I explore the cultural politics of yoga in relation to broader anxieties of Indianness that emerge through global capitalism. I draw on fiction and digital media from India, the United Kingdom, North America, and New Zealand to show how the imaginative power of yoga both conceals and potentially exposes exploitation in a new world of flexible work. While Indian state visions often link yoga to larger dreams of economic triumph, novels perform a critical self-study that calls attention to yoga's reliance on a global precariat. In a range of fiction and digital media, including the American web series *Om City* (2014) and Alexandra Gray's British novel *The Yoga Teacher* (2008), teaching yoga requires precarious labor that replicates long-standing class divides within twenty-first-century space and time. Drawing on the work of Farah Godrej, who sees the possibility for the practice to question the values of capitalism,[105] I explore evidence of this critique within popular culture. Yoga may relieve the pressures of neoliberal life for some, but these cultural texts reveal how the flexibilities demanded of those who teach can also be the cause of such stress.

This ambivalence in which yoga can be used to both ennoble and exploit workers speaks to cultural questions about how it has been integrated as a flexible Indian solution to Western crisis. I explore how yoga has become popular in the United States as an Indian-inspired antidote to the problems of technology in the new millennium at just the moment when Indian information technology workers in a gray market play key roles in whetting appetites for new technology. Visions of yoga in autobiography and media allow particular Indian bodies to seem powerful while deflecting attention from the exploitation of Indian technology workers. These spaces can conceal the racial divisions of labor that, ironically, enable them. Reading cultural representations of yoga against the often hidden histories of transnational Indian labor, I show how visions of yoga rely on, while they mask, inequalities and exploitations in labor markets. Exposing how this cultural logic may shape flexible personhood is an important project of this book.

Finally, this chapter explores the ambivalent yoking of the economic concept of "free" to the political concept of "freedom." I investigate the discourse of laughter yoga as described by its Indian founder Madan Kataria and portrayed in a documentary by the Indian American filmmaker Mira Nair. Laughter yoga reveals how the pursuit of freedom is shaped by the changing pressures wrought by India's economic transformations in the 1990s. That freedom sometimes comes at the cost of reiterating colonial and capitalist hierarchies. Although the Indian state's promotion of yoga bespeaks its desire to profit, Western fiction and memoir, such as the New Zealand novel *Heavenly Hirani's School of Laughing Yoga* (2014), depict India as a place of free spiritual healing. Just when the state is hoping to make money, these cultural fantasies indicate Western desires to view India as an endless supply of willing and virtually free labor. As these visions reflect the unintended consequences of India's political insistence that yoga is a "gift," they reveal tense histories shaping the idea of "free" and the ideal of "freedom." Through close readings of these texts, I inquire into the true cost of laughing freely.

In chapter 6, "Framing New Parts," I amplify the voices of those who are keen to use imaginative interpretations of yoga to forward more diverse representations of flexible Indian identity in a globalizing world. Using the lens of a remixed *svādhyāya*, I read these works as critical forms of self-reflection designed to illuminate structures of possibility for ideas of Indianness. The diasporic art of Chiraag Bhakta in *#White-PeopleDoingYoga* (2014) directs our attention to the stylistic power of framing, accumulating, and juxtaposing to critique an overbearing architecture of social power. Focusing on the gendered critique of yoga found in the essays and poetry of the Indian American writer Reetika Vazirani, I suggest that her works illuminate the significance of yoga as a search for ethical representation, social justice, and antiracism, against and over the pursuit of health, well-being, and national pride.

As these writers of Indian origin create visions of yoga that promote critical self-reflection, collaborations with Western groups without Indian backgrounds seek to portray yoga for productive cross-cultural connections. These forms use the instabilities of satire, irony, and even stereotype itself to critique limited ways of envisioning India. Focusing on diasporic satire in the Canadian web series *Yoga Town* (2013), I analyze how the series raises problems of white privilege and commercial exploitation, challenges the essentialist specter of an ancient Indian spirituality, and invites practitioners to participate in a form of *svādhyāya*. I argue that these forms of popular culture work to cultivate yoga as a practice of attending to the invisible assumptions that legitimate flexible ideas of India in the world today.

As a modern practice of transformation called into being through global encounters, yoga now stands at a moment of paradox. The more it is promoted as a cosmopolitan gift to the world, the more it can be used to reinforce selective visions of legitimate India. In the 1960s, my grandmother took up yoga to fight the diabetes that ultimately killed her. As far as I can tell, nobody in the family agonized about whether yoga was un-Islamic. Today, Muslims in India have begun to ask if performing sun salutations involves them in a chess move within a larger game to Hinduize the country. Cultivating the practice for a genuinely open pluralism, a robust space of cross-cultural encounter, and a meaningful site of Indianness—ideals I believe in—requires us to think about the changing political conditions under which so many people practice.

oooo

Inspired by the maps of yogic bodies in fragile manuscripts, I have aimed in the previous pages to sketch a microcosm of this book that illuminates it as a whole. Now I shift from the illusion of one hovering above to the eye that sees from a partial place, time, body, and past. This, too, is part of setting up.

Yoga's imagined flexibilities have called to me because I need them. Like those of so many people, my experiences have been shaped by interwoven perspectives on very different worlds. My mother was born in India in the coastal city of Khambhat. Centuries before her birth, European travelers wrote wonderingly of the bands of yogis who haunted the outskirts of town. Before it silted up, Khambhat was a port where men boarded ships to sail the Indian Ocean out to East Africa and beyond. Old Dutch engravings of the gulf show galleons, looking like finely etched pirate ships, muscling their way in and out of India.

My family were Shia Muslims who liked to trace their lineage back to Yemen. Since the 1870s, I'm told, my ancestors sailed out of Khambhat to make their fortune, then sailed back to marry and start their families. Some fanned out across Southeast Asia and the Pacific, finding themselves in Bangkok, Singapore, Japan, and as far east as Hawaiʻi. They formed part of the broader Gujarati mercantile diaspora whose lifeworlds spanned the Indian Ocean and beyond.[106] My great-grandfather first went west, to Aden, then shifted course to Hong Kong. Somewhere along the line, after World War II, the name Hussein Ali disappeared into English and resurfaced, newly sutured, with different spacings, scripts, and letters. Back in India, for others, the family name turned into one that marked them as people from China. My grandfather spent his youth in Hong Kong learning the family textile business. He stood tall in sunglasses between the counter and the wall of ornate bolts of fabric. With his brothers and cousins, he sold the kind of expensive silks you close your eyes to touch. "European cloth, not Indian," my aunt told me as she drove through the winding tree-lined streets of Singapore after teaching her last yoga class of the day. "Everyone wanted the latest French fashions." My family was formed through tangled trading networks of goods, people, and ideas.

During World War II, my grandfather couldn't travel home to see his wife and children in Khambhat. My grandmother took in laundry to survive. After the war, she announced to her husband that the whole family would move to Hong Kong; evidently she was like that. My mother was five when they left. Her connection to India has often been uncertain, composed of guest room drawers filled with seldom worn saris. She persuaded her parents, against their desires, to let her go to university in the United States. "You'll marry an American and never come back," they prophesied. That's essentially what happened. In Boston my mother met my father, who had made his own improbable journey from a small dairy farmer town in northeast Texas to write his dissertation on American politics at Harvard. My mother found his Sulphur Springs family of Methodists bewildering. "All your grandfather can talk about is football," she would say. "They think paprika is a spice."

One side of my family Indian, the other side white, I grew up in Reagan's America wearing jelly shoes and leg warmers. The school I attended was largely white and firmly Christian. Its mascot was the Scottish Highlander. By middle school I was earnestly approached for conversion to the Episcopalian church by my classmates. India came into our suburban ranch house as the sound of crackling, operator-assisted calls late at night. My mother would shout into the phone in a language I could not understand.

Every other year we traveled to Bombay to see our family. In the first story I ever published, when I was thirteen, I described roller coastering with no seatbelts in the dawn ride from the old Bombay airport to my aunt and uncle's flat overlooking the Arabian Sea. The city smelled of salt and heat, while the buildings looked like paintings, only crumbling. I remember taxi rides through the city with my cousins, hiding on the backseat floor so that the driver could pretend he drove only four children. Against the white cement block walls of my elementary school classroom, India seemed like a land of endless liberation. Yet it was also the land where I felt I was always doing something wrong, always out of place, my American accent strange even to my ears. As a university student, I resented automatic assumptions that I should study India. It has taken a long scholarly journey—through the study of Mandarin, a PhD in postcolonial literature, and a first assistant professorship in world literature to an eventual academic home in Asian and Pacific studies—to bring me back to thinking about the idea of India in the world.

Yoga has helped me join fragments of lived experience. It has offered a shared point of connection between my white American relatives and my diasporic Indian ones. It has yoked my love of reading to my sense of being in a body. My Indian grandmother's generation practiced yoga; my generation practices; my children love to show me their wheels and handstands. Even our cats like to tunnel under my mat. Yet writing this book has made me conscious that yoga can be used to conceal divisions, ruptures, and dreams that cannot be fundamentally reconciled.

Conceptualizing yoga as a committed practitioner but not an uncritical disciple has helped me come to terms with the fact that I may never fully meet the expectations of those I speak with in this book. Those who thrive within yoga's devotional traditions may feel I am too acidic. Those dedicated to academia's more esoteric discourses may feel I am too sweet. Some will look for more depth of experience, while others will wish I would simply go away. All of us together—readers and I—may need, as said in so many yoga studios, to sit with these discomforts.

———— ⚭⚭⚭ ————

This book yokes together three imaginative visions of yoga that frame the practice: the mat, the photograph, and the page. As Peter Morey and Amina Yaqin have argued, frames create narratives whose "parameters are defined by questions of belonging, 'Otherness,' and threat."[107] Noticing these boundaries reveals how they create conditions of possibility and mark areas of exclusion. The hard, angular lines push bodies into place, inviting us to think about the social discipline that has long marked yoga in many forms. Acts as different as the austerities of ascetics or the compulsive posts of social media influencers reveal the meanings of yoga made within often unquestioned borders. The flexibility projected onto yoga hints at relentless pressure from an unseen world. As a practice, yoga is always framed.

Yet yoga is also a framing practice in its own right. The American writer Elizabeth Kadetsky, reflecting on her immersion into postural yoga in *First There Is a Mountain* (2011), observes that "in our bodies, we made new frames in which to sit and live."[108] Tracking fluidity as well as rigidity in the making of flexible personhoods is one purpose of this book.

THE MAT

From the twenty-first floor, lit by the sun over the Arabian Sea, I can see a woman doing yoga. She is too far away for me to hear her teacher giving guidance or to catch what shape she has composed with her limbs. But I know it is yoga because, from twenty-one stories up, I can see the unmistakable form of a bright pink mat.

The mat is one of yoga's many frames. The mat offers a living page. We turn our bodies like alphabets in motion, slowly spelling out a kind of script we are just now learning how to read. The mat tells us how close we can come to another person. It defines individual space as it synchronizes collective action. On the first International Day of Yoga, Narendra Modi led a new rising India in its poses on a sea of mats. The next year, the country declared, those mats would not be made in China. The mat changes the crowd into a population under control.

The stickier the mat, the more likely it is made with PVC. Polyvinyl chloride is a plastic made soft with phylates. It releases carcinogens into the air and is thought to disrupt the endocrine system. PVC produces dioxins. So does the making of paper. Yoga's frames, the mat, the photograph, and the page, yoked in their link to slow violence. Today it is not the people who teach yoga who grow rich through the practice. It is those who control the mats.

THE PHOTOGRAPH

The twentieth century is the century of writing yoga with new light. When the cameras came to take pictures of young men under the tutelage of the yoga guru Krishnamacharya, they reshaped the practice of yoga from one concerned with invisible things to one meant to be seen. Lenses lingered on lights and darks, capturing what was perceived in colonial photography as the very essence of Indian difference. Cameras captured wild bodies while composing new ones. Once the body of the yogi in India was considered fearsome and superhuman, a body of warfare and ashes. Over time, images of unearthly figures capable of occult contortions gave way to clean musculature and geometric shots. In India and well beyond its borders, yoga has come to promise the perfect orderly body.

In the digital age of the twenty-first century, yoga offers a visual cipher for the dream of a perfect life. On Instagram, you can scroll endlessly through square frames of practitioners recording their moments of ideal practice.[109] Yoga influencers stage their practice with care. Bollywood stars like Shilpa Shetty share images of themselves practicing in ideal settings, such as a sea of grass below a bright blue sky. A luminous sunset glows on a lithe pale woman in an arm balance on a beach. An athletic white man practices a complex inversion on a park bench beside his bicycle. Many yoga influencers are fond of photographing themselves in what appear to be untouched—yet are also clearly touched-up—natural spaces. These worlds reflect the gaze of the middle class, the segment of society for whom lush fields and boundless seas are not places to work. In these photographs, yoga appears to bend the universe to its dream of perfection.

To produce these idealized images, frames exclude. Western social media feeds often repeat astonishingly similar body images, creating an echo chamber for white, thin, flexible female bodies. In parts of the world where Indians have migrated and often struggled, it can be especially galling for some members of the diaspora to see one of India's most popular cultural icons represented in this way. When practices from India are seen as uncool—as signs of unwelcome otherness—it is often people of Indian ancestry who pay the price. But when the appeal of such practices spreads, it can seem that the greatest benefits often bypass communities of Indian origin.

The frames exclude many of the globally shared challenges that shape the twenty-first-century world. Perpetually scrolling images of yoga in pristine natural spaces conjure life without the ravages of infectious disease, climate change, environmental pollution, political violence, or labor exploitation. These images, seen en masse, can appear willfully blind.

The edges of the photograph—the places that rely not on the unseen but on the unseeable—frame this order. Often women work beyond the frame. So do servants and people of castes not historically considered suitable for yogic cultivation. The sharp rectangles of the photographic paper slice away peripheral vision. In relating to photographs, we are called to practice a form of *svādhyāya* that requires cultivating attention to all points at once. "You do not look at your left hand," a teacher says. "But you must feel it is there. You must sense what you do not see."

THE PAGE

Like the mat and the photograph, the page offers yoga a box. As pages have moved across time from the delicate edges of a manuscript to the uniform sheets of mass-produced paperback to the glowing rectangles of a screen, they have served as spaces that both contain and liberate the practice. On pages, philosophical portraits of dizzying contradiction have taken shape. Maps of subtle bodies have been charted. *Āsanas* have been line drawn. Stories have been told. Yet when I read a novel, its rectangularity never strikes me. Not once do I ask why the book in my hands is not a circle, a triangle, a trapezoid. The frame seems natural, its shape inevitable, its right angles the only way to organize unruly words.

How do we find our way to the page? What are the streets we must cross, the doors we must open, the air we must breathe to find our way both inside and outside these frames?

Pages are the flattest of boxes where the inside exceeds the outside, yet the outside casts a shadow over what can be read. This tension between compression and liberation is not simply a struggle between repressive and productive forces. As poets often know, form pushes a poem to flower in full. In an *āsana*, I feel my body becoming a new kind of word, learning a new kind of language. Something turns, a knee or an elbow or a hip, and suddenly a secret room appears inside that opening. Spaces begin to unlock. Stories begin to reveal themselves. The frames close the doors on the practice, yet they also allow hidden exits and entrances to appear. Remembering what the door locks out, while following those secret tunnels, is the challenge of reading yoga on a page.

Writing in 1965, the philosopher K. J. Joshi suggested that "yoga" in its earliest uses could signal the connections that allow language to make meaning. "The word has appeared in this sense, in the *Ṛg-veda*," Joshi wrote, "where a Vedic seer asks as to who knew the *yoga* (i.e., connection) between the words of a verse."[110] In the pages that follow, yoga is my theme, but also, in Joshi's sense, it is my method. A remixed *svādhyāya* allows me to speak with concern about the politics of Indian identity, yet also to commit to a practice that reminds us that identity lies in becoming rather than in being. This book does not simply analyze visions of yoga. It also seeks to testify to yoga's imaginative power.

2

CONDUCTING MASS PRACTICE

India's Vision for Yoga

I n November 2014, my aunt took me to lunch in Singapore with a group of her friends, all advanced yoga practitioners. "Did you hear?" one woman asked. "India's made a ministry for yoga."

A ministry for yoga—it sounded like something Kafka would create. As I came to learn, India had had a department of yoga since 2003.[1] But the elevation of a basic department to a grandiose ministry indicated something new in the political landscape. It suggested a larger story about yoga's rising symbolic and material power for the Indian state in the new millennium.

This chapter explores the urgency with which the Indian state has promoted ownership over yoga at home and abroad. Under the tenure of Prime Minister Narendra Modi, yoga has drawn the focus of an intensified state gaze. The government has turned to a practice with roots older and broader than the modern nation-state to engage in a twenty-first-century project of nation making and identity politics that suits its ambitions in a globalizing world. I argue that the rise of yoga has been powerful because it produces the appearance of agreement for politically opposed visions, allowing Hindutva, or ideological visions of Indianness as fundamentally Hindu, to flourish while simultaneously projecting Indianness as expansive, open, and tolerant. Visions of yoga render these tensions more resilient.

This point of agreement—this "culture peace," as I call it—reveals how states recruit cultural practices to ease their national transitions into globally integrated economies. The Indian government, sometimes in partnership with private bodies, has created a set of stories and spectacles through yoga that seek to brand the practice as Indian and to leverage this vision of India for a globalizing nation. Yoga is not only the subject of philosophical treatises and practice manuals. It also, increasingly, comes to life in visual and verbal forms as different as national branding campaigns, social media, UN resolutions, trade agreements, and India's income tax act. These stories help to conjure a flexible India.

This chapter meditates on the state's controlled yet contradictory choreography of yoga through yoga diplomacy, the Incredible India tourist campaign, the making of a Traditional Knowledge Digital Library, and the establishment of an International Day of Yoga. I suggest that state-authored, state-commissioned, and state-inspired visions of yoga not only aim to inscribe new forms of political and economic discipline upon the bodies of their citizens. They also mark one place where a state, having moved away from a socialistic pattern of society toward neoliberal capitalism, seeks through spectacle to find emotional connection with its populace. It uses the language of cosmopolitan giving as a hidden language of nationalist regaining. Through the act of giving yoga to the world, India as a nation gets it back.

This project, by which gifts to the world affirm national ownership, potentially veils less generous histories. Yoga helps to figure India as flexible, turning its once burdensome Orientalist legacy of ancient spirituality into a marketable modern asset for a rising power. Yet this flexibility emerges through projects of fixity, silence, and potentially even injury. To turn yoga into a national project with legal, moral, and economic claims upon a global public, the government must transform the practice itself through codification and categorization, which requires exclusions and repressions. These create unseen frames for the new flexible India of state spectacle.

Although some of these initiatives predate the ascendance of Narendra Modi to national office, much of this political prominence was achieved in the years between 2014 and 2019 under his leadership.

Manmohan Singh, India's prime minister for the decade preceding Modi's first term, mentioned yoga in recorded public speeches only once—when he conferred the National Communal Harmony Awards to the Ramakrishna Mission in 2006.[2] In contrast, Modi in his first five years spoke of yoga in recorded speeches *ninety* times. This exponential surge in political rhetoric has infused the practice in India with new energy. This period has witnessed the beginnings of a transformation in the institutional landscape of yoga, as the Indian government seeks a leading role in defining the practice on a national and global scale. Yoga has helped to produce a flexible image of Modi that overlays the goals of Hindu nationalism onto those of pluralist liberalism, while overwriting narratives of violence that have haunted Modi's political reputation and histories of modern India at large.

Though Modi is vital to this story, the powers unleashed during his tenure go well beyond a single figure. Although I use the singular noun for simplicity, the Indian state is anything but singular. In weaving diverse representations together, I may appear to posit a unity to the state that does not really exist. But I am less interested in the state as a realistically described institution and more concerned with its effect in promoting ideas of the nation through diverse rhetorical projects. In reading the Indian state as a maker of words and images, I draw inspiration from Akhil Gupta's argument for "a perspective that sees the state as constituted through writing."[3] State writing and state spectacle may in isolation betray very little imaginative flair. Yet put together, these productions begin to compose larger cultural narratives that illuminate the emerging logics by which India asserts itself. My approach takes the state as a cultural creator, a force perpetuating words and images that—though produced by different people for different reasons—all draw upon an imagined central bank of Indian political legitimacy. In this chapter, I explore texts that bear the touch of the state and its aspirations. Some are state-authored; others are state-inspired; and yet others seek state blessing.

These state texts and theatrics come to life through the circulatory economies of English, where national elite and semielite discourses are yoked to international public spheres where English is used. In a complex multilingual nation, such discourses should not be taken as India's governmental totality. But this small slice of the state is a telling one. English has historically served as a key language of India's modern foreign policy, reflecting the legacies of colonialism, imperialism, and globalization. While by no means the only or even the most important language that circulates ideas of India abroad, English remains a privileged, if often ambivalent, outward face of the nation. English has also loomed large within Indian national discourse as a market advantage. Driven by growth in export-led sectors since India's liberalization in the 1990s, a growing class of citizens, part of the rising middle class that makes up "New India," has begun to use English as one of several meaningful languages in their daily lives. While only .02 percent of India's population are native speakers of English, 11 percent speak it as a second (or third, or fourth) language.[4] Portraits of yoga, I suggest, help India to imagine itself in English and to imagine the English language as Indian.

Such portraits also project particular imaginative power for the state of India. I trace the roots of this power to explore how the state in the twenty-first century establishes new frames within which yoga makes meaning. Through nation-branding campaigns, yoga is used to legitimate ideas competing within the nation of India's place in language, space, and time. Through international intellectual property regimes, yoga is transformed into Indian traditional knowledge. Through universalizing gestures, yoga is paradoxically reclaimed for selective nationalist ends. Through state spectacle, yoga is asked to erase Indian histories of violence.

In philosophy and folklore, visions of yoga have long pointed practitioners toward a world beyond everyday experience. The practice has promised entry to a realm of power that ordinary people cannot perceive, let alone control. The yoga of today offers a similar window into some of the unwitting alliances between pluralist liberalism and Hindu nationalism that help to shape India's image in a globalizing world. In exploring these connections, I join forces with scholars such as Andrea Jain, who contends that "the current Indian government and its allies instrumentalize the rhetoric of yoga as a unifier toward a neoliberal shift in 'lifestyle' for the sake of increased productivity, all while reifying boundaries between social groups and privileging a Hindu heteropatriarchal elite."[5] The culture peace of yoga masks, yet relies on, the turbulence and turmoil brought through violent and capitalist practices. These texts and theatrics do not simply describe state yoga. They shape yoga into a practice of imaginative power.

THE POWERS OF YOGA

Storytelling traditions in South Asia have long linked yogis to the pursuit of political and military might.[6] In diverse ways, leaders on the subcontinent have harnessed the practice to augment their political reach.[7] Modern Indian politicians have sometimes looked to yogis to help them win elections and wield influence.[8]

In part, yoga's allure endures precisely because its public image has changed. The yoga practiced globally in the twenty-first century is best understood as a product of late nineteenth- and twentieth-century transformation in a world of nationalist Hindu reform movements, Indian enthusiasm for Western sport and naturopathy, emergent public health initiatives, and colonial attempts to uncover yoga's philosophical traditions.[9] As many of these projects strategically amplified yoga's connections to diverse systems of thought and practice, they brought yoga into a new frame: colonial modernity and its discontents. Yoga is much older than the idea of the modern nation-state and certainly older than the independent state of India.[10] But modern Indian nationalism has used the practice to lend legitimacy to its search for a different political shape.

By the mid-twentieth century, a new international reputation for political peace and public dignity was inscribed, in the style of a palimpsest, over yoga's existing links to force and violence. Eighteenth-century yogis were often formidable warriors, and philosophies of yoga in the *Bhagavadgītā* were invoked to justify violent anticolonial struggle in the twentieth century.[11] Yet with time, yoga came to signal peaceful resistance. Gandhi, one of the primary figures who spearheaded this transformation after his return to India, suggested that yoga was ideally suited to shape healthy nonviolent workers in the independence movement.[12] He made the public performance of bodily discipline and meditation, including yoga, into a nationalist practice with political heft.

This new halo effect has not gone unnoticed by the Indian state. In modern India, Joseph Alter argues, "often body discipline is regarded as both the means and the ends of nationalism."[13] Indian leaders, exemplified in the newly independent state by Jawaharlal Nehru, drew heavily on the social capital sparked by Gandhi's bodily discipline to legitimate their foreign policy agendas. Nehru relied on what Andrew Kennedy describes as "moral efficacy," or a belief in India's capacity to persuade through nonviolent means, to shape his decisions about how India should best pursue its national interest.[14] Although Nehru was not as iconic a practitioner of yoga, he developed a leadership style that capitalized on Gandhi's reputation. An aura of moral authority and benevolence toward the larger world, crystallized for popular imagination through yoga and meditation, has offered political benefits to the Indian state beyond the independence struggle and into the twenty-first century.[15]

Many practitioners in India and beyond deepened yoga's peaceful image by integrating it within emerging regimes of health and wellness. As yoga developed in the late nineteenth century, it moved into a frame of physical fitness, mental health, and spiritual well-being.[16] In the late nineteenth- and early twentieth-century United States, spiritual entrepreneurs such as Swami Vivekananda, Paramahansa Yogananda, and Pierre Bernard used yoga to support grand mythmaking of India's spiritual prowess as well as to conjure an alternative space for Westerners to explore discontents with industrial modernity.[17] In mid-century Britain, Suzanne Newcombe has shown, yoga became popular with women as a practice that might liberate them from constraining gender norms of Western biomedicine.[18] Although it was still viewed suspiciously by many, especially before the late twentieth century,[19] yoga nonetheless began to take imaginative shape through a rhetoric of nonviolence, health, well-being, and authenticity in India and the West.

Frequently detached from the nuances of Indian religious or ritual practices, visions of yoga at the turn of the twenty-first century have come to exude an aura of transnationally exchangeable goodness. This reputation has helped yoga claim a place across the world as a practice suitable for diverse societies. Yogis have also continued to play their cultural role from folklore as figures of threatening political influence. Indira Gandhi was notoriously dependent on her yoga teacher, known as the "Indian Rasputin," and the figure of the charlatan yogi became a recognizable villain in twentieth-century popular culture (as seen in the works of V. S. Naipaul and John Updike).[20] In later chapters, I explore the ongoing vitality of these sinister traditions. Yet yoga's reputation for charismatic, mystical control has also been recalibrated through new regimes. Yoga has thus been appropriated to bolster diverse ideas of the good—good bodies, good minds, good spirits—in many parts of the world.

Yet yoga has simultaneously renewed its link to politically controllable power—a distinctly different approach to goodness. In India, some strands of yoga have become integral to Hindu nationalist groups seeking to develop strong and militant bodies through techniques presented as ancient and Hindu.[21] Postural yoga, along with other forms of self-strengthening, was used to cultivate new forms of masculinity for Indian men who longed to escape colonial charges of effeminacy. Throughout the twentieth century and into the twenty-first, Raphaël Voix has argued, "renunciant activism has mostly been associated with the dominant Hindu nationalist discourse."[22] Such visions of yoga have inscribed ideas of India as fundamentally Hindu upon individual bodies.

Twenty-first-century yoga can thus appeal to Hindu religious authorities to expand their influence—making the practice seem like a ministry of a different sort. The success of Baba Ramdev, India's most visible yoga superstar on a domestic and increasingly global stage, illuminates this appeal at work. Ramdev began his career as a Hindu ascetic, and his popularity, as Joseph Alter argues, "is rooted in the conflation of wisdom and power manifest in the physical embodiment of classical world renunciation."[23] He advocates practices that aim, grandly, at what Chandrima Chakraborty describes as "healing modernity itself."[24] This project promotes conservative heteronormative gender ideologies as integral to its moral vision.[25] Ramdev has effectively used charismatic authority, business savvy, and digital presence to spread his vision across India. As Arkotong Longkumer reveals, this has been seen as a way of imposing Hindu practices and hierarchies onto minority groups, such as Christian communities in Nagaland, who are perceived as "un-Indian."[26] The equation of particular Hindu lifeworlds with the identity of India marks Ramdev's initiatives. He launched the Bharat Swabhiman Trust, which asks its members to commit to "100% voting, 100% nationalist thinking, 100% boycott of foreign companies and use indigenous products, 100% unite nationalist people, and 100% construct yogic india" [sic].[27] Ramdev was reported to have told followers at a mass yoga camp, "There are two things I have to do. Make all foreign companies do *shirshasana* (a yoga headstand) within five years, and put Mother India on the throne of the world."[28] Foreign companies' yoga practice is imagined as subservience to an expansive and even imperial Indian worldview. Yoga has come to signal the cultivation of an ideal nationalist and modern body that can suit the values of Hindutva.

Precisely by seeming beyond and before capitalism, such visions of yoga have shaped new Indian consumers. In contrast to expensive and time-consuming approaches, Ramdev was one of the first to make yoga nationally accessible through mass media and mass yoga camps.[29] His presentation as a lower-caste person has helped to recruit a diverse range of people.[30] At the same time, Ramdev has also been seen to disparage Dalit communities in ways that reinforce hierarchies of caste.[31] While these mass camps challenge capitalist exclusions by offering yoga at low cost, they have also helped to recalibrate attendees into potential consumers for the emerging market of goods and services that Ramdev's enterprises can provide. As my cousin said to me, as we sat around the glass dining table in her parents' Mumbai flat, "They've now realized they can charge more, not less, for these traditional things."

Ramdev's popular promotion of yoga has become a walking—or bending—advertisement for lifestyle products that merge a transnationally circulating logic of health-conscious consumption with an aura of ancient Indian spirituality and asceticism.[32] This builds on the work of earlier figures such as the Maharishi Mahesh Yogi, who began to market such lifestyle items in the mid-1980s.[33] As Ramdev's political allies in the Hindu nationalist Bharatiya Janata Party (BJP) have come to power in the new millennium, they have used state institutions to expand this consumer-making potential. India's Defense Research and Development Organization, for example, developed herbal products that entrepreneurs like Ramdev can market.[34] Buying Indian-made household products continues the Gandhian legacy of *swadeshi*, or national production of goods, in a postsocialist context. Yoga is thus used to shape new consumers for the Indian state's twenty-first-century campaign of "Make in India," because its image can merge a rhetoric of indigenous power with the neoliberal circulation of goods, rewriting capitalist consumption as political work.

This rewrite also expands capitalist practices by concealing some of yoga's capitalist potential. Seen in one light, the economic value of yoga is greater than ever before. Figures for the global industry circulate at USD $88 billion, with India's market share put at Rs 490 billion.[35] Market mechanisms appealing to India's growing middle class have helped to create "yoga millionaires" like Sarvesh Shashi, whose Sarva brand appeals to young millennials in India's urban centers.[36] At the same time, the Indian state under Modi has revised key national texts that make yoga more lucrative for Indian entrepreneurs by downplaying its economic potential. The 2015 Finance Act freed yoga from service tax, and in 2016, yoga was specifically mentioned in Section 2 (15) of India's Income-tax Act under the rubric of "charitable purpose."[37] Although Ramdev oversees a large international commercial enterprise, the technical beneficiary is the charitable trust Patanjali Yogpeeth. In 2017, the trust successfully gained tax-exempt status under the argument that the provision of yoga in India officially constitutes medical relief and education.[38] Modi's government has thus begun to reconfigure structures and free yoga providers to pursue entrepreneurial gains under the legal framework of offering charity. Yoga thus assumes a flexible form within a cultural and structural narrative in which economic capital is at once desired and disavowed.

Through the changing economic ecology of yoga, the state and its allies cultivate citizens' bodies and minds, create a new set of consumers, and sponsor the development of products for them to buy. A lifestyle narrative of continuous self-improvement and transformation oils the workings of India's expansion from a postindependence, quasi-socialist "License Raj" to the glamorous entrepreneurialism of "New India." Yoga helps to integrate citizens within capitalism because they can think of their spending as aligned with noncapitalist ideals.

Yoga has also ascended to new heights within India's higher education boom. In 1947, India had 19 universities and 695 colleges. By 2019, universities numbered 900 and colleges more than 40,000.[39] As earlier forms of yogic education under the tutelage of a guru have given way to bureaucratic credentialing, yoga has become a subject at the tertiary level. In this sector, a massive influx of private and religious money has come to fill conspicuous gaps in opportunity for India's enormous youth population. In the early 2000s, the Indian government bestowed the status of "deemed university" upon two yoga training institutes that offer advanced degrees in yogic sciences.[40] At yogic institutions like S-VYASA, headed by Modi's key advisor H. R. Nagendra, students are recruited into bachelor's and postgraduate programs with the promise that "the wisdom of the ancient Indian scriptures will help in dealing with issues from management strategies to corporate governance in today's highly competitive world of business."[41] As Meera Nanda has shown, state governments have favored the growth of yoga institutions by awarding them valuable land and infrastructure.[42] By authorizing and subsidizing schools that can turn out large quantities of Indian yoga instructors within reliable time frames, the state bolsters Indian material control over the production of the practice. This work of state-conferred legitimacy creates both a cultural rhetoric and a material basis for a narrative of yoga as Indian.

Beyond the tertiary level, state intimacies with yogic organizations are poised to reshape broader discourses of Indian education. In 2016, the school education department encouraged Mumbai schools to work with Ramdev's organization to offer monthly yoga to students.[43] The government has explicitly bolstered the practice of yoga by making it advantageous or mandatory in many state schools. "If you do yoga in school, you get extra marks," an old family friend in Mumbai assured me over a cup of tea. In 2017, the Central Board of Secondary Education announced that "yoga . . . must be encouraged in the schools to create a sense of physical fitness, discipline, sportsmanship, patriotism, self-sacrifice and health care."[44] In 2019, the government entrusted Ramdev's Patanjali Yogpeeth Trust with oversight of India's first board of Vedic education, education based on principles attributed to authoritative texts in Hindu traditions that offer visions of ideal social order. As a private entity that pledged sizable sums to the board, the trust can create standards for the teaching of Vedic knowledge that expand the remit of schools run by Hindu organizations such as the Rashtriya Swayamsevak Sangh (RSS), the Arya Samaj, and Ramdev's own organization.[45] Yoga, often presented as a practice aligned with Vedic values and knowledge systems, stands to gain new prominence. These incentives may shape a new generation of practitioners who experience yoga through an expression of Indian public citizenship aligned with Hindutva.[46]

The national privileging of the practice emerges in a global landscape where yoga has been extremely successful. By the 1990s, as Andrea Jain has shown, yoga had moved into mainstream popular culture in many parts of the West.[47] It also dramatically grew in popularity in Asia, exemplified by more than 10,000 yoga studios in China, where practitioners have sought new forms of physical and psychological capital.[48] Yoga has gained popularity in societies facing the new risks and precarities of capitalism, especially where health care systems lack durable solutions to emerging health hazards, such as lifestyle disease and mental illness. Indians, as Jain argues, find yoga newly meaningful for these same reasons.

For the state of India, yoga's global popularity represents both a resource and a threat. As yoga's value has risen around the world, India appears to have missed out on many benefit flows in terms of economic capital, cultural recognition, and national branding. Recapturing those flows has become a priority for the state. In this pursuit of lost benefits, India draws on many pre-existing strengths. Yoga is seemingly everywhere, in a way that India's small foreign service, roughly the size of New Zealand's, simply cannot be.[49] It is beloved, and thus can leverage a large body of unpaid ambassadors. Yoga is also largely perceived as nonthreatening. Unlike such practices as Falungong in China, it does not claim a central site of authority that unnerves state power. Indeed, India has made sure that yoga will develop hand in hand with the state.

The only thing yoga is not, in many parts of the world, is Indian. When I shook in my first warrior pose in a university basement twenty years ago, I didn't associate it at all with Indian gurus or subcontinental spirituality or a search for my roots. I did it just like everyone else I knew: to put off my writing. When people asked me what kind of yoga I practiced, "Stanford yoga" was the most honest answer.

India does not have to do much to export yoga to many parts of the world. But to capture its benefits, the state does have to rebrand yoga as an icon of India. It thus seeks to craft a story that can reconcile national heritage with global participatory culture. It is this work, partly authored by state agencies, partly created by willing partners in multinational media, and partly crafted by individuals who have sought the blessings of the state, to which I now turn.

NATIONAL POSTURES

They catch your eye when you're not expecting them. On buses turning a corner in Australia, pinks and yellows stand out against the eucalyptus greens and dry ochres. On screens in international airports, pearly Taj Mahals soar up to greet the crumpled clothes, unbrushed hair, and wailing children of tired travelers. On a billboard in New York's Times Square, a woman lies supine in front of a fuschia border shaped to resemble perfectly packaged ocean waves. Incredible India strives to be everywhere.

In the early twenty-first century, the Indian government embarked on an ambitious and expensive rebranding of the nation through the tourist campaign known as Incredible India. Under the leadership of Amitabh Kant, joint secretary of the Ministry of Tourism and Culture from 2001 to 2007, the campaign adopted a high-end, experience-oriented approach that fit into India's larger efforts to use public diplomacy to influence global elites.[50] Launched in the mid-2000s, a time when India enjoyed a high economic growth rate, the campaign was aimed at both international and domestic markets. The government outsourced much of its work to public relations and advertising firms. Earlier Indian nation-branding campaigns of the new millennium had encouraged Indians to spend money in new ways by envisioning what Ravinder Kaur calls "largely middle-class investor-citizens" who "lay claim to their citizenship rights and entitlements through investment and consumption."[51] Incredible India's imagery modulated this logic one step further: the campaign invited its audience to invest in personal growth and spiritual exploration in ways that subtly encourage flows of money to and within India.

The broader twenty-first-century historical forces shaping this approach, as Kaur has shown, lie in "the capitalist transformation of the nation-state wherein the logic of capital is the glue holding the nation and state together. The *nation* in this scheme," Kaur contends, "is imagined as a vast enclosure of production, its territory a reserve of untapped natural resources, its population potential producers/consumers of goods and services, and its cultural essence a unique nation brand that distinguishes it from other investment destinations."[52] Visions of yoga have been used to shape a cultural logic that renders India market ready, rewriting the nation's ghosts of colonial extraction and vulnerability into opportunity and advantage. In concealing potential contradictions, images of yoga in advertising render the contradictions more resilient.

Modern tourism turns a profit from strategic fantasy making. Tourism inherits the ghosts of imperialism in multiple ways, trading on stereotypes of a place filled with inviting resources but also extracting resources, charming tourists out of their cash for national benefit. Yet tourist campaigns are not simply about economic relations in unequal and sometimes exploitative sites of exchange. They also have roles to play in the creation of national identity, pointing to the site where the canny dreams of marketers meet up with larger political aspirations about what a nation is and can be.

As a multiyear mixed-media campaign targeted at multiple audiences, including Indians, the Indian diaspora, and non-Indians, Incredible India sought to articulate India as a rising power. Its nation-branding program resituated the country in geopolitical terms and constructed diverse, even contradictory, images of it.[53] Produced to announce the arrival of a "New India," capable of confident self-representation, the campaign was very much a product of "New India's" paradoxes. Although underwritten by the wealth made possible by India's entry into the neo-liberal global economy, Incredible India in its early years largely invoked traditional images of preindustrial ways of life. The Taj Mahal, women in tribal dress, and elephants abounded. As the campaign evolved, it experimented with new, alternative ways of imagining an India that could nonetheless be seen as traditional. To consolidate the national brand, the campaign aimed to leverage yoga's existing international popularity to make it more Indian. In doing so, it reinvented the idea of "India" through intimacies with the English language, the spatial discipline of a new order, and a politically powerful logic of time.

Central to this effort was the long-standing idea of India's distinctive capacity to provoke transformation. The images produced for international promotion were visually sophisticated, often aiming for a form of photographic realism touched by a dash of magic. The campaign played with visual transformations of the English language, prefigured by the ! that replaced the I of India. This transfigured "I" became a place of visual focus in many advertisements: in some, it was replaced by the spire of the Taj Mahal. Playing on the fluidity among the "I" of "India," the "I" of the viewing self, and the dramatic vertical lines found in the Indian landscape, the campaign anchored itself in the concept of surprising substitution.

Yoga figures as an alphabetic join that makes a connection, through English, between India and the world. In one image, the missing "I" of India is replaced by the upright posture of a yoga practitioner.[54] English becomes part of Indian landscapes and bodies, while Indian landscapes and bodies become part of English. Yoga iconography helps to give

English deepened purchase as a language both outward facing and yet, in the visual logic of the advertisement, essential to India itself.

The body of the yoga practitioner forms a pillar of "India" in literal and metaphorical ways. In 2004, the filmmaker Bharat Bala produced videos for Incredible India that featured practitioners working within the tradition of B. K. S. Iyengar. They were filmed in stunning locations in diverse parts of India, ranging from Ladakh to Agra to Rajasthan. In these early stages, the advisor who directed the practice on the campaign, who identified herself as "a direct senior disciple of Yogacharya Shri BKS Iyengar," had a great deal of creative control. She used real yoga practitioners, not body models, and was able to direct them in keeping with the values of her tradition. Costumes were kept simple—a bare chest for the young man, a black leotard for the young woman—for a classic look that aimed to emphasize natural continuities between people and landscape. As the advisor put it, the aim was to show that "Yoga has grown from this soil and is a gift from India to the world."[55] In the process of filming, this yoga for the camera received an unexpected benediction from another Indian practitioner: "[The young woman being filmed] was on the steps doing an asan with leg behind her head, and a yogi passed by and touched her and took her blessing. A yogini is considered a manifestation of Shakti which is why the sadhu took her blessing."[56] These representations of yoga resonated positively within India as a validation of the inner precisions of the practice.

As the Incredible India campaign developed, it took new risks. Prathap Supan, then the creative director of Grey Worldwide (India), oversaw the creation of a very different set of yoga-oriented visual narratives. Unlike the photographs featuring human bodies, this series brought a cheekier tone to the representation of Indian heritage. According to Supan, the images were the first billboards from the Incredible India campaign to reach Times Square, New York.[57] Brightly colored, featuring jewel tones of fuchsia, green, turquoise, and yellow, they play with the energetic dynamism between the visual folkloric traditions and the witty, knowing voice of the English text. Captions include imperatives such as "Perhaps it's time you learned to breathe," "Get to know yoga from its mother" and "Get rid of 21st century stress. Change the way you

stand," placed between images of practitioners in inversions.[58] The advertisements resituate yoga within an imagined past, while the color pal-
ette and verbal tone insist on the stylized cool of postmodernity.

This series is notable for its strong use of geometrical discipline. The
"Perhaps it's time you learned to breathe" and "Get to know yoga from
its mother" advertisements are broken into orderly horizontal triads,
while others are divided into quarters or nest images and words in separate boxes. This framing stands in sharp contrast to stereotypes of India
as the land of uncontrollable excess. While the images in Incredible India
are visually energetic, they are controlled through quadrilaterals, much as
practitioners are defined through the rectangle of a mat. Yoga's discipline of body and mind creates a form of cultural authority for India that,
in the minds of the tourist operators, Westerners desperately crave. Yoga
offered an important source for political authority making when India
was not politically strong, as exemplified by the global image of Gandhi
and his meditative practices with moral purpose. In the twenty-first century, the Incredible India tourist campaign restructured this form of
authority to sell it within global capitalism.

While yoga has allowed India to remap itself in space, it has also
enabled the nation to reap the benefits of inhabiting a palimpsest of time.
To locate India within a nineteenth-century logic of civilizational grandeur, Incredible India riffs on a common popular assertion that yoga is
five thousand years old. In one advertisement, the caption reads, "Get
rid of 21st century stress. Stand for 5,000 years."[59] That figure appears
in advertisements sponsored by the India Brand Equity Foundation, a
government trust to promote the "Make in India" initiative. The microsite that accompanied this campaign tells readers to "Stand on your
head. Breathe in deep. And let 50 centuries of science, spirituality and
civilization cleanse your stress away. Get a dose of Yoga."[60] The presence of a deep past is key to this power.

The five-thousand-year claim, as many scholars will quickly point out,
is historically dubious. Some of the earliest pieces of evidence for what
looks like postural yoga, such as Indus Valley seals, lend themselves to
inconclusive readings.[61] Talismanic texts, such as the *Yogasūtra* attributed to Patañjali, are not five thousand years old and contain few direct

references to poses. But those making the claim are less interested in India's past than in what such a past might imply for India's rightful future. Such campaigns attest to what Manjari Chatterjee Miller and Kate Sullivan de Estrada describe as "India's exceptionalism," which draws upon the concept of "India as a unique civilization-state."[62] In this logic, modulated through imperial administrators and taken up by Indian thinkers, India—along with China—constituted one of the great ancient civilizations of the world. Although India had weakened and decayed, making it vulnerable to imperial management, it could identify a grand past that might return. Such thinking underlies Indian efforts to be seen as powerful by the world, especially prominent in the twentieth and twenty-first-century growth of the Hindu right, where the idea of an ancient Hindu past before the Mughal empire or British colonialism nourishes assertions of twenty-first-century Indian strength. This numeric fantasy further supports Indian desires to supersede China—which often claims a five-thousand-year history—as the foremost rising power of twenty-first-century Asia.

Though I suggest this is its subtle implication, the tag line of the advertisement does not actually say "Yoga is 5,000 years old." It reads, "Stand for 5,000 years." This is actually much truer to the history of yoga as a pursuit of immortality and supernatural power. The twenty-first-century reader is likely to take it as hyperbole. But the implied five-thousand-year past and the promised five-thousand-year future constitute the cultural logic of the Indian state's deferred recognition project, in which Indian power and global recognition in the present rest on these mythical time horizons. This vision of yoga appears to be before the present and yet of the future, before and yet within global capitalism, and before the rise of nations and yet the essence of India as a modern-nation state. Yoga offers useful imaginative powers to the Indian state for this flexible recognition project, which is anchored in a barely graspable past and a continually deferred future.

This palimpsest of time controls the visual vocabulary of the image, which appears at once ancient and hypermodern. The sculptural qualities of the English typeface subtly echo the visual qualities of Devanagari script, while the illustrations invoke premodern pictorial traditions.

(In contrast, influential mid-twentieth-century Indian guides to postural practice tended to favor photographic realism and simple line drawings.) At the same time, the images are meant to be read as modern. They make far more use of negative space and solid coloring than many of the older pictorial traditions they reference, and they represent what their creator has referred to as a "kitsch" style. The spatial order superimposed here contributes to the hypermodern temporality. Given the pervasive reputation of India as the land of chaos and crowds, the geometric visual ordering and individual separation of the bodies hints at a future India of regulated individualism that is nonetheless the conduit of tradition. In short, these illustrations are not meant to be taken as old—they are a fantasy of legitimating antiquity wrenched through a brightly colored hypermodernity. What demands recognition here is a state-sponsored and commercially produced vision of an India that stakes its claim to the now in the unreachable past and future.

As these outward-facing vocabularies ostensibly address international audiences, they recruit these audiences as unexpected potential allies for the Hindu right. Incredible India 2.0, which launched in 2017–2018, placed particular emphasis on spiritual and wellness tourism.[63] One of the new sites featured was Goraknath, traditional base of the Nath sect of yogis. Replacing Bollywood stars as the central ambassador for Incredible India was none other than India's Prime Minister Narendra Modi. Both of these choices, in different ways, marry Hindutva sympathies with neoliberal aims. Both author India's search for constantly deferred recognition on a global stage.

HOLDING THE POSE

While the Incredible India campaign articulates one expression of yoga's imaginative power, the Indian state has also sought to reclaim yoga for India through the legal mechanisms of an increasingly interconnected trade order. As with the tourist campaign, international legal conventions have created new frames to define national intellectual property.

Codification projects aspire to create the kind of stable borders that enable claims to ownership, yet they are also continually contested from within and from without. It is within these contests that flexible imaginative powers for yoga, as well as for India, are produced.

India's entry as a founding member into the World Trade Organization in 1995 brought with it new obligations on member states to develop compatible forms of intellectual property protection, and the Indian state was out of step with many other countries. The WTO's Agreement on Trade-related Aspects of Intellectual Property Rights placed India among patent-oriented legal economies, and India, which allowed patents on processes but not on products, was not well equipped to compete. Aligning itself with international norms, the government sought to establish legal ownership of yoga, based on the United Nations Convention on Biological Diversity, which India signed in 1992. The convention set out under Article 8(j) the concept now known in abbreviated form as "traditional knowledge."[64]

If the convention obliged its signatories to protect traditional knowledge, perhaps a greater spur to India was the fear of losing out to international patents. In 1995, U.S.-based scientists received a patent for the wound-healing properties of turmeric, a traditional folk remedy in India. Alarmed by the thought of losing control over traditional forms of healing, with benefits unlikely to flow to India, the state began documenting such practices. This project, which relied on evidence from historical texts, allowed the Council for Scientific and Industrial Research of India to successfully challenge the U.S. patent on the grounds of prior art.[65]

Emboldened by this legal success, in 2001 the state began to create a Traditional Knowledge Digital Library (TKDL), designed to help patent offices block new applications under the concept of prior art. The database was a joint project between the Council on Scientific and Industrial Research and the then Department of Ayurveda, Yoga and Naturopathy, Unani, Siddha and Homeopathy (AYUSH). The TKDL has been recognized as a pioneering institution for its legal innovations against biopiracy and its more philosophical role as the crucible where older holistic systems of South Asian practice take new shape through the vocabularies of national modernity.[66] It exemplifies, as Pradip Thomas argues, "a national accent on computerization and the digital" that has marked India's aspirational identity in the twenty-first century.[67] In other words, nothing says "traditional knowledge" like a website.

The chief architect of the TKDL, Dr. V. K. Gupta, declared that "using information technology tools and a novel Traditional Knowledge Resource Classification System (TKRC), the TKDL has converted and structured ancient texts into 34 million A4-sized pages along the lines of a patent application."[68] Indian textual diversity of language, script, pictorial tradition, and page size now achieves standardization of the highest order. Through a complex coding process, information about each entry is automatically translated into multiple languages through a knowledge-based conversion.[69] Classificatory systems have often been read as the arm of colonialism, ordering an unknown world to make it most usable for exploitation; this classificatory gesture has taken on new life as a nationalist construction of indigenous knowledge. Standardization, moreover, effectively makes the holder of traditional knowledge into the nation-state in what Allison Fish describes as "a critical turning point."[70] It is not a specific yoga school or geographical community that serves as the traditional owner; instead, the idea of "tradition" or "collective ownership" is effectively abrogated to the government.[71] As they codify, agents of the state create new imaginative powers for yoga to serve the nation.

Paradoxically, it might seem, yoga is not highly visible on the Traditional Knowledge Digital Library. This partly reflects the fact that most entries in the database are available only to the international patent offices that subscribe to it. Other absences probably reflect disruptions in funding or differences in administrative vision. As the World Trade Organization has cautioned, documentation of traditional practices is precisely what can render them open to abuse by nontraditional owners.[72] Yet beyond practicalities of revenue flows, local politics, and awareness of the dangers of making knowledge public, this invisibility actually signals one of the techniques by which yoga becomes an Indian national endeavor.

To make yoga fit the category of "traditional knowledge," the database works to remove yoga from its most internationally familiar

Anglophone discourse. On the TKDL's public website home page, a basic screen that contrasts with the slick graphics of the Incredible India campaign, the word "yoga" does not appear. Nor is yoga a prominent category despite globally high-profile yoga intellectual property cases in the new millennium.[73] Instead, yoga postures and breathing practices appear under the category of "Siddha," which the TKDL defines as an Indian system designed to achieve bliss and perfection.[74] This system, traced to a complex set of medieval traditions, links yogic practices with alchemical pursuits in the search for semidivinity.[75] In the 1920s, Siddha was presented as a specifically Tamil contribution to Indian systems of indigenous health care.[76] Elements of this narrative shape the rhetoric of the TKDL, which notes its Tamil origins as well as its links to Shaivism. Although the word "yoga" has entered different languages ("yoga" in English, "yujia" in Chinese) and thus potentially lost its edge of difference, "Siddha," with its strong link to Tamil textual and medicinal traditions, brings a guarantee of subcontinental authenticity. The word choice of the database works to defamiliarize the idea of yoga, offering instead an italicized *Astanga Yogam* that expresses a symbolic resistance to the idea of "yoga" as a word in English. Whereas the tourist campaigns aimed to make yoga eminently translatable across language and beauty standards, the TKDL provides an imaginative project in which yoga becomes *less* translatable—and thus more deserving of the "traditional knowledge" designation.

This rhetorical framing of yoga also places it within a philosophical lineage connected to the rise of the Hindu right in the twenty-first century. To David Gordon White, the heirs of medieval Siddha traditions are to be found in the Hindu World Council (VHP) and, in softer form, in the BJP.[77] As White describes, the leader of the Nath Siddha tradition sat on the board of the VHP when it authorized the razing of the Babri Masjid in 1992, which led to national communalist riots in 1992–93.[78] This tradition continues its political influence in India. Since 2017, the successive leader of the Nath order, Hindutva icon Yogi Adityanath, has held power as chief minister of Uttar Pradesh. The national textual production of yoga therefore takes on a Janus face to speak to two audiences. One audience is the international patent officer, who aims to respect

Indian traditional knowledge and may need some rhetorical markers that secure "yoga" within non-English, non-globally circulating signs that make it seem indigenous. The other audience, in the background, is the saffron tide, which may be politically pleased by a national project that places yoga in this philosophical lineage. "Siddha" can serve as a bureaucratic codification that ironically produces a flexible India.

How do we reconcile such projects with the often-heard claim—made by Indians—that yoga is "universal" and "belongs to the world"? This rhetoric is the basis upon which a new globally savvy nationalism asserts itself. The "nation" asserts its borders precisely at the moment that it appears open to the "world." "World" has become a language that justifies certain forms of exclusion precisely through its seeming denial of any limitation. This paradox creates the cultural logic that unites India's codification projects with its universalizing projects, to which I now turn.

GIVING AND GETTING

The most powerful imaginative tool that India may have to assert ownership over yoga is not nation branding, nor legal mechanisms, nor even a small army of teachers. Instead, it is the act of appearing to give it away.

In 2014, India's Prime Minister Narendra Modi made international headlines when he successfully bid the United Nations General Assembly for the creation of an International Day of Yoga. Resolution 69/131 passed uncontroversially to proclaim June 21, the summer solstice in the northern hemisphere, as a special day to spread ideas about the practice. In 2015, the first International Day of Yoga was celebrated to much media fanfare. The resolution was uncontroversial because it framed yoga as a secular contribution to global health. The language of the resolution deployed the selective frame of wellness, resonating with UN statements on preventing disease, noting "the importance of individuals and populations making healthier choices and following lifestyle patterns that foster good health." It lent formal recognition to the idea that "yoga provides a holistic approach to health and well-being."[79] The United Nations thus enthusiastically supported an idea of yoga that had become popular in India's early twentieth century. This internationally sanctioned yoga was also, as the UN rhetoric shows, fully compatible with a neoliberal approach to health as individual responsibility. As opposed to public health approaches requiring comprehensive and expensive investments by the state, such as national health insurance, structural changes to working conditions, or communities that promote active lifestyles, yoga promises the political narrative of a free or relatively cheap state lunch. This fantasy forms part of yoga's new imaginative power across more and more of the world.

Yoga could be understood as an acultural, secular, and technocratic "best practice" that could be spread globally—the point, indeed, of the International Day of Yoga for the United Nations General Assembly. But it was arguably not the key point for many in India. There this technocratic language of universals became the coded way for different political interests to advance their causes under the banner of "world" and "universal." As Peter van der Veer argues, "[forms of yoga are] often described . . . as 'gifts to the world,' but that does not mean the givers have lost them."[80] Perpetuating a logic of Hindu universalism that van der Veer suggests has shaped India's religious modernity, this rhetoric enacts bids for identity and ownership. By "giving" yoga to the world, India was really pursuing the project of getting it back.[81]

I encountered this logic in action in the south Mumbai bookstore of Kitab Khana, where on the second floor, hidden away from the crush of college students and parents, I found a heavy hardback volume entitled *Yoga: Bharat's Invaluable Gift to the World* (2015). It was written by V. Ravi Kumar, whose author biography identified him as a youth worker in the service of the RSS, India's foundational Hindu nationalist association since the 1920s. The book cost a shocking 995 rupees—easily three times the price of many other books in the store. I bought it. Endorsed by such figures as Prime Minister Modi and Sri Sri Ravi Shankar, it had been brought out for the International Day of Yoga in 2015.

The book highlights its connections to Hindutva organizations and worldviews as it articulates its ambitions for India on a global stage.

"Bharat," often used as an aspirational name for "India" and a fantasy of an uncolonized Hinducentric original civilization, in the subtitle indicates how useful yoga can be for that political vision. The author's other books, listed in the back, included *Glimpses of Hindu Genius* (in both English and Hindi versions) and *Hindu Resurgence in South East Asia*. Kumar lists his "Books in writing (to be published later)," which include *India's Resurgence in 21st Century* [sic] and *Great Indian Muslims—Role Models for Indian Muslim Youth*. The former aimed to celebrate the rise of India and its diaspora; the second appeared to be, in the guise of multireligious commendation, a disciplinary tactic to steer Indian Muslim youth away from potentially threatening behavior.

The book reflects an attempt to harness digital material on yoga for a flexible Hindu nationalism, offering an undigested synthesis of yoga in English in the digital age. According to the author's note, "most of the content and the photos in this book have been taken from various free websites, and from my personal experiences and travels around the world."[82] While the chapters ostensibly give references, some material in the book is copied without attribution.[83] The volume yokes together lists of unattributed quotes about yoga; jerky shifts between historical theories of yoga and modern physiological benefits; and accounts of how yogic concentration helped Vedic seers gain insights into the universe. On the cover, the "Y" of "Yoga" is figured by the silhouette of a yogi performing a handstand with legs spread in a split. Within this landscape, its nationalist ambitions are clear: "one small yoga stretch in Mohan-Jo-Daro 5,000 years ago has become one large Yogathon across the world."[84] Though the production values differ sharply from the slick professionalism of the Incredible India campaign, the book's design reinforces the same logic by which yoga embodies intimacy between India and English.

Within overtly nationalist projects that bear such a distinct Hindutva ideology, what are we to make of the opening statement "Yoga now belongs to the world" (author's note) and the first chapter titled "The Universal Appeal of Yoga"?[85] This diplomatic gesture invites us to consider Marcel Mauss's classic theory of gifts, which distills the hidden ambitions of giving. "The form usually taken is that of the gift generously offered," Mauss argued, "but the accompanying behaviour is formal pretence and social deception, while the transaction itself is based on obligation and economic self-interest."[86] In this light, those giving yoga to the world may well be expecting to gain something in return—international status, economic benefits, or sympathy for Hindutva causes. Now "the world" and "the universal" are invoked precisely to forward political claims for visibility and recognition on behalf not only of India but also, in some cases (as with Kumar's book), a soft Hindutva. This rhetoric aligns with the social transformation of neo-Hinduism in a global age, where increased integration with global networks has gone hand in hand with a revival of political investments in India as a nation defined by a Hindu essence.[87] Routing yoga away from India as a "gift to the world" recaptures the practice for selective national visions.

This cultural logic informs India's attempts to remap and redefine yoga in the world. The state has eagerly sought the universalist imprimatur of institutions such as the United Nations and the World Health Organization to validate India-centric visions of how yoga might spread. In 2019, the Ministry of AYUSH sponsored a New Delhi meeting of international experts through the World Health Organization to review a draft document setting out benchmarks for yoga training.[88] Working through the WHO's Traditional Medicine Strategy 2014–2023, the Indian government has promoted an India-centric approach validated by a scientific health care framework. Leveraging the universalism associated with such international associations has become an increasingly important tactic.

What India hopes to get is what it appears to be giving: the cultural ownership of yoga. Unlike in a purely economic exchange in the market, where full ownership passes as soon as money changes hands, the identity of the gift is more bonded to the identity of the giver than to that of the recipient. The more enthusiastic the claim to give the practice to others, the more indissoluble this bond becomes. Through the rhetoric of the "world," India under Modi instantiates the nation as the proper steward of yogic tradition. This shift pulls yoga away from specific historical lineages of practice, the names of prominent gurus, and the branding operations of commercial studios. The act of giving solidifies the inalienable properties of the gift. In this sense, there is no real contradiction between expansive, generous claims for yoga's universality and contracting, codifying claims for its proper practice.

MASKING VIOLENCE

The most provocative form of yoga's imaginative power lies in its potential to mask and overwrite narratives of violence. Yoga has been used to recalibrate the international Anglophone reputation of Narendra Modi, the most prominent political practitioner of yoga in India since Gandhi. Modi came to national power as the leader of India's Bharatiya Janata Party (BJP), a right-wing party associated with Hindu nationalism that, as of 2015, has been considered the largest political party in the world.[89] He was re-elected for a second term in 2019.

Modi claims a long history as a practitioner of yoga. As a full-time worker for the RSS in the 1980s, he sought out instruction from the institute of H.R. Nagendra, who now heads the accredited Indian university S-VYASA. Nagendra consults with Modi's government on yoga policy and oversees influential Indian government initiatives to regulate yoga through international institutions.[90] Modi has cultivated a persona in which his reputation for daily practice bolsters his claims to dedicated national service. Yoga has become part of his signature style, as visible as his remaking of the Nehru jacket.

Modi's political style has often invoked the ideology of Hindutva.[91] Before he assumed national office, Modi served as the chief minister of the state of Gujarat with a platform that emphasized neoliberal economic reforms. But he was also known within and outside India in relation to major communalist riots, considered some of the worst in India's recent history, that broke out in Gujarat in 2002. Sometimes described as the Gujarat Pogroms, this period of religious rioting began with a train of Hindu pilgrims (including children) set ablaze, an act recalling the legendary train violence when India and Pakistan were partitioned in 1947.

Angry Hindus retaliated against Muslim communities for these attacks. In the ensuing weeks, around a thousand people were brutally killed (again including children). Modi's government was accused of failing to stem the tide of communal violence, and there remained widespread public suspicion that the BJP and other Hindu nationalist groups (such as the World Hindu Council) permitted or even actively incited the attacks on Muslims. Modi lent little comfort to the state's Muslims and declared that his only regret was that he had not handled the media better.[92]

These chilling events inspired prominent Indian intellectuals to place Modi within a linguistic frame of criminality, political manipulation, and fascism. In essays that were published in the Indian magazine *Seminar* after the riots, Modi was described as presiding over violence, accused of serving as a patron for the rioting gangs, and critiqued for his manner of responding to the public.[93] In the same issue of *Seminar*, other essays similarly described his tactics as cynical plays for power that used religious discourse to seek to consolidate his position among religious believers.[94] Modi faced lengthy court challenges in India and beyond for his role. Although he was given a clean chit by a special investigation team in 2012, he then faced a decade of appeals to this decision before receiving a clean chit from the Supreme Court in 2022.[95] A narrative of questions regarding complicity has thus shaped his rise in Indian politics.

Modi's international image has also been shaped through such questions. In 2005 the United States imposed a visa ban on him that remained in effect until 2014. Britain imposed a diplomatic boycott that lasted until 2012. In 2014, just before Modi visited the United States as prime minister, he received a U.S. court summons to account for his role in the riots. Although Modi was immune to such summons as a head of state, the publicity generated before a major U.S. visit served as a keen reminder of this narrative in the Anglophone public sphere. In 2023, shortly after Modi's receipt of a clean chit, the BBC released a documentary, *India: The Modi Question*, which investigates Modi's part in the Gujarat riots. Although critiqued by India as a "discredited narrative,"[96] the documentary presents enduring questions about Modi's ethical credibility, his control over right-wing Hindu agitation, and his ability to represent all Indians in good faith.

What has worked to offer an alternative to this narrative is not simply Modi's pro-business stance nor his legendary digital savvy; it is also yoga. Since he came to national power as prime minister, Modi's image and that of India have been linked through an intensive focus on the practice. In November 2014, he raised the ministry that regulated yoga to a national level, a move that brought dramatic attention to India's "yoga ministry" (technically the Ministry for Ayurveda, Yoga and Naturopathy, Unani, Siddha and Homeopathy, or AYUSH). Alyssa Ayres notes that "yoga made it to the short list of diplomatic priorities Modi outlined to a gathering of India's ambassadors in February 2015."[97] He has frequently promoted yoga in his talks with world leaders, offering books on yoga as formal state presents. On his diplomatic visits around the world, yoga has enlivened his encounters with such figures as Xi Jinping, Tony Abbott, Vladimir Putin, and Barack Obama, and the resulting publicity. This pattern has contributed to an underlying cultural logic by which yoga has helped Modi appear more human, as well as more superhuman.

Modi's new reputation as a global leader found spectacular opportunities through his proposal for the International Day of Yoga in 2014. Senior Indian diplomats have described it as very much Modi's initiative, a proposal that initially surprised both the United Nations and members of India's own Ministry of External Affairs (the branch of the public service tasked with public diplomacy).[98] The resolution passed easily, leading to the first celebration in 2015. For Modi and his government, the International Day of Yoga tells a triumphant story about rising India. Through yoga, India could appear as ancient yet contemporary; as above capitalism yet at its vanguard; as centrally Hindu yet broad-mindedly secular; as powerful yet peaceful. Through this celebration, Modi could be perceived by the world as both the nationalist prime minister and a capitalist world guru.

These alignments are made possible through explicit and implicit contrasts with populations who are simultaneously embraced and excised from sight. Anusha Lakshmi argues that "Modi's International Yoga Day has further entrenched the binary of the tolerant, 'civilised' Hindu and the intolerant, 'irrational' Muslim Other within the Indian national imaginary."[99] Andrea Jain, Sunila Kale, and Christian Novetske have described yoga in such a context as a form of "political theology" and "political ritual" that integrates conservative and neoliberal perspectives on the intimacy between individual personhoods and national bodies.[100] The International Day of Yoga has thus produced a large global platform that rebrands both the political leader and the nation on a global stage.

The International Day of Yoga lends itself to dramatic visual representation that serves political ends. Indian and Western media, through their internet coverage, have created a visual archive of photographs that portray India and Modi in new and sometimes unexpected lights. Many of these images emphasize the dramatic scale of bodies as a figure for a hypermodern India. Modi led 35,000 people in practice at Rajpath in New Delhi, which also serves as the site of India's Republic Day festivities. The ability to mobilize large masses doing yoga—and the dramatic wide-angle and aerial photographs that they inspire—present Indian power as authoritative, disciplined, and peaceful. The human geometry on visual display, guided by a political leader, lends the politician the aura of a guru. The nationalist resonance of the site is amplified by aerial visions that show large, uniformly clad, and highly ordered Indian practitioners.[101]

Visualizing large numbers of people in India is of course nothing new. India has long been cast as the land of crowds. But what makes these images different from the long-standing stereotype is the visual organization of the bodies.[102] These are not crowds; they are mathematically constructed groups in grids. The bodies aligned in practice, in the aerial view, mirror the vertical lines of the colonial arch that focalizes the picture and creates its vanishing point. The orderly geometry of human bodies in yoga emerges more vividly in closer photographs that fill the frame, conjuring magnitude.[103] This kind of framing has a history within Indian representations of yoga; as Joseph Alter shows, twentieth-century yoga groups have used photographic techniques to imply expansive memberships (which are difficult to document statistically).[104] The grid lines of the mats resonate with the sharp geometric boxes of yoga in one stage of the Incredible India campaign, where bodily curvatures are both energized and disciplined through color and space. The mass ordering of bodies also echoes, while it reworks and silences, the choreographic signature of Bollywood dance scenes where crowds perform synchronized movements. Whereas Bollywood films are often suffused with multisensorial excess,[105] the photographic archive of mass practice captures an ideal in which sights, sounds, and bodies are under control.

In such visual imagery, yoga appears endless. It also embodies a highly controlled mass order. Unlike in conventional crowd scenes, bodies do not touch or blur into each other. Even as the extended elbows overlap the visual field of other bodies, we know that the practitioners are rarely in contact: the image evokes interconnection without tactile corporeality. The embodied humans in these photos come to resemble the highly stylized human bodies emblazoned on the logo of their identical International Day of Yoga t-shirts. The people have become the brand.

State-orchestrated visual spectacle in the twenty-first century is ironic in India, which gave up state control over influential media such as television after the 1980s. Now, state theater cannot simply impose itself upon a nation with only one channel. It must compete for attention both domestically and globally in a world dominated by what Douglas Kellner calls "media spectacle."[106] Since the deregulation of media industries in the 1990s, spectacles have had to become ever more spectacular to claim attention. The strategic brilliance of yoga as a site of public diplomacy in some ways is not simply its spread as an embodied practice or its potential to increase tourist dollars to India, but its ability to claim for the Indian state an interface where it can become intimate with the public.

In June 2016, I found myself part of this intimacy. On a stage in the grandest room of University House at the Australian National University, I watched the wooden paneling soar upward like the adornment on a fine coffin. A group of kind, energetic middle-aged Indian men in suits bustled about. They pulled out banners. They set up microphones. They hovered, like anxious parents over a sleeping newborn, above the laptop from which cords and drives and cables dangled. This was my first meeting with the local chapter of GOPIO, the Global Organization of People of Indian Origin. In partnership with the Indian High Commission in Australia and UNESCO, they had been tasked with an event to celebrate the second International Day of Yoga. We sat on stage and looked out at the room. It was almost full, the audience only slightly diminished by the winter rain.

I asked polite questions of the panelists and thought of all the things about yoga that could not be said at this event. I had become part of a state spectacle that was in part legitimizing a personal brand and its larger worldview. In 1992, many miles away, watchmen in my aunt and uncle's apartment building had taken down my family's surname from the signboard of residents. They didn't want to reveal where Muslims lived in the building. But the mobs broke into my family's workshop where, on better days, artisans painstakingly smoothed the chipped edges of carved wooden furniture and mended old rugs. The rioters broke the pieces already broken. These unspoken stories rained down, softly and silently, behind the stained-glass windows.

The solicitous group of GOPIO organizers left me with a thank-you bag. Inside was a heavy, colorful book created for the first International Day of Yoga, commissioned by the Ministry of External Affairs and Public Diplomacy Division. I let it sit, wrapped in plastic, for six months beneath my desk at home before I opened it.

It's the eyes that strike me first. The cover image of the book, *International Day of Yoga*, shows Modi sitting in a half-lotus pose. His eyes are open. He gazes straight ahead at the camera.[107] His face is the perfect rectangle, white hair and cropped beard seeming as symmetrical as the left and right halves. It visually echoes the hazy gray rectangle of India Gate, visible in the distance far behind him. Though Modi reportedly was not originally scheduled to practice with the crowd, he unexpectedly took his place at the front.[108] In doing so, he gave himself a public role beyond measure.

The long scarf he wears, like a stylish version of the Indian flag, bears the tricolors of white, green, and saffron. It is one of the few times that Modi, who usually prefers variants of saffron, wears the dark green associated with Islam.[109] The hues match the colors of the International Day of Yoga logo. Though the logo marks a United Nations Day, the colors are India's colors. They radiate out from a blue human silhouette like the petals of a lotus and the aura of a halo. Modi, as always, is stylish. Tailored by the fashion designer Troy Costa, his clothes walk the line between India and the world. While many Indian men working internationally have adopted Western fashions of capitalism, such as suits, Modi's look harkens back to the distinctive Indian tailoring made iconic by Nehru. But for all the traditional homage, the cuts are fresh. He has won the hearts of millions of Indian youth this way, including those from Muslim communities. While Muslims old enough to have lived through decades of communal riots are often wary and unforgiving, many young Muslims dismiss this history. They see in his stylish persona, his brash temperament, and his love for corporate capital a model of their own desires. Modi rules by cool.

Modi's eyes look straight ahead. They see the camera, yet they also seem directed inward. In contrast, the eyes of the yoga practitioners sitting behind him move in many directions. Most of the visible practitioners are girls and women. Most hold their hands in a prayer position, while Modi's fingers shape themselves in a mudra. The young women's eyes, mostly, are closed. Many of their faces show the parted lips of intense focus. It is the expression in every photo of my daughter's face when she was two, lips poking out unconsciously as energies are absorbed in shifting sand, running water, flowing ink. Who controls the forces that flow through this practice?

In the third row, I catch three young women who look anxiously to the side. One seems wary, watchful, as if concerned she isn't doing it right. Another looks almost critical of her fellow practitioners. The third, the only one who has not put her hands in prayer position, appears afraid. Behind them all, off to the side, is a young bearded man with eyes open. He is smiling, cheekily. Such are the multiple imaginative possibilities of the International Day of Yoga. A political leader appears to command the devotion given a guru, but behind this image are multiple gazes and multiple perspectives. Even a highly ordered and regulated visual India, it seems, is of many minds about this enterprise. A meditation, a performance, a bad idea, a joke: these are the possible stories pushing against the singularity of an Indian state narrative.

In story and spectacle, the state simultaneously speaks and denies. Inside the commemorative volume, readers receive two warnings: that the opinions presented in the book do not represent the views of the Government of India, and that no material can be replicated without the consent of the Ministry of External Affairs. Both disavowing and controlling, invoking a participatory world heritage while simultaneously drawing upon intellectual property protections, the warnings reveal anxieties about what the state can and wants to own.

In the moments when such political tensions are least evident, they are most powerful. In a digital photo essay series on the International Day of Yoga in the *Daily Mail*, Modi lies supine in *śavāsana*, or corpse pose.[110] Yoga quite literally allows him to be seen from a new angle. Reversing his features, turning his face upside down: this is precisely the sort of transformative effect that yoga promises. The photograph lends Modi the authority and centrality of geometry, placing him in the foreground of the frame, while the supine pose implies the egalitarian inclusiveness of a democratically elected national politician. This image, and many others like it, circulated broadly through international mainstream media. They have helped to create a new social profile for Modi.

But these images also come with shadows. The power to orchestrate large groups, to synchronize their movements, and to direct their thinking is uncannily similar to the power that allows political groups to create, mobilize, and direct rioting gangs. Indeed, the alignment between the two images—yoga class and gang riot—comes together in the history of Hindu nationalism, in which the physical and mental disciplines of yoga can and have served as a foundation for martial political strength. In the image of *śavāsana*, we can begin to see grimly ironic echoes. These practitioners are playing visually at death, but behind them, in history, lie the dismembered and burned bodies of people killed in communal violence. On the International Day of Yoga, corpses have given way to corpse pose.

Yoga is sometimes described as alchemical, an art of transformation. Here that transformation is not just physical, psychological, or even spiritual: it is also political. Through these images of Modi leading International Yoga Day, yoga is used to transform the historical context in which he is read as a national, and even world, leader. The spectacular visuals of yoga, through highly orchestrated mass events, work to displace international frames of chaos and religious violence. Yet these exclusions, these terrible pasts, haunt the photographs. Seen from one angle, they may be one reason these photos exist.

CONCLUSION

India's campaign to promote the nation through yoga informs new visions of Indian leadership that draw cannily upon the iconography of the past as they aspire to material power in the present. They expand the symbolic and material touch of the state over a practice once seen as outside dominant social systems. Through visions of yoga, the body of the state and the body of the populace are made into one at the place where coercion and consent converge.

Yoga's narrative of transformation, of seemingly endless possibility, has also become a potential way for politicians to say no to material reforms in the lives of Indians. In Modi's second International Day of Yoga speech in 2016, he was reported to declare, "We did not have health insurance in olden times. But Yoga is a practice which gives health 'assurance' with zero spending."[111] His exemplary role as yogi has been used to justify working conditions that are associated with public health crises. In 2015, India's "yoga ambassador" C. M. Bhandari extolled Modi as a "selfless Karmayogi" whose use of yoga and meditation enabled him to work the grueling hours required of a prime minister. Challenging studies that linked medical problems to an increased workweek, Bhandari used Modi as his example to argue that yoga allows time devoted to labor to grow, not to shrink: a canny recasting of yoga as a capitalist tool that justifies the increasing expansion of work hours in the global economy.[112] This is precisely the logic, as Sarah Sharma has shown, behind the rise of corporate yoga worldwide, which seeks to "extend the limits of capitalism via a limitless body."[113]

As a practice that has been widely promoted for all through capitalism, regardless of gender, caste, or religion, yoga can be imagined by the state in ways that conceal and perpetuate histories of social exclusion. Seen in relation to caste, yoga's past is complex. Some strands of yoga's history show the making of upper-caste Hindu selfhood, while others suggest its capacity to bring different castes and religious groups together. Yogis in the Nath tradition during the colonial period, for example, rejected caste and gender hierarchies and challenged the Brahmin orthodoxy of their day.[114] Yet in the twenty-first-century, Nath political figures like Yogi Adityanath have been reported as saying that those opposing yoga should "leave Hindustan" or "drown themselves in the ocean."[115] Yoga thus serves as an ambivalent site of cultural incorporation for India's Muslims, Christians, and other religious minorities. Some BJP politicians have used it to reach out to Muslims by describing Muslim practices of prayer as forms of yoga. But many Muslims remain skeptical that the government's fondness for yoga is not a way of promoting Hindutva in disguise. They worry that the BJP trades politically on the interpretative possibilities of the practice, so that a sun salutation that looks like exercise to some will look like Hindu devotionalism to others. The uniformity of the orderly crowds promoted through the International Day of Yoga conjures up an India without difference, where all bodies must conform to the universalizing logic of the human silhouette on the t-shirt logo.

This chapter has traced the emergence of one form of yoga's imaginative work: its cultivation to produce a flexible India in the twenty-first century. Yoga's political profile can work to support democracy, yet it can also offer images of crowds under the control of spellbinding charisma. In these crowds, India's complex hierarchies of social control become invisible. We see no caste, no rich and poor, no religious markings. In the state's political spectacle, the neoliberal mandate of individual welfare for bodies matches the state's desire for a strong population under its control. Through the practice, the state reflects its own need to remain emotionally relevant to the citizenry that now faces the choice-making imperatives of neoliberal individualism. Yoga marks a place where those efforts help to create a flexible narrative for the new India, which looks old and new at the same time. India's leaders may not be able to fly, enter other people's bodies, or steal people's souls, like the yogis of folklore. But they too desire yoga for its powerful magic.

3

ALIGNING BOTH HANDS

Yoga in Indian Fiction

My hands reach out. The shelves unfold before me, heavy with stories yet to be touched. I pull out a book, just as I did when my father took me to The Happy Bookseller on Carolina summer evenings, just as I did in the Mission bookshops in San Francisco, just as I did on the second story of the old Strand when Mumbai was still Bombay.

When I was ten years old, the difference between America and India was measured by the difference in the smell of bookstores, the heft of pages, the nature of ink. In America, the crisp pages shone creamy white and the print stayed put in its place. In India, letters traveled in all directions. Their blurred edges bled into the grain of the translucent pages. When I turned a new leaf, the words stayed with me, the back sides of the letters throwing gray shadows across the next page of writing. They troubled and confused me, these three-dimensional ghostly words, written in a language I loved and yet whose mobile life I could not fully comprehend. As I read the stories of Ruskin Bond and Enid Blyton, sprawled on my cousin's bed back in the Bombay flat, I could not shake the sense that the pages in my hands were haunted by shadowy reversals.

In the Fort bookstore, the air conditioning hums. Gone are the slowly circulating ceiling fans of 1980s Bombay, where the blades moved in unison with the clerks behind the counter. The threshold leading to the crisp interior of the store is guarded by men in uniform. Outside, on the pavement, booksellers call in loud and wild voices to anyone who catches their eye. Inside, tones are quieter, and many of the clothes (including mine) could have been bought from the folded stacks of expensive woodblock-print *kurtas* at Fab India next door. The bookstore belongs to and defies the chaos of the city, full of openings and closings, replete with secret passages and locked doors.

In the twenty-first century, the bookstore bustles. Within this world of imaginative life, a realm not under the direct hand of the state, what new visions might rise to confirm, challenge, or complicate the meaning of yoga in India today? How do these visions of the practice inherit, interweave, and interrogate much older traditions? In this world of readers and reading, I seek the imaginative power of the practice. What I find are apparent oppositions that reveal themselves as political flexibilities: fictional visions that support state-sanctioned ideals, novels that profess the state's disavowed fantasies, and stories that critique the violence within the dream of yoga's power to bring peace.

———— ∞∞∞ ————

All over the world, it seems, bookstores are closing down. I can map each city I've lived in by the ghosts of vanished places. Yet in India new bookstores have also opened their doors. You can feel a confidence in the air, the image of the "New India" as it would like to see itself. The polish belies barely concealed anxieties. Frowning parents in Mumbai browse beautifully printed retellings of the *Mahābhārata*; six-year-olds tug their hands and point toward the walls of brightly colored comics. The children's shelves aren't just packed in the B and D sections with the complete works of Blyton, Bond, and Dahl. They've also expanded with last names like Arni, Murthy, and Kapadia. College students crowd the aisles with Chetan Bhagat's latest book about young Indians struggling to define success beyond good marks and a job in IT. These are India's growing readers of English, hopeful that the language will carve a passage into another world. Not only elites but also lower-class and Dalit communities have projected onto English the hope, perhaps illusory, that they might move more freely within and beyond India's complex social hierarchies.[1] These readers, their anxieties, and their aspirations have done what once seemed impossible in India: they have turned English into a language of bestsellers. If the shelves offer insights, it is that these new generations of urban readers seek not so much the playful torment of India's metafictional magical realists as what Ulka Anjaria calls "livable futures"[2] for their lives and their nation.[3]

This thirst for a fantasy of the real goes hand in hand with a need for a glorious past. India's mythic thrillers pack the shelves and tables of urban bookstores, reaching back to envision a time of heroism when Indian technology, medicine, and culture were the envy of the world. Flying chariots, magical herbs, and fantastical militaries abound. Mythic thrillers often lend comfort to the idea, promoted by India's Hindutva right wing, that the glory of ancient India lies in a past that can be presented as fundamentally Hindu.[4] India's politicians, including Narendra Modi, have traded on this idea, offering up images from India's textual traditions as signs that ancient Indians really did pilot airplanes, conduct surgeries, and reach the moon.[5] These imagined pasts offer guidance and consolation for India's twenty-first-century struggles. Linking the realist with the mythic, visions of yoga join these modes of imagining India.

Portraits of the practice take shape within a long history of written reflection. Not far from the tables piled with bestselling thrillers, but set in the shadows, are stories of India's gurus. Quietly, as if not to scare the stories away, I flip through autobiography after autobiography. Each book reminds me of the history of religious cosmopolitanism I've learned from Srinivas Aravamudan. Since the eighteenth century, Indian religious figures, novelists, and poets have created a language of their own that Aravamudan calls "Guru English."[6] This English guides, babbles, and flows across borders. It has helped Indians loom large on the global stage, shaping them as authorities even and especially when India was not politically strong. It has woven its way into the imagination of Western writers as well as Indian ones, creating the tight confines considered stereotypes,[7] yet also inventing new possibilities for expanded connections. Sometimes through complex coauthoring processes, gurus who wrote or published books for international audiences, such as Paramahansa Yogananda in the 1940s and B. K. S. Iyengar in the 1960s, used stories to elaborate their own authority; as Suzanne Newcombe has shown, bookstores formed central spaces where specific ideas of yoga were shared and codified for transnational audiences.[8] In the twenty-first century, stories help to project a guru's authority across time and space to direct the course of life when followers may not be able to meet face to face.[9] Readers form markets for spiritual empires.

Not all such new visions can be found on the shelves before me. The twenty-first-century world of code has allowed them to proliferate within digital discourse. Downloading a yoga-themed novel by a writer of Indian descent, I'm struck by how close I feel to the Incredible India campaign. Offering yoga as a gift to the world, and offering it to figures capable of high status in the West, are two projects that braid together the dreams of the Indian state with the approach of this novel and others like it. Interweaving a universalized language of yoga with sectarian interpretations of Hindu philosophy, such fiction reveals some of the broader sympathies between the two. This strand of Indian popular culture can serve as the right-hand man—and, I find, it often is a man—of the Indian state's imagination.

As I browse through the shelves in the Fort, pulling and flipping and scanning, I find a black book. The paper and the binding are not the kind used in the New India by Penguin or HarperCollins or Rupa, and from my fingers I know that it is self-published. On its cover glows a full moon over a mountain. A man hooded in black, completely covered except for his eyes and hands, lunges across the illustration. When I come to read it in full, back in the room where my grandfather used to listen to scratchy tapes of Koranic chanting, I find myself catapulted into sinister traditions of yogic folklore. In this novel, published in the wake of 2008 terrorist attacks on Mumbai, yogic philosophy propels a search for Indian justice and order that goes beyond what the state can openly allow: yogis condone torture, killing and chemical weapons to keep an imagined India safe.

My final discovery appears in Crossword. Unwisely, I go on foot to Kemp's Corner. I sidle up to Mumbaikars for a hint of pedestrian solidarity when I need to cross the road. By the time I make it safely across Crossword's threshold, I am in no hurry to leave the orderly grids of books in rows. Yet this safe, cool, aboveground haven takes me through a portal into an underworld of occult feminist fantasy. In the Tantric mystery novels I discover there, yoga feeds on female energies through sex and blood. These visions invite us to ask prickly, uncomfortable questions about the gendered foundations of yoga's left-hand history, and to question whether those sinister stories can spark revolutionary, self-reflective questions about yoga's capacity for exploitation.

In the pages that follow, I hope to apprehend yoga in Indian and Indian diasporic fiction in English through both left and right hands. I show how this twenty-first-century fiction draws strength from diverse religious genealogies, including the Vedas, Tantric sources, and the medieval *Bhāgavatapurāṇa*. Exploring these reanimations allows me to trace how intertwined discourses of yoga promote particular ideals of Indianness in the world. This quest often throws me off balance, calling to mind Purnima Mankekar's idea of "unsettling" India.[10] One of yoga's imaginative powers, I suggest, is its ability to inhabit not only India's perceived center but also its borders and margins. Yet whereas Mankekar works with the metaphor of "unsettlement" to illuminate India's renegotiation of borders, visions of yoga invite us to consider the complementary possibilities of flexibility. Precisely because the practice can stretch in such seemingly different directions, from seemingly peaceful quests for health to bloodthirsty battles for power, it renders more resilient the underlying intimacies between these different journeys and destinations.

These flexible visions reveal twenty-first-century links between historical ways of conceptualizing yoga. Although there is limited evidence for yogic practice in the Vedas, yoga is often imagined in "right hand" ways by the state and popular fiction as a practice used to bring about a perfected society, attributed to the Vedas, of peace, justice, and contentment. Although historical scholarship on Vedic society links this period as much to imperial violence as to idyllic social life,[11] the word "Vedic" in the twenty-first century is often used to figure a harmonious cosmological ideal that demonstrates a glorious Hindu past. This political fantasy is important to some parts of the Hindu right, who project onto the rhetoric of Vedic society the image of a powerful, original Hindu India (often referred to as Bharat) to which twenty-first-century India should seek to return. Aligned with this project are religious visions that are not themselves strictly traced to the Vedas, yet can be considered compatible with the broader political fantasy. Yoga is often called upon as a tool to enact this ideal. In contrast, yogic traditions linked to non-Vedic practices, such as Tantra, have often been perceived as the dark, magical, sinister "other" to the supposedly upright Vedic universe of peace and devotion. Although these divisions help us to understand historical differences in goals among yogis,[12] Indian popular culture of the twenty-first century, as in centuries past, reveals interwoven cultural logics that join the "right hand" and "left hand." Although they may appear to be at odds, they haunt each other's presence.

In the first part of this chapter, I explore a "right hand" vision, Mohan Ashtakala's speculative fiction *The Yoga Zapper* (2015), which brings to life a Vedic-inspired world of sectarian cosmology through persistent recruitment of non-Indian white subjects—resonating with the Indian state's Incredible India campaign. In the middle section, I investigate a vision that interweaves right and left. Atul Merchant's thriller *Taskari* (2014) yields insight into twenty-first-century battles over the meaning and purpose of yoga by openly celebrating the violence necessary to bring about a harmonious Vedic world order. In the final section, I turn to a feminist Tantric vision, Shweta Taneja's urban fantasy *The Rakta Queen* (2018), to explore how the "left hand" capabilities of yoga may offer a form of *svādhyāya*, in the remixed genealogy I have offered, to critique exclusive, gendered, and violent state practices. These morphing visions of yoga create the welcoming gateway to India, the security guard evicting the unwanted, and the surprising portal to new worlds when it seems that all borders are closed. Such flexibilities reveal a complex and contested grip on the meaning of Indianness today.

RIGHT-HAND IMAGINARIES: THE READER
AND THE TOURIST

Authority over yoga is changing in the twenty-first century. India's internal regimes of dedicated practice, with authority conferred through charismatic benediction, are gradually giving way to transnational bureaucratic regimes of hours-based certifications and employment qualifications.[13] In the new millennium, India has sought a leading role in shaping how yoga can reproduce as it spreads. In the late 2010s, the Indian state moved assertively to work in the protective shadow of international bodies like the World Health Organization and the United Nations to create new regimes that inform how yoga can be taught in the twenty-first century.[14]

At stake is whether the practice will foreground Indian histories and cultural identities as it grows globally popular. Though the state has energetically assured the world that all are welcome as practitioners and convinced bodies like the UN that yoga is a holistic health practice best understood through deracinated scientific rhetoric, the state does not want to abandon key connections between yoga and ideas of Indian cultural, moral, and technological prowess. The Ministry of Ayurveda, Yoga and Naturopathy, Unani, Siddha and Homoeopathy (AYUSH) begins its "Guidelines for Organizing of Yoga Fest/Utsav in States/UTs" with the statement "Yoga is a system of holistic living, having the roots in Indian tradition and culture."[15] As the state seeks a stronger voice in how yoga is taught globally, it must at once deny and proclaim that yoga is culturally intimate with India.

Fiction plays a key role in this quest because it offers an alternative pathway to authority over and through the practice. When I read Mohan Ashtakala's self-published *The Yoga Zapper* (2015), I found myself hailed as both reader and tourist, invited through yoga to affirm particular and selective ideas of India. I had the uncanny sensation that the logic of Incredible India was speaking through the novel. These ideals unwittingly resonate with soft Hindutva images of an indigenous India designed to comfort an embattled Hindu majority, an idea of indigeneity invested in forgetting anything that came before Hindu lifeworlds and disavowing anything that came later. In my reading, I build on Patrick McCartney's work on "the ways in which non-Indian consumer-converts of yoga potentially become enculturated into banal, affective, vicarious support and tacit endorsement of Hindutva through the coercive consensus-building involved in adopting a yogic way of life."[16] This political ideal of a Hindu-centric India is both a domestic project and a way of selling India to foreign tourists, especially those who can be read through the category of white racial identity. Although the novel draws on South Asian religious discourses more complex than simple political propaganda, its fantastical worlds turn readers into tourists. Such fiction offers popular culture's unwitting right-hand man to the Indian state's imagination.

Mohan Ashtakala, a writer of Indian origin based in North America, describes himself as "an initiated Hindu Vaishnava priest" who "has lived in yoga ashrams across India."[17] Ashtakala locates his source of authority over yoga in a key sectarian Hindu tradition marked by devotion to the god Vishnu and his avatars. Charmingly self-deprecating on his website, Ashtakala offers a list of nine interesting things about himself: "Mohan has a degree in Accounting and worked in that field for several years while indulging in his passion for writing. As an accountant, he was a pretty good writer of fiction."[18] His novel emerged through the new digital channels offered by self-publishing and explicitly directs itself to U.S. audiences.

The Yoga Zapper tells the story of two white American brothers, Jack and Steve, who travel to India and discover a special yoga shastra that "zaps" them to different moments in time. This journey takes them into a cyclic cosmology of four ages, or *yugas*. In the perfect first age of Satya Yuga, beautiful people meditate in village sunlight; in the degraded fourth age, Kali Yuga, monstrous cannibals devour the beauties of the planet. Portrayed as a world of unfettered capitalism and dictatorial power, the fourth age figures fears that resonate with the twenty-first century. The brothers must fight an epic battle to destroy the evil forces of the Kali Yuga, preserve Vedic and yogic teachings for humanity, and restart the world afresh in the first age. Embracing its capacity to explain India to non-Indians, this novel is resolutely anti-subaltern. It blends twenty-first-century realism with faith in *siddhis*, or special powers; presents yoga as a key technology for liberation; and features protagonists whose journeys resonate with the spiritual tourism promoted by Incredible India and its ideal vision of a Hindu past. Yoga is envisioned as a practice whose flexibilities reconcile, and thus render more resilient, claims to universalism invested in hierarchies of race and gender.

Ashtakala articulates his novel as a gateway to Indian philosophies and mythologies:

> Yoga is not just a grounded physical practice (though it can be taken as just that), or a deep spiritual philosophy (which adds depth to the practice), but also has its own legends and mythic origin stories—a view of humanity's future (and past), of society's moral evolution and a view of yoga's own rise, diminution, demise and eventual rebirth—all wrapped up in an exciting and engrossing tale.[19]

His ultimate goal is "to expose the authentic narratives of the Yoga tradition through the medium of modern, page-turning novels."[20]

Ashtakala aligns "the Yoga tradition" with the *Bhāgavatapurāṇa*, a tenth-century set of narratives from medieval South India in the Vaiṣṇava tradition with which he identifies. The *Bhāgavatapurāṇa* is usually understood as a collection of stories that emerged within post-Vedic *bhakti* traditions of devotional theism that privilege emotional intimacy with the divine. Such traditions are often seen as at once egalitarian and hierarchical, challenging caste divides in their insistence on direct devotion to the divine yet also compatible with the dominance of Brahmins in social and political spheres.[21] Ashtakala cites the edition published by the Bhaktivedanta Book Trust, a publishing arm of the International Society for Krishna Consciousness (commonly known as the Hari Krishnas) that promotes texts from Vaiṣṇava traditions. This translation and its commentary are often considered to reflect a sectarian interpretation of the *Bhāgavatapurāṇa*. Yoga is thus read through, and in some ways merged into, a specific religious discourse of devotion.

Claiming the *Bhāgavatapurāṇa* as central to "the Yoga tradition" represents an unorthodox approach both to the *Bhāgavatapurāṇa* and to traditions explicitly centered on yoga. In many ways, "yoga" understood as a form of devotion in the narratives is quite different from the kind of disciplined and austere mental practices associated with earlier sources, such as Patañjali. It is fascinating that Ashtakala turns to the *Bhāgavatapurāṇa* to authorize foundation myths for yoga, because this text is potentially interested in making yoga less—not more—powerful. Scholars have argued that the *Bhāgavatapurāṇa* appropriates an earlier eightfold system of yoga into its Vaiṣṇava devotionalism and cultivates a yoga oriented toward sacred sound.[22] At the same time, Barbara Holdrege shows, the text gives an account of its own origins that stresses the inadequacies of yoga. Though the poet Vyāsa has become adept in the practice, he feels unsatisfied. To reach fulfillment, he is advised to sing the praises of Krishna, which leads him to create the *Bhāgavatapurāṇa*.[23] In these understandings of Ashtakala's source text, yoga is a good but insufficient start. Whereas the *Bhāgavatapurāṇa* wishes to applaud but also supersede yoga as an ultimate project, *The Yoga Zapper* gives yoga the last word in its final line: " 'Come,' said the old man, 'let us practice yoga.' "[24] While the source text of the novel runs on devotional energies, the novel's rhetorical stress on yoga offers a new, transnationally acceptable way to validate Vaiṣṇava Hindu cosmologies for nonsectarian audiences.

In drawing on the *Bhāgavatapurāṇa* as a source of legends about yoga, Ashtakala gives these narratives a new social role. In India and beyond, as McComas Taylor has shown, seven-day public recitations of the *Bhāgavatapurāṇa* are immensely popular gatherings where devotees create twenty-first-century forms of religious capital.[25] Unlike many of these recitations, which focus on stories of Krishna's life, Ashtakala concentrates on cosmology.[26] His novel is particularly concerned with the system of ages, found in India's epics and in the Sanskrit collections of religious stories, legends, and folklore known as the *Purāṇas*. As many religious and yoga-related texts have done since the first references to this system appeared around the turn of the Common Era,[27] *The Yoga Zapper* presents the age of destruction, the Kali Yuga. The novel thus links twenty-first-century understandings of yoga to ideas about the beginning and end of the world.

Ashtakala's use of the *Bhāgavatapurāṇa* ties his portrait of yoga more closely to broader ideals that have been important to visions of India as fundamentally Hindu. When the world restarts after the grand battle, Steve and Jack find themselves in the first, orderly age of Satya Yuga that resonates with soft Hindutva visions of political perfection before the perceived corruptions of Islam and European colonialism. In this ideal age, the forest dwellers speak in Sanskrit as a perfected language—a concept that has been important to Hindu nationalism in the twenty-first century.[28] This vision merges with Ashtakala's allusion to Buddhist political perfection as interpreted through the gaze of Western Orientalism, exemplified by the British writer James Hilton's portrait of the mythical valley of Shangri-La in *Lost Horizon* (1933). Ashtakala draws upon the Buddhist ideal of a hidden paradise designed to protect key spiritual teachings from the chaos of the world:

> The residents of Shambala smiled again, joyful and satisfied to live in their intimate spiritual community, taking care of each other in their simple, sweet lives. They re-established their rituals—those of waking at the brahma muhurta hour, yoga, meditation, japa and puja, performing their duties, gathering wood, cooking and singing the evening kirtans—finding in this both solace and structure.[29]

Alluding to macro and micro time found in the *Purāṇas*, the novel envisions a perfected, preindustrial, precapitalist "before" that is also an "after," a place where the corruptions of the Kali Yuga have been washed away. Yet the pastoral peace of that age can only be regained through the battle that ends and restarts the cycle of time. In this way, the mythical ideal is both perfectly peaceful and predicated upon massive destruction. These fictional pasts are at once grand and vulnerable, embattled and hegemonic.

Despite many liberal threads that run through the novel, *The Yoga Zapper* reveals visions of yoga that reiterate particular social hierarchies at its center. Although the gender transformation of yoga shifted it from a practice largely limited to men in the early twentieth century to a pursuit popular with women by the late twentieth, Ashtakala's novel aligns yoga with male desire. *The Yoga Zapper* invites readers to identify with heterosexual masculine longing as part of their journey into this imagined India. Steve, cast back to the first age of time, finds himself in an idyllic world in which he is immediately treated as an honored guest. These fantasies could be those of Incredible India, which works hard in advertising campaigns to assure Western subjects of special hospitality if they come as tourists. When Steve arrives unexpectedly from the future, villagers wash his feet and scatter his path with petals. He is taken under the tutelage of a fatherly rishi and falls in love with the rishi's exceptional daughter. Shanti's name in Sanskrit, "peace," makes her a cipher for the spirit of her idyllic age. Although Ashtakala tries at the very end of the novel to give her a more exciting role—she pilots a *vimāna*, or flying chariot, in the final battle and destroys the evil data collection center on the moon—by and large, Shanti upholds the ideal that women should be demure, faithful, and gorgeous. Through Steve and Shanti's attraction, yoga gains new imaginative power as a fantasy suitable for heterosexual men.

This feminized object of desire hints at the political and economic powers that shape such longing. Shanti calls to mind the forms of female beauty found in the Amar Chitra Katha comics and Indian children's mythic tales on my childhood bookshelves, yet also not out of place in Western fashion magazines: "a young woman in the prime of youth, she displayed slender arms and unblemished skin the color of freshly-pressed, golden olive oil. . . . Her breasts, though small, clung full and firm on her strong, yet supple, frame."[30] Flexibility is one of her key allures. Desirable by both Western and Indian beauty norms, which were historically shaped through interconnected colonial and capitalist circuits, Shanti is imagined as a perfect object for men to behold.[31] She exemplifies a particular ideal of Indianness validated as "Indian" through the gaze of a non-Indian man. "India's opening up to the world 'outside' in the current economic climate of globalisation," Vanita Reddy argues, "finds a symbolic parallel in the beautiful Indian woman who has become linked to the world outside through the global currency of her beauty."[32] Projected onto such beauty, yoga is used to secure the sign of India.

The novel's universalizing visions of yoga pull its image of India into unwitting alliance with racial hierarchies. The gifts of yoga are offered selectively. The novel asserts authority over the practice through the act of giving it to American men who can be seen as white.[33] These attempts to create an Indian cosmos populated by white Western characters resonate with the soft power strategies of Incredible India. Like the 2009 "Motherland" marketing campaign, which profiled Europeans and other foreigners who had chosen to make India their home, the novels aim to make India into an object of desire for white Western subjects.[34]

In India, as Shefali Chandra has shown, engagements with whiteness have often energized forms of Indianness, particularly those with high status.[35] In the spaces connecting India and the United States, which shape *The Yoga Zapper*, the relationship between Indianness and whiteness has a vexed and vexing history. Indians in the United States have been asked to map themselves on shifting ground in a world governed by the historical resonance of a white-black polarity, a set of racial categories that do not match major person-making categories in South Asia (such as caste, religion, or diet), and an ambiguous legal history of insecurity in relation to the changing construct of whiteness.[36] Before 1923, Indians of high caste and light skin were able to access the U.S. category of whiteness in states divided into "white" and "colored." Material benefits, such as eligibility for citizenship, rested on such classifications. In 1923, however, the famous case of Bhagat Singh Thind ruled that Indians could not be considered white.[37] Though Indians kept trying, they could not fully crack open that legal category.[38] Once affirmative action policies afforded material benefits to minority status, some Indian Americans were more willing to let go of whiteness. For others, inspired by anticolonial activism, civil rights, and racial pride movements, whiteness was something to dismantle rather than to desire. By 1980 Indians were counted as "Asian" for the first time in the U.S. census, and by 1990 the census included an "Asian Indian" checkbox. Pushed into and thrown out of historically shifting racial categories, Indians in the United States have experienced a form of citizenship in which they have been forced to be flexible: a strong contrast to the strategic opportunism exemplified by Ong's "flexible citizenship."[39] These uneven and ambiguous histories shape how Indian diasporic novels reach out to subjects who access the category of whiteness.

The logic of the gift entwines Indian identity more closely with whiteness. Steve in *The Yoga Zapper* exemplifies the myth of the American Dream, and at the end of the novel, he is joined with Shanti to become a progenitor—a " 'Prajapati' "—to repopulate the world.[40] As Mauss suggests in his theory of the gift, the act of giving strengthens the bond between giver and receiver.[41] In giving away the future of yoga to characters who can be read as white, the novel binds ideas from India more closely to the social privileges associated with whiteness through its image of a new generation who will carry both lineages in their bodies.[42]

These racial politics simmer within the novel's overt rejection of racism. *The Yoga Zapper* aims at many points to carefully offer a cosmopolitan portrait of yoga practitioners. The group of spiritual elect who carry the teachings of the Vedas and yogic philosophy through the ages and eventually repopulate the world are "twelve young couples, each from a different community, representing the different peoples from all parts of the earth."[43] The heroic warriors who aim to save the world from tyrannical destruction represent "diverse backgrounds, origins, and races,"[44] while the yogis reveal a wide range: "some had bodies the color of dark rainclouds, others came from desert lands and wore long robes, several, light-skinned and blue-eyed, appeared from the northern snows and a few, golden-hued with enchanting black eyes, journeyed from the southern seas."[45] As these passages reaffirm, the novel appears committed to precisely the mantras used by the Indian state in its presentation of the practice: yoga is a universal practice open to all.

Yet exceptionalism also marks this vision. *The Yoga Zapper* appears keen to deliver the future of yoga into the hands of white male Americans alone. Jack is told " 'This shastra is more valuable than you can ever know. Your life, the future of the entire world depends on it. You have to take it. Only you. No one else!' "[46] Exceptionalism, of course, is part of how fantasy works, and I do not think that Ashtakala in any way means to imply disparagement of other ethnic groups. (Indeed, Ashtakala's second novel, *Karma Nation* [2018], deals with an Indian-mediated vision of American interracial romance.) However, a cultural script working through liberal cosmopolitan visions suggests that a Hindu-centric world view is especially keen to attach itself to the power invested in figures who can be seen as young, male, and white.

At the same time, Indian cosmology is in charge. Visions of whiteness are contained within the cosmological structures attributed to yogic philosophy. This gives explanatory power to predominantly Hindu religious narrative while reaching out to show how this logic governs the experience of non-Indian bodies. Once, "Hindoos" in the United States had to negotiate legal definitions of whiteness; now whiteness must obey cosmological laws found in Vaiṣṇava texts such as the *Bhāgavatapurāṇa*. In such a vision, Indian writers seek to control the terms of representation of race—something that minorities in the West have rarely been able to do. Through the twinned frames of writing and yoga, Indian diasporic writers fantasize about a universe where the larger norms and structures—nothing less than the logic of the universe—are Hindu-centric and Indian. The novel thus both courts and disciplines whiteness in ways that resonate with the strategies of the Incredible India campaign.

Such fiction seeks to resolve tensions between the desire to give yoga to figures of high status in the world and the yearning to amplify Indian control over yoga's development. This doubleness in visions of yoga turns India's unsettlement into its flexibility. By offering such malleability, yoga helps to conceal key contradictions. By interweaving complex South Asian religious discourses, reinforcing gendered hierarchies, and appealing to particular racial ideals, novels like Ashtakala's align powerfully with the way India wishes to present itself through yoga to the world. These forms of popular culture join forces with the state, serving as its right-hand man.

UNSPEAKABLE STATE FANTASIES

Not all stories are so overtly well aligned. Yoga's presence in fiction does not always match the Indian state's projected image of health, wellness, and utopian society. It also lures us into spaces where the state may not want, or may not want to admit, intimacy with the imaginative work of popular culture. To such a story I now extend a hand.

———— ∞ ————

One November night in 2008, a group of men stepped off a black boat onto an almost deserted Mumbai beach. Their backpacks were blue, the small bags they carried red. They headed toward the Gateway of India.

Over the next few days, these kill teams fanned out across the city of Mumbai. They shot commuters, rabbis, and backpackers. They set fires and bombs. They killed police and children.

One of those children was in the Taj Mahal Palace Hotel. When I was not much older than that child, in the early 1980s, my family would take me to the Taj for ice cream and dosa. The curves and angles of its gray-and-white stone divided the sewage floating out where the sailboats moored from the cool glasses of *nimbu pani* and crisply fried delights inside. That November, the cool refuge for the elite became its blazing prison. One hundred and sixty-six people died, including a mother and her son.

That child had a friend, and that friend had a father, and that father was an aspiring writer. In the days following the attacks on Mumbai, he wrote a novel and published it himself. He named it *Taskari*, meaning "thief" in Sanskrit. The novel is Atul Merchant's answer to India's ago-nized question of how to face terror, especially Islamic radicalism linked to Pakistan. His solution is a Hindu-centric form of yogic warfare.

The yoga that weaves its way through this novel is far from the pos-tural practices found in the *shalas* near Merchant's home in south Mum-bai. Instead, as in *The Yoga Zapper*, it takes the guise of *bhakti*, or devo-tional, yoga. To reflect on how Merchant thinks about yoga as a response to India's twenty-first-century predicaments, we must step back through what he presents as his own gateway to the practice: north Indian clas-sical music and the yogic philosophies that resound through its notes.

Before writing fiction, Merchant tells his readers, he was a student of north Indian classical music. He studied with a sitar player named

Rooshikumar Pandya, who encouraged him to try his hand at writing. Pandya was a student and the second husband of the notoriously reclusive Annapurna Devi, one of India's masters in the north Indian classical tradition of hereditary musicians. Before she locked herself away from the world, becoming "the greatest surbahar player you never heard,"[47] Annapurna Devi was one of three luminary heirs in her musical world. The other two—her brother, Ustad Ali Akbar Khan, and her first husband, Ravi Shankar—became world famous for bringing north Indian music to global ears. All three were taught by Annapurna Devi's father, Ustad Allauddin Khan, who was considered one of the greatest musicians of India's midcentury. As a student, Merchant became close to the family. When a reporter from *Man's World* came in 2000 for the first interview Annapurna Devi had granted in fifty years, it was Atul Merchant who guided the reporter into the "forbidden zone" of her Mumbai flat on Malabar Hill.[48]

Merchant sets the second half of *Taskari* (2014) in an ashram where devotees practice *bhakti* yoga through music. The ashram resonates with the ideals Merchant credits to "GuruMa Annapurnadevi—the entire second half of my story and the philosophy behind it is based on the *sanskar* [imprint] she endowed us with by generously sharing what she inherited from her father."[49] Baba, the guru of *Taskari*'s fictional ashram, declares that " 'it is said that Bhakti Yoga is the easiest way to achieve salvation; and music is the easiest of all the available mediums. . . . Undoubtedly, music is a gift from India to the world.' "[50] Echoing the language that the state uses for yoga—India's "gift to the world"—the novel tells a similar kind of story. By giving music away, India can claim this approach to yoga more tightly.

For many ethnomusicologists, one of the virtues linked to Annapurna Devi's musical lineage has long been its religious cosmopolitanism. For many centuries, in Hindustani music traditions in northern India, Muslim musicians at court sang to Hindu gods. Until the twentieth century, most Hindustani musicians were Muslim singers and players who learned their arts from their families before them. For these hereditary musicians, sound offered a devotional path to the sacred that did not necessarily distinguish between Hindu and Islamic understandings of the divine. Ustad Allauddin Khan was known as "a devout Hindu and Muslim."[51] Annapurna Devi was born into a Muslim family (where she was originally known as Roshanara Khan) and became Hindu upon her marriage to Ravi Shankar.[52] Histories of music have celebrated this tradition's ability to bring musicians, patrons, and listeners together across India's tense religious lines.[53]

The story of north Indian classical music has also illuminated the rising power of communal distinctions in ways that have empowered Hindu middle classes at the expense of the Muslim hereditary families. India's emergent music institutes relied on Muslim hereditary musicians to train a new generation of middle-class Hindu musicians who would ultimately replace them.[54] In light of the broader marginalization of Muslim communities in twenty-first-century India, the story of classical music can be read in ways that lend comfort to soft Hindutva and even Islamophobia.

These tensions—Hindustani music as both the space of complex collaboration and the site of Muslim decline—shape the significance of yoga in Merchant's *Taskari*. The novel intervenes in a larger, anguished debate about how the nation should confront endemic issues of corruption and how it should approach the kind of security challenge posed by the young men from Pakistan's Lashkar-e-Tayyaba who blew up the Taj. The key theme is the idea of "thievery" as morally necessary in immoral times. "Although 'Taskari' in the Sanskrit language simply means theft, it has much deeper significance," the novel declares in its back matter. It authorizes this through reference to a text from the Black Yajurveda, a part of the Veda that intermingles ritual utterances with discussions of their meaning: "According to the Krishna Yajurveda Taittariya Samhita [*sic*], whenever someone steals, Lord Shiva will 'steal' it back."[55] Ustaad, Rani, and Raji, the main characters, are Shiva-like thieves who steal from the rich to give to the poor. The first half of the novel focuses on their thefts; the second half finds them hiding from the law in an ashram of devotees who pursue *bhakti* yoga through music. The thieves assume that wealth in twenty-first-century India is fundamentally black money (the assumption behind Narendra Modi's demonetization campaign of 2016). They see this corruption as a sign of the cosmological concept of the

"Kaliyug," which, like *The Yoga Zapper*, the novel defines as " 'the Age of Downfall or Spiritual Degeneration.' "[56]

The folkloric traditions of sinister yogis have long shaped Western perceptions of yoga.[57] In some, trickster saints, like the founder of the Nath yogis, Gorakhnath, are thought to blend the sacred with the profane in order to arrive at deeper spiritual truth.[58] Portraits of Hindu holy men beyond India's borders reveal a persistent tension between the benevolent guide to enlightenment and the charlatan trickster who preys on naïve searches for easy answers.[59] Yogis of all stripes can be seen as hypnotic beings, their mesmerizing force a metaphor for the intimacy between weaving and erasing deceptions large and small.[60] Yogic groups in India and beyond have sometimes advocated violence as a means to pursue utopian goals.[61] Anxieties about sinister possibilities aligned with larger pursuits of truth have fed broader fears about the potentially disruptive presence of India and Indianness.[62] *Taskari* draws on such legacies to celebrate the sinister as a path toward what the novel presents as the right way forward.

As part of a larger rise of cultural narratives in India that speak to threats of terrorism, *Taskari* presents an idealized view of an alternative. This land is a place of peace, a utopia of cultural and moral sophistication, and a realm of ideal warriordom governed by individuals unaccountable to anyone. Just as the novel draws directly upon the authority of the Vedas, this political ideal is identified with generalized Vedic rhetoric. The ashram, a " 'Vedic Lifestyle Resort,' "[63] resonates with broader soft Hindutva fantasies of "Vedic" as a synonym for values of justice and harmony that lend strength to Indian national branding.[64] *Taskari* speaks approvingly of key figures in the creation of Hindutva, such as Vinayak Damodar Savarkar, and shares Hindutva's yearning for strong martial leaders. Dismissing the nonviolent methods made famous by Gandhi and Nehru, as well as due process of law, *Taskari* advocates harsher methods. Ustaad advises the police on how to torture suspects to produce confessions and how to plant evidence to ensure convictions. These tactics, the novel assures us, are necessary to ensure that true justice is done. Because governmental institutions are so thoroughly corrupt, only those outside the law have any hope of promoting what they see as

102 ALIGNING BOTH HANDS

true social order. Under the sign of the Vedas, *Taskari* draws on its authority of revelation to lend strength to this political vision.

While yoga is often cast in Indian tourist discourse as a welcoming gateway to India, *Taskari* reveals how yoga is used to manage a very different kind of border problem for the nation. Set in the Himalayas, the ashram of *Taskari* is not a remote apolitical escape but a site of vulnerability for India's national security. Baba, the leader, puts the situation this way:

> "Please understand that we are on the borders of Nepal and China. Our Government has left the borders unguarded. Each day hundreds of people infiltrate through these borders. Dharchula has become a preferred pass for the terrorists on one hand and on other hand, there is a multifold increase in Kailash-Mansarovar pilgrims who halt here for food and lodging, and donate."[65]

Merchant's novel reminds us of the strategic significance of the ashram for India's control over its geopolitical identity, locating yoga at the heart of broader anxieties over its historical ability to define, claim, and maintain its northern edge.

Visions of yoga in *Taskari* thus construct an alternate border that reaffirms a soft Hindutva view of India against a distinctively othered Islamic Pakistan. Over time, it comes to pass that some of the visitors staying in the ashram are potential Pakistani terrorists who use the ashram as a base to plot new violence. Baba deciphers their phone codes to reveal a plan to bomb the office of Narendra Modi and the headquarters of the Nagpur RSS. Raji develops a plan to use hydrofluoric acid on the terrorists, eventually killing two of the three. India, a signatory to the Chemical Weapons Convention of 1993, officially declared its stockpiles and announced their eradication in 2009.[66] Raji's extrajudicial violence thus violates India's international agreements as well as its domestic military policy. Yet his attack finds unofficial sanction in the novel from the police, the Indian army, and the Research and Analysis Wing (India's foreign intelligence agency), who are grateful for an operative who can maneuver in ways they cannot be seen to do. In this vision, yogis most effectively manage India's borders and security.

Although India has used images of yoga to leverage the perception of benevolent peace in its foreign policy—which some believe has helped it buy uranium and conclude nuclear deals—*Taskari* reveals an unspeakable fantasy for the state. Interpretations of yoga lend moral authority to the extrajudicial use of internationally banned substances to defeat a perceived terrorist threat. Baba teaches: "'Ahimsa is only loosely translated as non-violence. Unlike the English word "non-violence," which is absolute in its meaning, ahimsa means non-violence in a relative sense. There are times when violence can also be considered ahimsa if that violence is used to stop greater violence.'"[67]

This interpretation resonates with early twentieth-century understandings of yoga in texts like the *Bhagavadgītā*, where Krishna's justification of violence to Arjuna was used to legitimate anticolonial visions of armed resistance to the British.[68] The flexibilities within this yogic concept allow violent practices to conceal their own status as violence. This vision of yoga animates alternate sovereignty that addresses the vulnerabilities of twenty-first-century India.

Though *Taskari* is particularly direct in its use of sinister yogic practices to fight a war on terror, it is not alone. Amish Tripathi's *The Immortals of Meluha* (2010), which became a bestselling novel and launched a popular series, envisions an enduring conflict between the Suryavanshis, or worshipers of the sun, and the Chandravanshis, or worshipers of the moon. Although their territorial control does not map geographically onto today's India and Pakistan, the symbolism lends itself to such a reading through a Hindu nationalist lens: the Suryavanshis practice customs associated with Hindu lifeworlds (such as caste) and are highly refined and virtuous, while the Chandravanshis bear a lunar symbol that resonates with the Islamic crescent and are described as terrorists. The Suryavanshis wish to convert the Chandravanshis to what they see as their superior way of life; only then, the novel implies, will peace reign. Within *Taskari*, as well, is a hint of coercive conversion. Those who accept India's "gift to the world" may be graciously embraced within universalistic norms of benevolence, but those who deny this gift—those seen as Pakistani Muslims, like the plotting terrorists who stay at the ashram but refuse to participate in yoga or music—lose any claims to due process, law courts, or life itself. Yoga sits at the heart of these emerging fantasies of Hinduized metaphysical, moral, and political power.

Books like this one invite readers to realize how the power of the left-hand traditions—the yogi as a figure of violence and black magic—remains vital within twenty-first-century Indian fantasies of yoga as an imagined solution to ongoing problems with border management, national image, and international terror. Although these images are exactly the opposite of the peaceful, health-giving practice that the Indian state promotes in public discourse, the left-hand traditions both challenge and underwrite the powers projected onto yoga. It's unlikely that many—or any—of the bookstore-goers I saw in Mumbai took home a copy of the book I bought, hidden as it was on the obscure second story, but the fact of its existence reminds us of the concealed currents and eddies that shape yoga's imaginative power. These anarchic, unauthorized stories may be disavowed by the state, yet they yield insight into the darker logics that continue to energize a yoga of peace, love, and tourist travel.

Such disavowed fantasy, visible in these uncensored fragments of popular culture, haunts the claims of the state. This yoga works under cover of darkness with banned substances toward what it sees as the liberation of India from foreign sources of violence. In this novel, the right hand, though it cannot admit it, knows all too well what the left hand is doing.

SINISTER QUESTIONS

In Haridwar and Varanasi, one finds many types: holy men, yogis, survivors of black magic. Some of them were willing to answer the strange questions put to them by Shweta Taneja, a woman from Bengaluru who wanted to write a novel. Out of that crucible came fantastical fictions that contemplate an alternative, underground India where a woman might be able to become a master of yoga.[69] In a world of warring supernatural powers, yoga emerges as the cause—and possibly the cure—for gendered violence and political strife.

Is it possible to turn the sinister energies of yoga against itself? Are alternative politics available through and within such a landscape of power? Yoga, in Taneja's Anantya Tantrist multivolume urban fantasy series, is not the low-cost health technology of Narendra Modi's public dreams, the aspirational wellness pursuit of India's growing middle class, or the Vedic fantasies of soft Hindutva. Instead, her fiction critiques the exploitative grounds on which particular kinds of yogic authority exist. This occult universe confronts key issues of gender, caste, corruption, and violence that shape India in the new millennium. In this sense, I read her work as a contribution to the remixed yogic genealogy of *svādhyāya*, or critically reflective self-study, as it scrutinizes the structures of power that inform what yoga means and how it works.

Speculative fantasies published in the 2010s, Taneja's books took shape in an Indian scholarly and publishing landscape where writers were encouraged to draw upon Indian mythologies and epics.[70] Taneja's work plays with the long-standing concept of yogic *siddhis*, or supernatural power, which looms large in India's folkloric traditions.[71] "I wanted to focus on Indian fantasy," she told *The Hindu* in 2017. "There are no ideas from Western stories in my book."[72] For Indian women writers, speculative fantasy offers potential precisely because it allows for what the queer Dalit writer Mimi Mondal calls "radical worldbuilding"—an opportunity to figure socially oppressed characters as powerful in ways that realist fiction renders difficult.[73]

Taneja's fiction draws on Tantra, a form of yoga with a sinister reputation. A broad set of esoteric traditions outside canonical and Vedic texts, Tantra is frequently understood to promise paths to enlightenment through sex, violence, and subversion. Although Tantra is often popularly presented as an "other" to a Vedic world, yoga historically developed through both Tantric and Vedic practices.[74] In the early twentieth century, Julian Strube argues, Bengali intellectuals brought such Tantric practices as kundalini and chakras into influential modern under-standings of yoga.[75] Hugh Urban traces a twenty-first-century vision of Tantra as a world of enchanted objects, ritual sacrifices, and murderous spells to a dynamic dialogue between British and Indian writers in the late colonial period, where Tantra inspired "fears of social degeneracy, the threat of sexual pollution, the paranoia of criminal or subversive activity."[76] Frequently portrayed as violent rebels plotting the overthrow of the British, fictional orders challenge the reach of colonial power and also threaten ideals of independent Indian nationhood.[77] Tantra may dis-turb, but it will always impress.

Within these visions, gender hierarchies shape the powers ascribed to yoga. Female figures can be considered vital and revered, yet male enlightenment demands instrumental sex with women of lower castes and classes. Over time, while many images of Tantra in the twentieth century have reveled in visions often seen as transgressive, erotic, and bloody, the practice has also transformed into a path to spiritualized sex-ual pleasure.[78] These new approaches have promised a radical escape from repressive social orders that support upper caste and patriarchal control, yet in reality they often continue to emphasize undemocratic and sometimes violent caste exploitation and gendered hierarchy.[79] These intertwined forms of everyday violence have haunted the politics of Tan-tra in twenty-first-century India.

In Taneja's *The Rakta Queen* (2018), the heroine, Anantya, is sum-moned by the head of the Association of Tantriks to solve a mystery plaguing an upcoming convention designed to make tantrism more understandable to nonpractitioners, called Tantri-Con. "It was a collab-orative effort between the Association and the human government to make tantrism more mainstream," Anantya declares.

> The Indian government had promoted the event as an indigenous sci-ence project, complete with advertisements and permission from the Green Tribunal to use the flood plains near the Yamuna for the con-vention. There was a series of tantrik duels planned to celebrate the power of tantriks and the magic science. The prime minister and some ministers from the cabinet were also going to attend the final night.[80]

The convention riffs on initiatives that have characterized Modi's tenure as prime minister, which have emphasized practices and products that can be marketed as indigenous. Anantya's job—among many—involves preventing a hostile black magic takeover of Tantri-Con and saving the life of the Indian prime minister. In doing so, she preserves the possibility of an alliance between the world of human politics and the supernatural forces controlled by the tantriks.

Yet Anantya is also a strong critic of how tantrism fundamentally exploits female energies. The novel portrays *maithuna*, the ritual intercourse for which Tantra is famous, as a highly instrumental practice designed to harvest female power for male purposes. Male tantriks in the novel need female energy to power their rituals, and they can get it through blood or sex. This gendered exploitation invites satire on the cultural contradictions that inform the Indian government's approach to Tantri-Con. When a well-meaning girl at the information desk declares, "We offer *vegetarian* tantriks who can—," Anantya cuts her off.

> "Vegetarian tantriks? What in Bali's name does *that* mean?"
> She looked at me, her doll-like eyes wide. "White tantriks who perform pure rituals, pure vegetarian rituals, ma'am. No violence. That's the only kind [the Central Association of Tantriks] approves."
> "Are you serious?"
> She frowned.
> "For horned-rhinos' sake! White tantriks use your, *your* vagina, to power up their rituals. How kinder is that than any other kind of tantrism?"[81]

Given the politics of vegetarianism under Modi's tenure, with its controversial bans on cattle slaughter,[82] *The Rakta Queen* invites readers to consider the contradictory ideas around what constitutes "no violence" in twenty-first-century India. In the novel, these indigenous sciences rely on forcible resource extraction from bodies who have little power over larger structures: infants, animals, and women. Tantriks, traditionally, are men: Anantya is unusual in being her own female tantrik. The extraction of vital forces from female bodies looks very much like the colonial extraction of India's resources for Western might. In a world where the quest for energy—mundane and cosmic—is a quest for power, the Anantya Tantrist novels use the tools of speculative fiction to motivate feminist *svādhyāya* of twenty-first-century Indian inequality.

This portrait of a hierarchical tantrik universe exposes how economic practices can perpetuate ongoing hierarchies of caste and class. Supernaturals, or sups, form a lower class of beings who cannot move freely in the human world unless they take maya potion, which disguises them as humans. Tantriks control the supply of potion and use it as leverage to dominate sups. While economic growth in postliberalization India has moved millions out of poverty, the rise of capitalist practices has also brought new anxieties about inequality and control. As more and more public goods are given over to private entities, these privatized systems can work to benefit particular social groups over others—a situation exploited by the makers of the maya potion. The allegorical world of Taneja's speculative fiction testifies to ongoing anxieties about the power of the marketplace and its ability to reinforce rather than reduce social hierarchies.

In the end, Ananyta remains unsure how female tantriks can find a way to access their own power without exploiting others, but the novel hints that writing may provide one path. The capacity to envision alternate worlds through fiction emerges as a new kind of yogic practice that taps into the imaginative power of a female writer rather than the extractive rituals of *maithuna* or blood sacrifice. Like the mantras that Ananyta uses to fight her opponents, the words of the novel fight their own battles against gendered violence and social discrimination.

Unlike many of the idealized guru autobiographies that dominated imaginative representations of yoga in India's English traditions in the twentieth century, newer and edgier fictions like Taneja's show awareness of the politics of spirituality. Although advocates of modern postural yoga sometimes suggest that it eludes the chaos of politics, the two worlds have never been entirely separate. Twenty-first-century fiction reveals the ongoing vitality of yoga's other side: a world of supernatural forces where power over others, rather than liberation, health, or well-being, may be the dominant prize.

This vision of the practice might surprise practitioners accustomed to a yoga of peace and love. In these novels, the rise of yoga supports competing political fantasies. Although historians have uncovered the long histories linking yoga to diverse religious traditions now seen as Hinduism, Islam, Buddhism, and Jainism (to name a few), twenty-first-century visions of yoga often present it as a fundamentally Hindu practice that must be either embraced or refused by religious others. This logic informs what E. Dawson Varughese calls the genre of "Bharati fantasy," to which many of these novels belong.[83] At the same time, imaginative confrontations with yoga's capacity for violence can also inspire critical projects of *svādhyāya*. Feminist novels like Taneja's work with the state's dreams of yoga as a unifying form of indigenous science, but they also call attention to the hierarchies that make these claims to universalism and indigeneity possible. In such fiction, yoga offers an untapped potential for female and nonbinary figures to confidently inhabit public space—often not easy in India of the new millennium.

The urban bookstore, the threshold linking national conversations with international dialogues, reveals yoga as a contradictory gateway between India and the world. The tensions speak to broader anxieties that India, as it becomes more globally prominent, may somehow become less Indian. Yoga works as a practice that promises the hope of indigeneity for many people, a portable form of connectivity that remolds the body in ways that allow flexibility in moving across geography and social class. Through yoga, bodies seem to become more invested in solidifying the borders of Indian identity. Yet in its passage into a diverse range of bodies, yoga itself is seen to grow more Indian. Under the guise of worldwide inclusion, visions of yoga are used to fantasize solutions to India's crisis in border management—Indians pouring outward, foreigners rushing in, and instabilities within the idea of the India they traverse.

Such novels say what the state cannot. They thus offer us a glimpse into an alternate world, a possible world in Debjani Ganguly's sense,[84] where we can find laid bare the cultural logics that bolster state visions and reveal the threatening currents the state's imaginary relies upon yet seeks to repress. These novels locate yoga within a sense of crisis around India's public institutions. Yoga offers the fantasy of an alternative moral, metaphysical, judicial, and political system free from lies and corruption—and yet it also relies on practices that might seem to be the essence of deception and exploitation. This flexibility is at the heart of the political work that these novels provide. They collectively imagine yoga as a new form of public good, all the more powerful because it is often paradoxically private, undemocratic, and unaccountable.

Such novels illuminate how yoga's flexible forms mask contradictions in competing views toward modern capitalism and violence. The stories are full of such tensions: tourist guides that lambast increasing privatization, as in Mohan Ashtakala's *The Yoga Zapper*; capitalist theft correctable only by yogic thievery, as in Atul Merchant's *Taskari*; and feminist tantriks who work in the pay of patriarchs, as in Shweta Taneja's *The Rakta Queen*. Right-hand visions of yoga for holistic well-being are never far from left-hand specters of physical violence, gendered hierarchy, and economic exploitation. Twenty-first-century yoga fictions pursue ends that can be read as unspeakable state fantasies. These disavowed projects thrive in yoga's imaginative life—and they give us a window into how the yogic world-making of official India may also rest upon underworlds.

CONCLUSION

I place my right hand in the center of the mat for *vasiṣṭhāsana*. The back of my hand looks like my mother's did when I was a child. The silver ring she gave me when I was a teenager—round at the bottom, straight at the top—shines like soft moonlight. My left hand stretches up; the skin along the inside of my tallest finger tightens. One hand the lowest, the other hand the highest.

I almost miss the book. I'm so unaccustomed to receiving university mail that I don't look in my pigeonhole until after two postal pickup notices have arrived. On one of them is the "return to sender" date. It's today. The parcel is wrapped in cling wrap. Beneath the wrinkles, I can see the handwritten address in blue ballpoint pen.

My uncle has sent me a book. It is a kind of yoga, he says, that I may not have seen before. It focuses on moving your fingers. He woke up deaf in one ear a few months ago, and after using this book, he has recovered 80 percent of his hearing. "Not bad for an opera lover!" he writes. It is an English translation of a Kannada treatise: *Mudras and Health Perspectives*, by Suman K. Chiplunkar. I remove the copious layers of cling wrap, like peeling an onion. When my uncle mailed this in August, it was monsoon season in Mumbai. The book is perfectly dry. It's ready for an Australian cold spring.

I try a mudra out. I choose jnana mudra, the one that I would assume if someone just said "Do a mudra"—thumb and forefinger touch to form a circle. I sit for ten minutes, breathing in the pattern the book prescribes. The book says to do this to increase my brain power, improve my memory, and attain peace. This all sounds good. My memory has broken into tiny pieces since my first child was born. Now my daughter generously helps me out when we play memory matching games. I can still best her younger brother, but I know it is only a matter of time. Is it coming back together, my memory, in the connected circuit of finger and thumb?

I have always talked with my hands. Various people have tried to break me of this habit, but they have not really succeeded. Hands do their own thing. The book tells me that if dance is a language, mudras are the words. When I look at my hands I see the small, careful strokes they made with pencils and paintbrushes in my childhood. My son, like me, has usually preferred fine motor skills to gross ones. My daughter teaches me to finger knit, her little hands looping into new and fast curves. We take yarn with us on outings; she finger knits bracelets and necklaces while we sip tea with our friends. Her hands are readying to write, her kindergarten teachers tell us.

My generation of Americans didn't do much with their hands. I was born in the 1970s in the midst of feminist scorn for old crafts. "Darn socks?" my mother said incredulously when I said I wanted to learn. "I will just buy you new ones." Handmade was unfashionable.

When handwork became my American generation's obsession, I felt both out of place and at last at home. I came to feel that all those punk knitters were onto something. Hands were tied to the soul. As I began to use my hands for more than just turning pages and typing, I found in the rhythmic endless beats of stitches the pulse of meditative breath. My children never played much with the felt starfish and whale and platypus I made for them, but I remember the up and down of my fingers and the expectant love that came out, like silver light, through my hands.

Fingers carry electromagnetic energy, my book tells me. You can even do the mudras while you sleep. One night, while I lie next to my son, I touch my forefinger and thumb in jnana mudra. The world is still, dark, filled only with stars and the breathing of my children. In the quiet, I feel a quiver. Between my fingers is a palpable buzz, as if my hands have completed an electric circuit. I think of my daughter's kindergarten, where all the children clasp hands around the table before they eat. I think of the energy passing through their fingers, scented equally with lavender and dirt.

Now I see mudras in strange places. It's part of the distinctive silhouette that begins Janelle Morae's "Yoga" hip hop video, both of and against the sexual party world that reshapes female bodies for male pleasure. It's the acronym for the Indian government's new microlending bank, Micro Units Development and Refinance Agency. MUDRA is there to make money. In these diverse hands, I witness strange new pathways of power. The energy circuits of popular culture, of gendered contradictions, of neoliberal capitalism.

I place my left hand on the center of the mat. My wedding rings glint as the light ricochets through the diamond. Taking my weight, left feels as strong as right. My right hand, freed of its usual burdens to carry and fetch, lifts skyward in lightness.

Yoga is the one place where right hand and left hand feel like equals. Muscles move in symmetry. The forms are full of rules. And through the rules, the body becomes its own alphabet. It writes a new language. In yoga, angles and lines open curves and flows. My hands reach out and return, filled with warm, glowing gems.

4

ASSUMING CORPSE POSE

Yoga in U.S. Popular Culture

In the days when I wore jelly shoes and leg warmers, India was the land of poverty and wildlife. At least, that's how it seemed to people around me. When my friend Anjali's father talked to our class about India, he said that American kids usually asked him where he parked his elephant.

Anjali moved to South Carolina in the middle of seventh grade. The middle school principal gave us twinned schedules. Anjali was tall and beautiful and wore a gold necklace with her name on it, which was helpful, because I had difficulty remembering such an unfamiliar name. The sky had sent me a kindred spirit. Anjali was the kind of person who did homework as if it were ballet. Our English class went up to the high school to write poems that didn't rhyme. In the advanced math class, we played endless games with M&Ms and wooden puzzles. We were expected to contemplate probability, likelihood, chance.

I did not question the probability, likelihood, or chance of sharing every single class with a girl named Anjali. It seemed obvious that I could take care of a new student. I listened to the problems of the popular girls on the gym bench. I French-braided everyone's hair on the bus. I did all my homework and did not cause trouble.

When Anjali invited me to her house for a sleepover, I rode the school bus well past my own stop. With each mile, the houses grew larger, as if we were traveling inside a time-lapse photo where the city expanded before our eyes. In her neighborhood, Wildwood, the cars glowed; no dandelions or clovers dotted the grass. I found this world awe-inspiring. The buzz of an electric garage door opener, the whispering of plush white carpet, the shiny black counters where Anjali's mother made after-school snacks, the corner statue of a Hindu god. All of it was a mystery.

It didn't occur to me until months later that Anjali and I had been assigned to the same classes because we both came from Indian families. It seemed like a mistake. I didn't know anything about Diwali or do pujas or speak Hindi. But by that time Anjali had begun to sit at a different lunch table, befriend the friendly Christian girls, and become a cheerleader. We still talked from time to time, but by the eighth grade we rarely slept over at each other's house, and the next year her family moved away. I got a postcard months later, telling me about her new life in another state. "And now I go by Angie!" she wrote. When I look back, thirty years later, it's hard not to read in our stories the casualties of the Indian diaspora. Even my fraudulent and fragmentary sense of Indianness, a sense mostly composed of getting things wrong, could be too much for someone on a teenage quest to leave India's poverty and elephants behind.

More than thirty years on, India has changed in the minds of Americans. From an unbearably hot country, it has grown cool. Sparked by the opening of India's economy and its willingness to work with superpowers, new—or seemingly new—ideas of the country have begun to circulate. Yoga has crystallized this fantasy of a rising India: a place powerful, peaceful, wise, and whole. The practice has been good to the idea of India. But where has it left members of the Indian diaspora? What does it suggest for the broader well-being of people like my friend, who felt that even ambiguous signs of Indianness might be too costly for them to keep?

This chapter tracks the shape of yoga across a diverse landscape of imagination in American popular culture. At some moments, yoga amplifies the presence of Indian culture; at other moments, it erases India from the picture. Through this uneven force, India is often lauded as the authenticating source for a powerful life technology, yet members of the Indian diaspora are not always able to claim the benefits of such power. As part of this amplification and erasure, India is often figured as a benevolent Hindu authority in sharp contrast to the twenty-first-century specter of Islamic terrorism. In just the moment when the United States cast intensified suspicion on its South Asian and Middle Eastern populations as potential terrorists, the newfound love of yoga has allowed Americans to think of themselves as cosmopolitan and open. This paradox has pulled the practice into complicity with soft Hindutva and U.S. military power—projects that many yoga practitioners in the United States might not wish to support.

Yoga is a cipher for cultural fantasies about an ideal life in an age of globalization. From twenty-first-century court cases to murder mysteries to news media to airport signs, these fragments of imagination suggest that as India appears to be rising, Indians themselves may be falling. To understand how yoga can frame India in this way, I turn to a murder, a trial, and a plane.

⸎

Yoga takes shape within frames. They might be the angles of a room, the edges of a photograph, or the lines of a page. Frames define insides and outsides, what belongs and what does not. They create conditions of possibility. Drawing on this idea, as Peter Morey and Amina Yaqin have done, I explore the ways particular imaginative visions of yoga are shaping stories of Indianness within U.S. popular culture. As Morey and Yaqin suggest, framing can be a morally ambiguous business.[1]

Histories offer us one set of frames. If you were an Indian coming to the United States in the early twentieth century, you might have been a Sikh farmer from Punjab who had fought in the British army.[2] It's likely that others were afraid of you. White Americans might have feared you'd take their land and jobs, just as they'd feared the Chinese and Japanese and other migrants from Asia.[3] The British might have feared you'd set up secret groups that would bring down their empire. By the 1920s, a web of laws began to seal up the gateways through which Asians had long entered the country. If you were living in the United States already, you might have been considered white, on the belief that ancient Aryans had settled India, and on that basis been granted U.S. citizenship. But you might have had that citizenship revoked when the government decided it had made a mistake. You might, like Bhagat Singh Thind, have gone to court to get your citizenship back, but like him, been told that Indians—or Hindus, as you might have been called regardless of your religion—simply could not count as white. By now, more and more acts would have blocked your path to entering the country and staying forever. For the better part of a half century, until the United States changed its migration laws in 1965, only exceptional individuals passed through the remaining nooks and crannies. If you were an Indian teacher of yoga, you might have found that yoga could move across regulated borders in ways that you could not. The practice could pack itself invisibly into a body of a different color with a different passport, a body that could stride with different powers down American public streets.

As yoga became available to new bodies, it was used to further diverse social and political ends through ambivalent relationships with India. Sometimes yoga's new mobilities worked to support and nourish the political struggles of America's minorities seeking justice and equality. Yoga helped Cesar Chavez work long days and longer nights in his quest to better the rights of workers.[4] Muhammad Ahmad's plans for a black nationalist liberation school included yoga.[5] As Stephanie Evans and Jana Long reveal, yoga sustained Rosa Parks and many other black Americans in their battles with pervasive injustice.[6] In some ways, yoga appealed to racial minorities because it could be understood as a practice with nonwhite origins. Ironically, that very logic could also work to keep yoga away from them. As Philip Deslippe argues in an analysis of yoga instruction in the pre-1965 United States, the yoga lecture circuit conspicuously excluded the American South, where Jim Crow laws created a hostile environment for traveling Indian swamis as well as for the significant black populations that lived in the region.[7] Access to yoga was thus always shaped by restrictive and discriminatory political structures.

At the same time, many ethnic minority practitioners sought to frame the liberatory potential of yoga through their own ethnic ancestries, such as African or Native American lineages.[8] Taking Harriet Jacobs as a nineteenth-century exemplar, Evans argues that "African American women's holistic relationships with their bodies was not solely the result of the introduction of Indian yoga or Asian influences in American popular culture."[9] These histories challenge the idea that yoga claims a singular source from the Indian subcontinent, offering strength for minority practitioners in the twenty-first century who wish to contest what they see as culturally appropriative dimensions within American yoga.[10] Jessamyn Stanley, one of the most influential black American yoga influencers in the first decades of the twenty-first century, argues in her memoir *Yoke* (2021) against a strong fixation on India: "Yoga naturally leads every practitioner to a deeper exploration of their *own* unique cultural identity. Sprinkling South Asian culture on your yoga practice doesn't make it more legit, it just makes it more appropriative."[11] Seen through this historical frame, deliberate movement away from the idea of India offers political potential for the social justice claims of non-Indian ethnic minorities and for critical reflection on diverse racial and cultural identities.

Ideas of India have also been supplanted for quite different political projects. Because of the vacuum created by racially restrictive migration laws, in many midcentury mainstream spaces the face of yoga gradually lightened. Many people came to yoga as a practice taught by a white woman on television, a media phenomenon that helped to shape the ideal American yoga body as thin, female, and white.[12] In the 1960s, yoga came to be considered "American" when it was promoted by white celebrities, even if they were not themselves American, such as the Beatles.[13] Over time, these perceptions have framed yoga within white spaces. Cultural symbols of South Asianness may appear, but the material powers afforded recognition, authority, wealth, and belonging flow most smoothly to those who inhabit the category of upper-class whiteness.[14] Though—or because—such frames may seem blank, neutral, invisible, or nonexistent to white practitioners, they stand out as border guards to others.

This is not to say that Indian practitioners did not find a way into American space. The enigmatic, possibly fictional Sylvais Hamati, a Syrian Indian, thought to have arrived in the United States in the nineteenth century before the tightening of the immigration laws, may have passed on hatha yoga and Tantric teachings to a white American who went on to found a spiritual empire. Swami Vivekananda, Parama-hansa Yogananda, Swami Satchidananada, and many others were able to establish ongoing presences, while others came on tours or set up practices run under their auspices.[15] Philip Deslippe challenges the idea that restrictive migration laws meant the absence of yoga in the United States in this period. His analysis of American early twentieth-century yoga documents the presence of a traveling swami lecture circuit where yoga was taught in ninety cities across twenty-six states.[16] Other Indian migrants brought yoga as a personal practice integrated with broader ways of living, passed down in oral histories and memoirs, but not for sale on the open market.[17] These histories testify to both presence and absence, exclusion and resilience.

By the 1990s, if you were an Indian coming to the United States, you probably had an H-1B visa to program computers. You might have been struck, perhaps baffled, by the yoga studios that seemed to pop up on every corner.[18] After the terrorist attacks of September 11, your chance of being attacked on the street might have risen because people thought you might harbor a commitment to Islamic radicalism.[19] In every corner studio, love, peace, and namaste would be on offer, while outside, men with brown skin might be put on government registers or disappear into the depths of detention under the Patriot Act. Women in South Asian families might hesitate to invoke the law when they were hurt by men in their lives, lest the legal system be used to wound them all.[20]

In the twenty-first century, the yoga deaths begin with a vengeance.

THE MURDERS

At first nobody believes me when I mention yoga murder mysteries. How can a practice of peace and love lead to mayhem and violence? But by 2020 you could order at least a dozen online. Tracy Weber writes "downward dog" mysteries for those who love yoga and pets. Authors such as

Neal Pollack, Diana Killian, Michelle Kelly, Greta Evelyn von Kirch-
mann, Julie Mulhern, and Meredith Potts have all published at least
one yoga mystery each. A few, such as Pollack, Killian, and Weber, have
even started series. Some of these books are aimed at yoga aficionados
and reviewed and promoted on yoga-themed sites; others hook unsuspecting readers in with other angles, in the hope that these readers will
be drawn to give the book, and yoga, a go.

Stacked up in piles on my desk, ordered into grids on my tablet, the
yoga murder mysteries take us through open doorways, darkened alleys,
and secret rooms. Murder mysteries, as a form of storytelling, are the
dream of mathematicians and architects. They begin in chaos and end
in order. They are geometric and fractal in nature, written to a formula
meant for adding and multiplying and repeating. Reading murder mysteries soothes readers in the style of solving crossword puzzles, lining
up Matchbox cars, or moving through sun salutations. Murder mysteries put people into place.

Like beer yoga or yoga with goats, yoga murder mysteries seem like
the height of ridiculousness: a fanciful quirk of Western, and especially
American, cultural elaboration and market branding. Yet the yoga murder mystery can also be read as a grand Indian tradition. Folklore is full
of sinister yogis bent on stealing souls.[21] Military history is replete with
killer yogis for whom "warrior" was not a metaphor.[22] Members of sects
devoted to Shiva in his fiercest form inhabited cremation grounds and
smeared themselves with ashes. For many onlookers in parts of India's
history, yogis might have seemed murderous, closer to the world of the
dead than the world of the living. Conquering death, an important goal
for many fictional and historical yogic sects, embodied the ultimate form
of power. It is thus especially ironic that some of these twenty-first-
century American cozy mysteries—in their way, the truest legacy of
this Indian approach to yoga—seem especially bent on putting India into
corpse pose.

The first to die is an aunt. Her name is Diantha, she studied yoga in
India, and her studio empire is now worth eighteen million dollars. In
Diana Killian's *Corpse Pose* (2008), the first in her series of yoga mur-
ders, the death of Diantha speaks to broader questions about the future

of yoga and its lineage in the United States. Diantha exemplifies the image of the white American countercultural student—the kind of person who travels to India in the 1960s, develops her own studio in the United States, rails against the evils of the dairy industry, and expands her own natural living product line. Her journey bespeaks the circular connection between the desire to critique capitalism and the desire to master its modes.

With the death of Diantha dies yoga's connection to ideas of India in the story. Though Diantha's Indian training legitimates her as an authority over the practice and helps make her a multimillionaire, the novel contains only one cultural reference to India: the parting gesture of "*Namaste*," which ends her will. By the twenty-first century, "namaste" was common enough as an opening and closing in postural U.S. yoga classes to prompt a mocking backlash of t-shirts with slogans like "Namastay away from me." But even this is too much knowledge to expect from the new heirs of Diantha's empire. When her sister hears the lawyer read "Namaste," she takes it as the name of an unknown person. "Who the devil is *Namaste*?" she whispers.[23] The comedy of the moment relies on the way it amplifies and erases Indianness in the same breath: even though readers are expected to know what "namaste" means, the word itself remains alien. The new heirs of yoga in the novel don't know anything about India and don't want to, even though they would like to have some of the eighteen million dollars.

The novel hands the future of Diantha's empire to her niece, A.J., whose favorite food is Pop-Tarts. A jam-filled biscuit that could be put in a toaster, the Pop-Tart was the kind of 1980s ultraprocessed food my parents refused to buy. (As the comedian Jerry Seinfeld so accurately observed, "They're never stale, because they were never fresh.") The antithesis of the stereotype of the whole foods, natural living yogi, A.J. can barely remember the postures her aunt taught her in her youth. When A.J. realizes that she must keep Diantha's studio going, she proposes to teach yoga for dogs. In many ways, she is in flight from the hipster, metrosexual, urban world where yoga has gained a visible following. Recently divorced after her ex-husband came out as gay, A.J.

appears to long for a world that is masculine, straight, and white. As she tries to solve the mystery of her aunt's murder, she falls in love with the tough-guy cop charged with conducting the official investigation. The new heirs of yoga, the book suggests, will be those, like A.J., who cannot tolerate anything that seems New Age, queer, or Indian.

Precisely because Killian's novels are written partly to bring new recruits to yoga, they offer prospective practitioners a cultural fantasy of a practice that has erased its connection to India. As I read them, I am dismayed, and more shocked than I should be, by how little Indian-ness the novel thinks its ideal readers can tolerate. In a way, much has changed between the United States and India since my 1980s childhood. But some parts still feel uncannily familiar.

I didn't expect to find such a vision at work in the writings of Neal Pollack, who probably surprised himself by becoming the author of yoga mysteries. In his memoir *Stretch* (2010), Pollack tells of his meteoric rise as the enfant terrible of the American literary scene, then his equally quick and self-destructive fall from grace: a fall cushioned by his new immersion in yoga.[24] How yoga remade him as a person and a writer is the theme, and Pollack's satirical sensibilities are trained on the emer-gent world of earnest multiethnic California yoga and its equally ear-nest contradictions. Pollack followed up with the creation of a yoga detective, the perfectly named Matt Bolster, who debuted in 2012 in a serialized novel (and with his own social media feed). A middle-aged white man addicted to marijuana and irony, Pollack's Matt Bolster roams Los Angeles teaching yoga classes and solving yoga murders. Great affection for the practice, coupled with self-satire, marks the tone of *Downward-Facing Death* (2013) and its sequel, *Open Your Heart* (2013).[25] To a certain extent, these novels suggest that India—in some ways por-trayed as the font of yogic wisdom—may really be the problem.

What fascinated me about Pollack's mysteries was that he had been reading the same emerging histories of yoga that I had. William Pinch, the author of a study on yogic militancy, must have been delighted that there was a yoga scholar in Pollack's novel who had written such a book—*and* that Bolster had loved it. And Mark Singleton must have been intrigued that his history of the making of twentieth-century yoga, a story of conversation between Indian innovators and Western physical culture, appears in new shape as a murderer's confession.

In *Downward-Facing Death*, Bolster investigates the grisly demise of a California guru named Ajoy Chatterjee. As a boy in India, Chatterjee was taught yoga, and eventually his guru sent him to establish yoga in the West. His path (except, hopefully, for his end) mirrors that of many historical Indian figures in the twentieth century who worked to export yoga to the United States: difficulty gaining traction, eventual success, then the overpowering forces of money and sex. (The novel insists that Ajoy Chatterjee isn't a fictionalized Bikram Choudhury precisely because the two seem remarkably alike.) Chatterjee's success in marketing, copyrighting, and selling a version of the yoga he was taught, along with his frailty in the face of new riches, attracts the censure and envy of his guru back in India. Through a falsified Sanskrit text, the guru tricks Chatterjee into committing ritual suicide. Proving a fake Sanskrit manuscript as a murder weapon, of course, poses courtroom difficulties. In search of justice, Bolster flies to India. When he meets the guru, Sri Charan, he learns that his suspicions were right. The guru, jealous of his student's fame and California real estate, did indeed provoke Chatterjee's suicide.

Even as Sri Charan condemns Chatterjee for corrupting yoga, he confesses to Bolster that the yoga he taught was a great con, not ancient spirituality at all.

> " 'I grew up during the Raj. We exercised so we could become strong and overthrow the British. We did the poses in our local gymnasium both before and after school. As for meditation, I learned it from my grandfather, who sat silently every night for twenty minutes after brushing his teeth.'
>
> 'So it's all a lie,' Bolster said.
>
> 'More or less,' said Sri Charan.
>
> 'And the Sequence [set of yoga poses, similar to the sequence made popular by Bikram Choudhury]?'
>
> 'How do you say it in the West? I 'pulled it out of my ass'? Well, I did. Yoga as you comprehend it came straight out of my old Indian ass.'

Sri Charan gave a little chuckle.

'It really is quite a prank,' he said. 'All these millions of people, stretching and grinding away, thinking they're going to achieve enlightenment, when in reality they're just doing poses from an old British physical culture textbook while reciting half-formed prayers to minor Hindu deities.' "[26]

Sri Charan has a good point. But historians of yoga don't see yoga's modernity—or its enthusiastic promotion within international twentieth-century physical culture—as a con. Though Pollack is of the ironic postmodernist bent usually skeptical of stable truths and earnest histories, his novel does not quite accept this version of yoga as a practice influenced by cosmopolitan innovations of the twentieth century.

So, after a visionary battle to " 'control the soul of yoga,' "[27] in which Bolster wars against Sri Charan's cynical nihilism and Ajoy Chatterjee eventually kills his guru, Bolster travels to an unnamed ashram beyond Lucknow. There he refreshes himself with what appears to be an unpretentious, pure, silent, and Indian yoga practice, led by "a portly middle-aged woman who had some cushions and a method and access to that most precious commodity of all: silence."[28] Then he takes this yoga back to California. In the last scene of the book, Bolster is conducting a class.

This ending fascinated me, because it captured so many of the larger patterns in the rise of yoga novels. Yoga in the West had problems. You can't add anything, let alone the allure of enlightenment, to a world awash in capitalist consumption, flashy sexuality, and image dominance without crisis. Yoga needed rejuvenating. In this logic, actual Indians—in India and in the United States—had messed it up. But white people might be able to set it right. They could offer American yoga, constantly claiming a mythical ancient tradition but also self-authored and self-authorized. I can't help but imagine that in a future installment Pollack will complete the cultural logic and allow Bolster to import this yoga back to India.

Though I delight in the undeniable wit of Pollack's work, it's hard not to feel some sympathy for Indian nationalists who see their country and its cultural symbols extracted for raw materials to enhance the spiritual cultivation of the affluent West. To be usurped by thin white women in Lululemon pants: Is this India's cultural fate? Is this any way to die?

THE TRIAL

Let us shift the scene from a murder to a courtroom.

In a new millennium May, the California town of Encinitas was so bright that the surfers might have drowned in the glitter of their reflection, the mothers with spandex leggings and lattes might have paused to pull out their darkest pair of shades, and the judge, walking from his car into the courtroom, might have paused to wonder at the power of the sun and the reasons one might salute it. Encinitas was a town composed of brightness. It glowed with expensive light that glimmered like champagne flowing into crystal. No wonder so many yogis came to Encinitas in search of meaning in that light.[29]

Encinitas was a place of water pulsing into cliffs, cars conspicuously not honking their horns, and instructions called out to packed rooms in shalas, churches, and classrooms. English consonants, and some Spanish vowels, and in one room in a public school district, Sanskrit syllables pronounced and mispronounced before the evangelical Christian parents began to ask questions. Why were their children practicing yoga at school? Was this not an unconstitutional mixing of church and state? Why could Eastern religions be okay when anything Christian was banned? The district decided that "surfer pose" would be safer. Down came posters with Sanskrit and postcards from India. Some sounds might be dangerous. Make the words English, make the walls white.

The year was 2013, a time when yoga had become popular enough in the United States for "Fuck Yoga" t-shirts to be sold. India too had become one of the United States' more popular partners. Five years earlier, the countries had signed a historic treaty to share nuclear technology—a sign, it was said, of two democracies growing closer in a world shaped by concerns about international terrorism and the rise of China.[30] Although neither India nor Pakistan had signed the nuclear nonproliferation treaty, India was seen as a trustworthy partner in a way that Pakistan was not. Perhaps, as some analysts speculated, the yoga of Gandhi had conjured India as a place of peace.[31]

But India, and Indianness, were not always trusted. A battle over their meaning took place in the coastal town of Encinitas. But the battle is not the one we might assume from the local newspapers and the national coverage that followed. It's not the drama between the Christian right, convinced that teaching yoga in Encinitas public schools threatened the religious rights of families and the religious establishment clause of their state, and the school district, adamant that their program was simply one of stretching, breathing, and stress relief. Nor is it the battle between academics called on to say if yoga is religious, pitting those who argued that this yoga owed much to secular physical culture against those who held the view, shared by the Christian right and some Hindus, that yoga is a ritual from a lifeworld where religious practice is not what you believe, but what you do. These contests all occurred, and they weave their way into the story. But the real trial I seek to explore is how, through yoga, anxious ideas of India have been put to the test in American law about public space. Through yoga's flexible forms, how and where can ideas of India belong?

A court decision cuts, excerpts, adjudicates, and frames. As a collage, a decision assembles and reassembles testimony; it bolsters some ideas and undercuts others. In the ruling of *Sedlock v. Baird* in June 2013, Judge John S. Meyer from the San Diego County Superior Court had to determine whether yoga could be taught to children in California's secular public schools. The particular way he chose to tell this story—his cuts, excerpts, adjudications, and frames—expresses ongoing American discomfort with India, even as the court decision invites yoga into the American classroom.

When the calls came about the legality of the yoga program, the fundamental question the district faced was whether yoga advanced the establishment of religion. California's state constitution, Article I, Section 4, reads, "The Legislature shall make no law respecting an establishment of religion," a law seen by the California Supreme Court as effectively identical to the U.S. national First Amendment establishment clause.[32] A practice that gave students the impression that they were participating in a state-supported religious activity would not be legal.

Yoga in the Encinitas schools was paid for by the K. P. Jois Foundation, an organization founded by Sonia Jones, the Australian wife of a hedge-fund billionaire, who had been transformed by the teachings of the Indian guru Pattabhi Jois.[33] Jois's approach, like that of many other yoga teachers, linked physical to spiritual transformation.[34] A student of Tirumalai Krishnamacharya, a master in the Vaiṣṇava tradition, Jois taught yoga at the Sanskrit college of Mysore University from 1937 until 1973. In the 1970s, he began to teach his methods internationally.[35] Jois was known for a physically intensive form of practice that became known in Western contexts as Ashtanga, or eight-limbed, yoga. "Ashtanga" referred to the eight limbs of yoga found in classical sources used by many yoga masters, but it also became a synonym for the kind of dynamic postural approach—"99 percent practice, 1 percent theory," as he would famously say—that Jois taught. Jones's foundation helped to shift Jois's yoga toward a new branding of "Jois Yoga." Though Jois was based in Mysore, he had taught in Encinitas on his visits to the United States, and teachers working in his lineage had taught in a shala there since the 1970s. In 2010, money from the foundation opened a second shala in a different style—a gleaming boutique space with a clothing store—that cost a million dollars to build.[36] Was the Jois Foundation a religious organization, and did the teacher it funded to instruct children in yoga bring religious practices into public schools?

What is striking, in the court narratives, is how the law sought an answer to this legal question by transforming it into a question about cultural connections to India. The court decision notes that the initial teacher in the K. P. Jois Foundation primary school program, Jennifer Brown, "was trained by Jois and taught at the Jois shala."[37] Since the court was trying to decide if the Jois Foundation represented a religious group, understanding the links between it and the teacher clearly mattered. But the court narrative proceeds as follows: "Jennifer Brown has an interest in India, and has studied Sanskrit. Jennifer Brown traveled to India over the summers, sent postcards that were put up in the students' classroom [sic]. She based the class loosely on the Primary Series of Astanga Yoga, and used some Sanskrit words."[38] In selecting this kind of information as relevant to court judgment, the narrative implies that not only particular models for yoga practice but also travels to India and the use of Sanskrit may by their nature contain hidden religious agendas.

This fear that South Asian cultures may be inherently at odds with Christian beliefs can be felt in the anxieties of the families bringing the suit. According to the court decision, one of the offended parents who "thought the program conflicted with his faith" was "very concerned about the use of Sanskrit" and "heard that his daughter drew something called a *mandala* [italics in the original] in an art class a year before yoga was taught at her school."[39] Although the families who brought the lawsuit never (according to the court narrative) actually observed one of the school yoga classes, they were troubled by their children's exposure to language and visual practice from the subcontinent.

The history of Sanskrit is indeed one of vast promises. Sanskrit claims a long history as a liturgical language through which upper-caste Brahmins have asserted spiritual control over others. Spiritual gurus like Osho have promoted the idea that the language offers an integral connection to the divine.[40] Hindu nationalists have idealized Sanskrit as a utopian language that will bring about a perfected spiritual world.[41] In this sense, Christian anxieties dovetail with specific Indian ideas of Sanskrit as a sacerdotal language with political aspirations.[42]

Sanskrit and mandalas bear strong links to ritual and symbolic work within Hindu, Buddhist, and other religious traditions (and mandalas can also denote forms of political governance), but the court narrative leaves unclear exactly how the father understood the conflict with his faith. The concerns of the parents and the school do not seem to have been rooted in sophisticated investigation into the metaphysical status of Sanskrit, its theorization of divine sound, or its counterhistory as a language of scientific discovery. Fearing yoga's religiosity through Sanskrit seems to have emerged from a much easier equation: Sanskrit is rooted in Indian culture, Indian culture is seen as highly religious, and thus Sanskrit must serve as a conduit for Indian religiosity no matter where or in what context it appears. The obvious association with India (in the case of Sanskrit) and with India, Tibet, and other South and

Southeast Asian geographies where mandalas have traditionally been used seems to have become the self-evident logic for this opposition. In court testimony, cultural practices linked to India are feared as inherently devotional and cast as incompatible with Christian beliefs within American public culture. "India" becomes a shorthand for "religious."

According to the court narrative, the school district accepted this equation:

> The District responded by removed [*sic*] anything considered a cultural components [*sic*] or that could be arguably deemed religious. Jennifer Brown's Ashtanga tree poster was removed almost immediately (and that was her personal poster). All Sanskrit language was removed. Jenn Brown took down the postcards from India. The names of the poses were changed to kid-friendly, kid-familiar poses. The so-called "lotus" position was renamed "criss-cross applesauce."[43]

In short, anxieties about yoga as a religious practice inappropriate for a public school were almost instantly transformed into anxieties about yoga's visible or perceived connection with India. In the court's logic, only signs of Indianness are seen as "cultural," whereas the replacement phrases, like "surfer pose" or "criss-cross applesauce," common within norms linked to whiteness in California, are not. This contrasts with earlier cases, such as *Malnak v. Yogi* in 1979, where the question of religion was approached in more philosophical terms (asking, for example, if students were required to acknowledge a supreme being).[44] As Sunila Kale and Christian Novetske suggest, the court case in Encinitas reveals the paradoxes latent within American understandings of secularity.[45] One of these paradoxes, I suggest, is the persistent racial and cultural assumptions that shape what counts as nonreligious.

The court decision cut and framed the words of expert witnesses to conform to this logic. Mark Singleton, who testified as an expert witness, is recorded in the statement of decision as saying, "The essential point is that yoga, as it has developed in the United States in the past 150 years, is a distinctly American cultural phenomenon. It is rooted in American culture as much and sometimes more than in Indian culture."[46] In the logic of the court narrative, the word "American" has to be understood as code for "nonreligious," or this comment (however historically accurate) makes no sense as an "essential point" for a ruling that aims to determine if a particular style of yoga violates the prohibition against establishment of religion in public schools. Many aspects of American culture are deeply religious; indeed, in the twenty-first century more than 75 percent of Americans identify with a religious tradition.[47] But the court framing of the comment equates "American culture" with lack of religious affiliation and "Indian culture," implicitly, with religiosity, which is particularly ironic given that Singleton's nuanced historical work does not support this idea. The framing of Singleton's comment in the narrative amplifies this logic, by which yoga, in order to be understood as suitable for American public schools, must banish any cultural reference to India. "Religious" versus "nonreligious" metamorphoses into a different contest, one marked by cultural categories that should not be mutually exclusive: "Indian" versus "American."

When the case went to appeal two years later in 2015, such a vision of yoga—authored and authorized by India, but also severed from it—animated the amicus curiae brief of the U.S. trade group Yoga Alliance. The brief begins with the claim that "the modern practice of yoga generally involves a series of physical movements (poses), combined with breath work and mindfulness practices, none of which is inherently religious or tied to either of the two different established Eastern religions that contributed to the historical development of yoga: Hinduism and Buddhism."[48] In this phrasing, "modern" yoga means postural, breath, and mindfulness practice. While this particular use of "modern" might be plausible—if not comprehensive—as a description of practices found in many commercial studios in the West, it leaves out the soteriological and devotional practices of yoga in many Indian, transnational, and increasingly U.S.-based contexts. In this reading, the numerous followers of Sai Baba, Baba Ramdev, Sri Sri Ravi Shankar, Jaggi Vasudev, and many others are not considered modern. Approaches to yoga that are vital in South Asia and among the transnational followings of Indian gurus thus are rendered invisible as modern yoga—even though they are thriving in the twenty-first century.

The brief repeats the often-used, but historically dubious, claim that "Yoga developed some 5,000 years ago."[49] This is a claim echoed by Indian state nation-branding campaigns. However, while the Indian state aims to use this figure to elevate India's stature in the twenty-first-century world, the brief grounds yoga in the authority of India's antiquity (one claim that the U.S. nation-state cannot make) and also banishes Indianness to the past. Hinduism and Buddhism (Jainism, Sufism, Sikhism, and other religious philosophies are not mentioned) are acknowledged as historical roots but denied any place within this definition of "modern" yoga: "none of which is inherently religious or tied to either . . . Hinduism and Buddhism." The Yoga Alliance brief thus depends on a cultural history of rupture. Yoga may have South Asian roots, but those are in the past. As scholars have noted, the rush to locate yoga within particular U.S. institutions by denying complex South Asian living traditions can seem extractive.[50] These omissions speak to the subtle operations of larger anxieties about the place of Indianness within public culture.[51]

To its credit, the Fourth Appellate District court, in its 2015 verdict on the appeal, explicitly refuted the idea that "Indian" was a synonym for "religious establishment." The higher court finding, which upheld the judgment that this particular kind of yoga could legally be taught in Encinitas public schools, stressed that the de-Indianizing process described and implied in the earlier court narrative was not required. "For example, the District eliminated the teaching of Sanskrit names for various yoga poses, yet we see no possible establishment clause violation arising out of the fact that yoga teachers had previously been teaching children the Sanskrit names for yoga poses."[52] The appellate court decision cut and framed the words of expert witnesses differently. For example, Mark Singleton's perspective appears anew: "Dr. Singleton stated, '[Y]oga as it has developed in the United States in the past 150 years is a distinctly American cultural phenomenon. . . . Many of the elements which contributed to its current form are in no way inherently religious.'"[53] While this statement resembles the quotation from Singleton recorded in the Meyer ruling, it is much clearer in presenting the concept of yoga as "American" as a descriptor, not an "essential point" about the establishment of religion, and much more explicit in its argument that the American contributing elements are nonreligious (as opposed to non-Indian).

Yet the consequences of the first court decision had already rippled beyond the page. In July 2013, the CEO of the Jois Foundation renamed the organization the Sonima Foundation. As the *San Diego Union-Tribune* reported, "At the conclusion of the Superior Court trial, Jois Foundation CEO Gene Ruffin announced that his organization was changing its name to reflect a broader mission about health and fitness. Sonima combines the names of foundation founder Sonia Jones and Ruffin's wife, Salima Ruffin."[54] The purging of Indian signifiers, beginning with Sanskrit, required erasing signs of Jois and his family from the name of the foundation originally established to honor his work. This yoga had to be stripped of any association, not just with Hindu philosophies and practices but with Indianness itself, in order to claim a proper role within American secular institutions. The home page of the Sonima Foundation now features a toned white Australian woman, bright hair blowing in an invisible coastal breeze.

Reading the court narratives, I'm haunted by hints of a different frame. Sometimes I see the principal of my elementary school, a former Episcopalian nun, stopping me on the boardwalk that led up to the trailers that housed her office. Our principal was known for piercing glances that brought our lower school assemblies to uneasy silence. "I like eyes," she would say coldly, waiting until we could show she had our attention. Now icy blue eyes that usually stared at troublemakers were trained on me. Without any preamble, she asked, "What religion are you?"

I blinked. "My father is Methodist and my mother is Muslim," I said. Somehow this seemed more acceptable than saying that nobody in my house believed much of anything they had been raised on.

The principal nodded. She walked on. I had passed a test, but I wasn't sure how. Why had I felt that saying "none" was not an option? What back room conversations about students like me were troubling this former nun? Did religion make Indianness more acceptable, or less?

THE GETAWAY PLANE

Yoga murder mysteries may be violent, but they are mostly fictions.[55] Not so the detentions of men of South Asian descent without due process in the aftermath of September 11. The Islamic extremist attacks on the World Trade Center and the Pentagon in 2001, which roiled the United States, were particularly traumatic for many who claimed subcontinental ancestry. In their homes they might weep in compassion for those who died, but outside their homes, they might be attacked for the turbans on their heads or the color of their skin or the mosques where they prayed.

As Sunaina Maira shows in her moving book *Missing* (2009), it has not been easy to be South Asian American in the first decades of the twenty-first century.[56] Widespread popular imaginaries have tended to blur religious, national, ethnic, and sectarian complexity into a view of brown-skinned people from the Middle East and South Asia as potentially dangerous. Sikh men were particularly visible targets for popular violence, since their turbans were often confused with the headgear worn by Islamic religious authorities widely shown on television. Muslim communities from India, Pakistan, and Bangladesh were placed under public suspicion. Vijay Prashad, reflecting on his own targeting as well as that of many others, points to the ironies in this practice: "A terrorist does not announce him or herself. That would defeat the purpose. But the visual sign is precisely what the racist would like to focus on, exactly what the terrorist would like to deny. The bodies of so many are stripped bare by this contradiction."[57] With the passing of the Patriot Act in 2001, when protections against privacy were suspended, more and more communities with links to South Asia came under surveillance or had good reason to believe they might be. While terrorist acts in the United States led by white men (such as the Oklahoma City bombing in 1995 and the storming of the Capitol in 2021) did not result in wholesale panic toward white communities, terrorism from Islamic extremists did inspire fear of a wide range of people who seemed, suddenly, even more foreign than ever. Men from Muslim-majority countries, such as Pakistan, were asked to register with the state; many disappeared into the darkness of U.S. detention. These xenophobic forces took a new turn in 2017, when Donald Trump's Executive Order 13769 banned travel by citizens of specified Muslim-majority nations. Despite the repeal of the order by Joe Biden in 2021, the twenty-first century has been marked by state anxiety about, and violence against, perceived terrorists who are imagined as brown.

In the decades after 9/11, when people of South Asian ancestry in the United States could be detained, spied upon, or publicly assaulted and mainstream media frequently figured South Asian bodies as objects of terror, yoga grew ever more popular. Yoga offered a form of masculine authority that was imagined as Indian, Hindu, and venerable—a stark contrast to the terrifying and unstable masculinity of an imagined young Muslim suicide bomber. It was also distinctly different from the militant Hindu, RSS-informed masculine yoga body long cultivated in India, as well as from Orientalist specters of sinister gurus. Yoga gained imaginative power in this period because it created an American frame for a safe subcontinental body.

In the first few years of the twenty-first century, just as being South Asian in the United States became dangerous in new ways, narratives emerged that began to sanctify postural yoga masters in American space. In part, this was because some of these masters were reaching the end of their lives. At the time of September 11, Tirumalai Krishnamacharya had been dead for more than a decade; Pattabhi Jois and B. K. S. Iyengar, students in his lineage, were both in their eighties and in the last stages of their teaching careers (Jois passed away in 2009, Iyengar in 2014). They could claim to have trained large numbers of students in India and the West (many personally, more through the institutions they established). Narratives began to spread not only through yoga classes but also through documentaries, oral history collections, and mass media. To be sure, yoga was not seen as completely safe, even in this historical period. Yogis could be still seen as charlatans, extortionists, and predators. In the wake of the revelations of sexual violations that eventually appeared after the rise of the social media hashtag #MeToo in 2017, many teachers were reevaluated in the harsh light of sexual violation in

American yoga communities.[58] Yet despite these significant challenges, a powerful, resounding image of Indian yogic benevolence had begun to take on new authority within the United States.

This public persona of the benevolent, if strict, father, bent on helping Americans (and everyone else across the globe) cope with the ills of their harried capitalist lives, came to lend a new patriarchal authority in the world of fitness. In 2004, *Time* magazine listed B. K. S. Iyengar as one of its most influential people in the world, presenting an article on his impact under the category "Heroes and Icons."[59] The highly photogenic Iyengar—still capable of extraordinary vitality in his eighties—was routinely figured in American media through a visual language that stressed both his Indian alterity (he was usually shown shirtless, with a red stripe running down his forehead) and his benevolence (he was often photographed smiling). On Iyengar's final tour of the United States in 2005, the *New York Times* reported that "although he can appear fierce, even forbidding, he has an impish, ready laugh and a quick wit that befits a man who can still perform a full backbend and stand on his head unsupported by a wall for more than an hour."[60] One of the most iconic images appears on the cover of his 2005 book *Light on Life*, in which a magisterial Iyengar, with flowing white hair and distinctive red stripe, is caught in an infectious laugh.[61] He became the face of yoga as Indian, Hindu, and graced with the wisdom of elders that carried popular currency in the post-9/11 United States.

This image of yoga in mainstream media emerged in a period when cultural symbols associated with Hinduism, broadly speaking, began to appear as regenerative spaces that could cure American anomie. The bestselling success of Elizabeth Gilbert's 2006 travelogue memoir *Eat, Pray, Love*, which recounted Gilbert's search to recover from divorce in Italy, India, and Indonesia, portrayed the life-giving effects of her immersion in yoga in India. Although the ashram remained unnamed, it was widely thought to be based on the Ganeshpuri ashram of Gurumayi Chidvilasananda, heir to the lineage of Swami Muktananda.[62] (Chidvilasananda also ran an ashram in upstate New York; this did not feature in Gilbert's book.) The book, followed by its film version in 2010 (released in both the United States and India), inspired an "Eat, Pray,

Love" phenomenon in which Western tourists flocked to India in search of spiritual enlightenment. American companies rushed to design tour packages built around the spiritual search figured in the book and film, while the film was promoted through Lonely Planet, the popular publisher of guidebooks.[63] Travel agencies promised to package Gilbert's narrative as an efficient experiential commodity.[64] This surge in spiritual tourism not only brought more Westerners to India's meditation centers but also inspired Indian ashrams to develop more Western-centric infrastructure.[65] The book and film opened up a lucrative market niche in rewriting, for a new generation, yoga's possibilities as the central point around which an American life transformation might pivot.

Reading *Eat, Pray Love* on a rainy day, I am transported in fits of giggles. Gilbert makes me laugh. At the same time, something in me wants to cry. Inheriting and energizing old tropes of an otherworldly and spiritually replenishing India, the book speaks to a larger cultural impulse in which, as Shefali Chandra argues, "whiteness will fortify itself through India."[66] This fortification, Chandra suggests, is possible only because of key elisions. Hinduism, in these narratives, is simplified by the conspicuous erasure of Islam. Keen to cast yoga as Hindu and benign, memoirs like *Eat, Pray, Love* are determinedly uninterested in the more ambivalent relationship between yoga and Hindu fundamentalism, especially when it might work to the detriment of Muslim, Christian, Dalit, and other communities in India. Although *Eat, Pray, Love* appeared during the war on terror, in which American military violence ravaged parts of the subcontinent, American whiteness is invited to see itself through the book's charming narrator as "wounded and innocent."[67] Given that the stereotypical yoga practitioner in the United States leans toward the pacifist left, it's especially ironic that yoga is used to frame these absences. We might read this as another consequence of yoga's move into the world of consumer capitalism, in which it absorbs, reflects, and amplifies larger trends in the popular imagination.

The very safety of the imagined yoga body offered an American (and more generally Western) entry into a comforting narrative about the United States' relationship to India and South Asia. This frame exacerbates the starkness of the stereotype of the Muslim terrorist while it erases the presence of the Hindu fundamentalist body. It soothes an American conscience, allowing the United States to imagine itself as a cosmopolitan nation open and welcoming to South Asia, while it conceals the specter of U.S. military violence against civilians in Afghanistan and Pakistan. This narrative of a benevolent Hindu Indian yoga has also been useful to the Indian state in its doubled quest to seem peacefully authoritative and aligned with the United States as the victim of terrorist attacks. Such an idealized image conceals much darker forms of representational and physical violence against people of South Asian ancestry. In this respect, the very veneration with which yoga has been treated ironically underpins an unwitting violence of its own.

In 2015, passing through the San Francisco airport, I encountered a sign for a yoga room. Yoga in the airport—what could be more wonderful for travelers weary of body and depleted of soul? I welcomed this idea. Indeed, the airport seems to be the very endpoint of American capitalist modernity: the expensive, mobile, technologized, and paradoxical nowhere that nonetheless feels all too familiar to those of us passing through. It is the epitome of the social condition that has made yoga so popular, and so necessary, as a way of coping with the precarities and injustices of modernity.

Yet the more I looked at the sign, the more it looked at me. The designers had gone out of their way to evoke highly abstracted shapes yoked to the idea of India: a body in lotus pose, the top of a mandala. These lovely, calming shapes, promising an Indian-inspired order in a chaotic United States, appeared in one of the places where people of South Asian descent are subjected to the most intense state and cultural suspicion.

In the first years after 9/11, I flew across the country many times. Almost every time, I was asked to step aside and open my carry-on bag. My white fiancé would stand and wait patiently for me. I'm multiracial, light-skinned, and more commonly taken for Latina or white than South Asian in the United States. But the name on my ticket is common in Pakistan. I would speculate, only half in jest, about the databases scanning through tickets for signs of Islam. Once I opened my bag next to another passenger who'd also been pulled aside. He looked to be of South Asian descent. He was also about five years old. The airline officials looked apologetically at his mother. I did not mind the inconvenience of opening my bag. But I did mind the fact that we, the passengers, the citizens of the airplane, were not asked to share this burden equally: we were made to perform a racialized division of labor to soothe anxieties around South Asian names and bodies.

The airport is not a comfortable space in which to be South Asian. Routine racial profiling was banned in the Bush administration in 2003, and the ban was extended and expanded under the Obama administration in 2014, but it explicitly excluded security screening in airports.[68] As Charu Chandrasekhar writes:

> Since 9/11 airlines have racially profiled passengers of South Asian descent in the name of passenger safety. They have subjected such passengers to heightened security screening and denied them passage based solely on the belief that ethnicity or national origin increases passengers' flight risk. . . . Airlines have also forced South Asian passengers to endure humiliating and degrading pre-boarding searches and interrogations.[69]

In 2013, two Indian American men and a Jewish Arab woman were summarily pulled off a plane on the tenth anniversary of September 11 because passengers alerted the pilot that the men had gone to the restroom.[70] This exception was protested by the Congressional Asian Pacific American Caucus, who wrote to the Justice Department that "the current exemptions in the profiling guidance effectively authorize discrimination in the name of national security, domestic surveillance and border security."[71] Airports are one of the last places in the United States where it is legal for law enforcement officials to stop someone based on their looks.

The criminal suspicions around otherwise ordinary behavior have shaped flying while brown into a recognizable experience. In a 2014 essay for "The Weeklings," reprinted in the popular digital magazine *Salon*, Sayantani Dasgupta shares the story in "The Perils of Flying While Brown" of how her multiethnic family—Indian and European, with different skin tones—experiences American security screening. "My nine-year-old daughter has developed a fear of the TSA [Transportation Security Agency]," Dasgupta writes. "She has a faraway look, as if she's remembering all the times that she has been yelled at in security, many more times than her fairer skinned older brother. Or perhaps she is remembering how often I, her dark-skinned mother, am 'randomly' stopped to have my hands coated with bomb-detection liquid. Random or not, this has never happened to her European father."[72] Dasgupta's story echoes and powerfully amplifies my experience. The narratives that we shape to make sense of these encounters align with long-standing cultural ideas about the perpetual foreignness of South Asians in the United States.[73] Now we are not only seen as different; we are also seen as dangerous.

In the name of protecting the body politic from terror, airport screening practices perpetuate their own subtle form of civic violence. They rip apart social fabrics of trust that have only recently, gingerly, and with great effort been woven. These practices—experienced by many first-hand, and more widely through the stories they provoke—work against a healthy civil society where people of all bodies and religions feel they belong. They proliferate the myth that certain names and bodies are safe. And they create a world in which suspicion comes to rule the day, both for security screeners and for those who feel targeted. Being singled out was, as Tariq Ali said of his detention in 2001, "a tiny enough scratch but, if untreated, these lead to gangrene."[74] Such infections can spread.

I look again at the inviting sign for the San Francisco Airport's yoga room. In the layered concentric rings, their full circularity implied but also hidden by the interruption of the rectangular side, cultural signs of South Asia have been stripped from South Asian bodies. It's no wonder the image seems so safe and relaxing. The abstract, rounded outline of the human figure in lotus pose could be anyone. It's also white.

Yet when I look even more closely at my photograph, I'm struck by how many ghosts appear reflected in the glass of the sign. There I am, taking the picture. Behind me are passengers crossing, and behind them is an airline pilot, or perhaps a TSA security screener, in his white button-down shirt with official insignia on the shoulders. We haunt this picture;

we trouble its promise of peace and repose. We complicate, even as we are enveloped within, an American frame for yoga.

CONCLUSION

Visions of yoga draw imaginative power from American cultural contradictions, spinning new stories for India, Indianness, and Indians in the United States today. The more healthy and life-giving the practice appears in the studio, the more capable of murder it seems on the page. Five years after the Encinitas school district banished Sanskrit from sight and hearing, the State of California began to court India's tourists and foreign direct investment.[75] Yoga rooms make airports seem more like home for some, concealing the way that they have become less safe for others.

Who benefits from these flexible frames? This question prompts another that has arisen anew, inspired by many of these contradictions: Does someone not of South Asian background practicing yoga count as cultural appropriation?

When the language of cultural appropriation circulated in the 1980s, it troubled me. It seemed to imply a separation between cultural worlds that didn't fit with my experience, and a confidence that didn't fit with my own awkward silences, my fifth-grade hand shooting into the air to answer a question about the India I did not really know. In the late 1990s and early 2000s, I became an academic through years of thinking hard about the need for models of cross-cultural engagement that did not result in crime and punishment. I believed—and still do, though this belief is tested each day—in the project and the possibility of writing across borders without doing irreparable damage.

As the new millennium has deepened into its third decade, the language of cultural appropriation has come back with a new force. This time around, I don't think of it as a directive for everyone to place themselves in tight little boxes, or to stop being curious and compelled by worlds different from the ones they grew up within. Now it prompts us to recognize a different problem: when cultural practices can be valued more than people. When the benefits of those cultural practices can be enjoyed by all but their costs are paid by only a few, we need to ask questions. I am glad that people of all bodies, colors, and ancestries come to yoga and find themselves transformed. I learn from and with such people. But tracing the ways yoga's imaginative powers at once amplify particular ideals of India and erase them from the picture matters for the Indian diaspora, and people of South Asian background more generally, as complex questions of rights, recognition, belonging, and authority continue to shape the flexibilities demanded of us every day.

I lost touch with my childhood friend Anjali, the only Indian American friend I had. It is a story of continental drift, of how the expected solidity of "India" and "diaspora" can melt into something thin and ungraspable. Certain costs of being Indian were paid in our American childhoods. Today, Indianness pays new wages, but not always to us.

5

BENDING OVER BACKWARD

Yoga's Precarious Work

Yoga is India's gift to the world.

—PRIME MINISTER NARENDRA MODI

Yoga is an $88USD billion industry.

—WELLNESS CREATIVE CO., "YOGA INDUSTRY GROWTH,
MARKET TRENDS & ANALYSIS 2021"

"How much do you make a class?"
"It depends."
"On average."
"Like $50, $60 a class."
"$50? That's insane."
"Shut up."
"You've got to value your time more than that."
"Maybe I should just deal drugs."
*"Yeah! Do you think that I would have time to write
if I had to go to some office job?"*
"Have you been writing?"

—TOM O'BRIEN, "EPISODE 2: 'SOMETHING GREAT,' "
OM CITY: THE SERIES

On the garden level of my aunt and uncle's apartment building, in a dark room in the Mumbai dawn, I join four other residents. In sunlight, the instructor works in a corporate office. In the shadowy hours, he teaches yoga. He leads us with expertise and conviction through a series of poses. To my right, two regulars inhale with ease. To my left, two muscular men strain and stretch. As we move into the final poses, my mind slips back in time to my seventeen-year-old self off to university, worried that I won't pay correctly for a taxi ride from the airport to campus. As we come out of *śavāsana*, I walk over to my bag, anxious to settle my debt with the teacher. I have prepared the cash amount specified on the flyer posted by the building lift. Then I notice that everyone else is seated for a final full prayer.

Yoga assumes form in a world shaped by the anxieties of economic life. How can yoga be free, profitable, and exploitative all at once? Where does the exchange of money fit within the complex negotiations and competing norms that frame the practice? In this chapter, I explore imaginative visions of how yoga works within economic structures since the turn of the millennium. These visions may seem incompatible, yet they gesture toward interconnected cultural logics that testify to expanding gendered, racial, cultural, and class hierarchies. As Andrea Jain, Verena Schnäbele, and Sarah Sharma have shown, yoga's increased global popularity reflects the rise of capitalist practices and their accompanying neoliberal logic, defined as the assumption that individuals seek freedom and flourishing through the market.[1] Yoga helps to make life under capitalism more bearable.

Visions of yoga help to recruit subjects into cultural logics of capitalism, both as consumers and as workers, precisely because many people see the practice as transcending the values, norms, and disciplinary regimes of exemplary capitalist spaces such as factories and offices. Yoga, I argue, can be imagined as a set of practices that promote self-making within capitalist structures because this often creates the illusion that yoga is outside capitalist values of exchange. Such visions reveal how the practice can be used to construct flexibilities and resiliences within capitalist life logics.

Yoga might thus be understood as an exemplar of "affective labor," a form that takes new shape in the shift from industrial to information economies. "This labor is immaterial, even if it is corporeal and affective, in the sense that its products are intangible: a feeling of ease, well-being, satisfaction, excitement, passion—even a sense of connectedness or community," Michael Hardt writes.[2] Such affective labor sits at the crux of a tension between capitalist and anticapitalist values. "On the one hand, affective labor, the production and reproduction of life, has become firmly embedded as a necessary foundation for capitalist accumulation and patriarchal order," he argues. "On the other hand, however, the production of affects, subjectivities, and forms of life present an enormous potential for autonomous circuits of valorization, and perhaps for liberation."[3] Attention to the diversity of stories and spectacles of yoga helps to chart where and how yoga recruits new bodies to neoliberal conceptions of labor under capitalism, and where and how it promotes alternative ways of thinking and feeling. This multiplicity helps us gain a clearer sense of how visions of yoga both reinforce capitalist logics and introduce notes of critical dissonance.

The dominant metaphor I lean on to understand yoga—flexibility—speaks to economic and labor transformations of the turn of the millennium. Two of the most vivid twentieth-century architectures of paid labor were the factory and the office, organized around the assembly line or the 9-to-5 day. The end of the twentieth century and the beginning of the twenty-first have seen the rise of flexibility as a new ideal for capitalist production and labor conditions. Factories with fixed overheads gave way to just-in-time production lines aligned with the vicissitudes of market demands. This required a more flexible labor force that could be increased in times of surge demand and released when market needs were low. Workplaces like offices also came under new economic and political pressures to offer more flexible forms of work to meet market demands for expanded communication and engagement. These forces intersected with feminist critiques of the rigidities of traditional labor markets, where, although high levels of factory or office work were performed by young women in globalizing economies seeking catch-up growth, norms around the workplace often assumed an ideal worker with no significant social obligations, such as childbirth, child care, or elder care, which continued to fall disproportionately to women.[4] Flexibility has been imagined as a response to these different demands.

While flexibility appears to allow everyone to have it all—markets to function more efficiently and workers to balance competing commitments—its flipped position is precarity. Precarity has become a keyword of scholarly investigation, often understood, as Clara Han puts it, as "the predicament of those who live at the juncture of unstable contract labor and a loss of state provisioning."[5] This condition assumes new prominence in a period marked by changing geographies of inequality. Although between 1990 and 2016, inequality rose in some countries and diminished in others, the United Nations argued that "countries where income inequality has grown since 1990 are home to over seventy percent of the world's population."[6] By the twenty-first century, as countries like India had moved more deeply into neoliberal economic reforms and countries like the United States had begun to rely more heavily on gig economies of independent contractors, the idea of "flexible labor" had become important in diverse cultural contexts.[7] A survival good masked as a liberatory ideal, this idea may in some ways expand the freedom of workers, yet it can also shackle them more tightly.

The entanglement between flexibility and precarity shapes the forms of affective labor that emerge through yoga. Like many other forms of labor involving care, reproducing yoga is often politically difficult even to perceive as real work. In many yogic institutions, the concept of *sevā*, or selfless service, has been an ambivalent economic sign.[8] Whether understood as service to a guru or to a broader community, *sevā* mobilizes, channels, and rewards unpaid labor. It can offer diverse alternatives to capitalist logics of profit and wage, especially in the context of devotion. Yet it can also figure an illusion through which unpaid labor is exploited for capitalist benefit, sometimes violating labor laws and displacing paid labor.[9]

Growing in popularity in an era of economic transformation, yoga attracts many people because it appears to remake the vulnerabilities of precarity into the strengths of flexibility. Yet at the same time, the practice is imaginatively caught within, and even constituted by, the problem it is said to address. Flexible labor for many people has gone hand in hand with precarious forms of economic existence beyond previous stable, if often also repressive, social structures. The flexibilities offered through yoga, for consumers and workers, rely on the structures of stressful life that yoga is thought to resolve. In this chapter, I draw on film, fiction, self-help narrative, and media from India, the United States, Canada, the United Kingdom, and New Zealand to show how yoga's imaginative power both conceals and potentially exposes key contractions in a new world of flexible work.

I begin by exploring how imaginative work calls attention to the economic precarities that shape the social meaning of yoga. While Indian state visions often link yoga to larger projects of economic triumph, exemplified by its role within "Brand India,"[10] novels perform self-studies of yoga's reliance on a global precariat. In a range of fiction and digital media, such as Alexandra Gray's British novel *The Yoga Teacher* (2008), teaching yoga to the upper classes is presented as the modern version of a nineteenth-century world of servitude. This pattern emerges in a range of North American yoga-themed cultural expressions, such as the web series *Om City* (2015), Tracy Weber's *Murder Strikes a Pose* (2013), and Rain Mitchell's *Tales of the Yoga Studio* (2011). The structures that have popularized yoga, such works reveal, rely on labor forces of flexible personhood. Although the practice may relieve the pressures of neoliberal life for some, the flexibilities demanded of those who teach can be the essence of such stress for others.

This ambivalence, in which yoga both ennobles and exploits workers, speaks to larger cultural questions about how yoga has been integrated as a flexible Indian solution to Western crisis. In the second part of this chapter, I explore a contradiction in which Indian workers support technology-dependent American lifestyles while Indian cultural practices ameliorate the problems caused by that dependence on technology. Reading the cultural history of yoga in autobiography and media against the migration history of information technology workers allows us to apprehend broader stories that tend to diffuse positive forms of authority across majoritarian subjects while concentrating exploitations within minority positions. Yoga takes on new meanings in such a double bind. The benefits of yoga may depend on, while they also conceal, inequalities and exploitations in worlds of work.

Finally, I explore the ambivalence within representations of yoga that link the economic concept of "free" to the political ideal of "freedom." Laughter yoga, a variant of the practice that became popular in India and globally around the turn of the twenty-first century, exemplifies this ambivalent relationship. Juxtaposing the autobiographical writings of the Indian inventor of laughter yoga with a documentary by the Indian American filmmaker Mira Nair, I argue that the discourse of laughter yoga gives new meaning to the Indian state's rhetoric that yoga is India's gift to the world. Although such language is meant to inspire economic activity while softening the harsh edges of capitalist exchange, Western fiction, exemplified by the New Zealand novel *Heavenly Hirani's School of Laughing Yoga* (2014), takes the Indian state's words literally. Novels like this one project cultural fantasies of India as an endless source of spiritual riches, reinscribing colonial hierarchies of servitude in a twenty-first-century transnational landscape. The ideal of laughing freely, I suggest, may turn out to be unexpectedly expensive.

Are these imaginative visions of yoga politically provocative critiques or neoliberal facades for changing economic structures? I suggest that both possibilities remain alive. Holding together contradictions is precisely the technique rendered resilient through the flexibilities of yoga. These works of art and media do not envision yoga as a secure exit from capitalism. But they may selectively expand collective interpretative resources for readers and practitioners to think about the social significance of yogic flexibility in precarious times. In this sense, they contribute to the critically reflective project of a remixed *svādhyāya*.

HOLDING SPACE, KEEPING TIME

" 'Holding space' is something we often first encounter in our yoga community. It's hard to describe."[11] "To hold space is to create and maintain a place where things can exist, expand and grow."[12] "Yoga teachers hold space for their students."[13]

Space that requires holding turns out to be surprisingly heavy. After a day of teaching my students and chairing meetings, directing and redirecting the pulse of ideas, exuding energy and absorbing emotions, I'm reeling from an introvert's hangover. I long for a yoga class where someone else will tell me where to sit and what to do. In yoga studios around the world, people come in search of a milieu where someone else will hold energies that cannot be seen. For many yoga teachers, the idea of "holding space" encapsulates an unspoken and intangible, but also essential, part of their work.

Yet the space teachers hold, often so gracefully and gently, is rarely their own. This work, like many other forms of care, eludes metrics of profit. Although yoga is a billion-dollar industry, few of those billions flow to the grassroots teachers whose bodily and emotional labor makes the practice possible. The American web series *Om City* (2015) points to the ways teaching yoga requires long hours and emotional intensity, yet rarely leads to economic security, let alone wealth. The opening scenes portray the flip side of the serene holding of space. Grace, the protagonist, lurches down from an inversion with the realization she's running late to teach a class. Dashing out the door, assuring her housemate that she'll soon pay her share of the rent, Grace races through the streets of New York as the flipped, ironic form of the leisurely male flâneur of centuries past. Her day requires her to travel the space of the city, moving from studios to lavish apartments to brownstones to teach the practice. Shows like *Om City* bring to light the labor involved in holding space in a tenuous, demanding geography. To hold space still for others, exhausting mobility—literal and metaphoric—is needed.

The work of care often takes place on borrowed ground. The world of yoga in many urban environments has been shaped by the pressures of meeting the rent. The idea of paying for someone else's ownership exemplifies spatial flexibilities that are also precarities. Money spent to rent will never return to the one who paid it. As a way to occupy space, rent can signal chronic indebtedness, a place of belonging that is simultaneously of nonbelonging. In Tracy Weber's Seattle-based American mystery *Murder Strikes a Pose* (2013), the controlling power of rent shapes the condition of possibility for a small independent yoga studio. "The neighborhood around Serenity Yoga seemed trapped between the forces of decay and renewal," the narrator says.

> Frozen by a poor economy and various environmental factors, the Greenwood business district sandwiched ghetto-like empty buildings in between trendy new construction. . . . I chose to open Serenity Yoga in these unusual surroundings for two very simple reasons: the rent was cheap and the studio's mixed-use building was only a ten-minute drive from my home. . . . I even ignored the empty storefronts of several recently failed businesses. I should have known better.[14]

Yoga offers a strategy for gentrification, revitalizing neighborhoods that will then price the yoga studio out. Matthew Remski argues that because yoga in capitalist contexts is often established within rent economies, yogic institutions exist in precarious modes. Rent leaves studios on the brink of viability: *"Many of the 10K/month [rent] club studios have been open for close to a decade, and they have zero equity to show for it,"* he argues.[15] In diverse geographies as distant as Hong Kong and Rishikesh, yoga studios have shuttered for failure to make their rent.[16] In this sense, the rent economy of yoga is especially painful: the investments seem to flow to everyone but the laboring body of the teacher who holds the space for students to inhabit and for landlords to profit from.

The desire to monetize space marks the extractive logic of big corporate chains that have come to dominate North American studio offerings. In the novels of Rain Mitchell, the owner-operator protagonist who cares about transforming lives must battle the predatory practices of big corporations, where bodies on a mat are simply resources to be extracted. Set in multicultural Los Angeles, *Tales of the Yoga Studio* (2011) explores a world defined by Hollywood image making, status-seeking anxieties, and ruthless pursuit of a bottom line. In the big corporate studios, yoga is simply an excuse to pressure, shame, and inspire practitioners into spending more money.

"You'll be happy to hear," [the attendant] says, "that you won't need your mats. . . . Oh, and we'd like to encourage you not to bring plastic water bottles into the studio. We sell reusable metal YogaHappens containers out front. They're coordinated with the color scheme of the studios."

. . ."How much are the bottles?" Graciela asks.

"Forty-two dollars," he says. "But there's unlimited filtered water throughout the Experience Center at no charge."[17]

This imperative to buy is concealed as free choice. "If you don't want to use [your plastic water bottles] today, I'll be happy to keep [them] here until after class," the attendant assures new students. "[One student] hates being told what will make her happy, especially since using her own mat and drinking from her own plastic (!) bottle is what would please her *most* right now."[18] As the rhetoric of the corporate studio defines happiness for its students, it dramatizes the corporation's hegemonic aspirations.

If consent fails, then coercion prevails. Teachers, surveilled via video camera during classes, are expected to increase the pressure on students to buy. "In the future," a new teacher is told, "you go over and remove the [plastic] bottles and put them outside the door. All very discreet and supportive. . . . You very softly say: 'Don't let that happen again.'"[19] Manipulating ideals of what it means to be a good citizen, the teacher is expected to transform her students into aspirational, docile consumers whose financial commitments lock them into loyalty and whose objects of desire are always kept just beyond reach. "And you might tell them," the studio representative continues, ". . . that if [students] want to do the more complicated and sexy poses . . . that they should think about private lessons. One hundred and twenty an hour."[20] The corporate exploitation satirized in *Tales of the Yoga Studio* shapes the racial and class contours of yoga in U.S. space, favoring upper middle class and white subjects through pricing structures and disciplining gazes. Through these regimes of manipulation, *Tales of the Yoga Studio* dramatizes how the illusion of choice is created to conceal coercion. The YogaHappens studio is a disciplinary space of biopower, where every suggestive detail conceals an extractive process. Making a body more flexible also entraps it within rigid social and economic demands.

As affective labor, holding space is vulnerable to the invisibilities that have often marked other forms of care work in market economies. The world of yoga has shifted from a practice dominated by male authority figures to a highly feminized corpus of teachers, and its flexibilities and precarities speak to gendered assumptions about labor. In the Western contexts portrayed by writers like Weber and Mitchell, yoga teachers are likely to be women. In some respects, the rise of flexibility as a workplace asset has offered feminist potential. As Kathryn Cady argues, "in the 1980s US context, flexibility became thought of as workplace justice, a feminist solution to help women balance paid work with unpaid household work and child care."[21] Yet the solution has not always materialized real results. "Regardless of the positive press," Cady reveals, "flexibility often failed to help women workers in the 1980s and 1990s."[22] Significant tradeoffs became associated with flexible work, both tangible, in reduced wages or benefits, and intangible, in reduced recognition or career mobility. For many female protagonists in Western yoga-themed fiction, the flexibilities that often draw them to teach also confine them within gendered hierarchies that limit prestige and security. Novels and films register these contradictions, holding out hope that the virtues of flexibility will transform the pressures of precarity yet also despairing of the ways flexibilities can be used to extend, rather than correct, spaces of precarious nonbelonging.

The resilience promoted through yoga is thus not simply a story of the psychological resilience of individuals facing often untenable demands. It is also a portrait of how capitalist precarity itself gains resilience as a flexible employment structure that can withstand the demands of labor politics. Although yoga teachers in some North American contexts have pushed toward collective bargaining,[23] putting a new spin on the trope that "yoga" signifies "union," the models that historically led to the creation of traditional labor unions are increasingly difficult to implement within the growing gig economy. The ideal of flexibility has placed many people in the category of "independent contractor" rather than "employee"—a change that can exclude them from key benefits and securities.

In this light, it is instructive to think of what it means to hold the space. Welcoming, guiding, and directing energy; creating atmosphere and environment; managing emotions and body parts; offering presence to students and asking it of them as well—teachers modulate a form of energetic awareness designed to produce new meanings, insights, and transformations in their students. Like Atlas bearing the weight of the world, teachers hold the space. But, balanced precariously in their own poses, they rarely own it.

While many yoga teachers are asked to do the work of holding space, they are also expected to perform the job of keeping time. The work of modulating time, as Sarah Sharma has argued, can allow yoga to perpetuate the temporal sovereignties of global capitalism. "The yoga instructor is a roving infrastructural technician of time maintenance who extends the sedentary tradition through recalibration, a form of temporal regulation and disciplining of labor," she writes.[24] "The sedentary body is both a sped-up subject of global capital who needs to slow down and a slowed down body who needs to get up to speed."[25] In addition to making workers more productive, yoga teachers are asked to testify to the effects of yogic time. "Mindful labor," Melissa Gregg argues, "refers to the degree of work involved in producing and maintaining affective composure in the absence of collective labor politics."[26] Yoga teachers are expected to embody affective composure, to testify with their bodies and words and presence to the transformative effects of the practice.

Fiction and film expose this labor as real work. "People expected me to be calm and collected at all times," confides the narrator of Tracy Weber's *Murder Strikes a Pose* (2013). "I wasn't allowed to be mean, or even irritated, for that matter."[27] Such pressure eventually leads to the breakdown of a yoga teacher in *Om City*, for whom the burden to perform and produce a totally calm environment for his students—an impossible task in New York—leads to anger and assault against a man who refuses to lower his voice in the hallway. "I'm teaching too much, and don't have time to practice myself," Des admits. "I'm tired all the time, I'm on edge." Yet even in the aftermath of this explosion, he still feels the need to testify to yoga's transformative capacity. "I am a tad bit worried about your anger," Grace says. Des straightens up. "You should have seen me before yoga," he replies.[28] Moments like these dramatize the pressure for an embodied testimony to yogic time that must be continually performed to keep up with the present moment.

The laboring body of the yoga teacher is expected to conform to the time needs of students. In some models, yoga teachers respond to this pressure by digitizing themselves, creating recorded classes that can be watched on demand. In other models, for more affluent clientele, teachers are treated as commodities whose time belongs to their employers. In Alexandra Gray's *The Yoga Teacher* (2008), her protagonist (also named Grace) must make herself flexible to fit into the temporal regimes of her employer.

> "Grace, we want to maximize our yoga time, so we'll have a yoga class before dinner the day you arrive."
> "Don't worry, Grace, you'll have time for a shower before we begin, won't she, Jackie?" Princess Elizabeth interjected.
> "She can jump in the shower, why not?" said Jackie.[29]

Reluctantly conceding needs that Grace herself might have, Jackie, as an employer, operates on the assumption that Grace will conform to the schedules of those whom she teaches. The work of flexible time modulation, performed across elite and corporate spaces, is part of larger disciplinary regimes that shape productive workers and enforce employment hierarchies. As a yoga teacher, Grace is not an authority figure but a servant.

Although yoga is often thought to direct practitioners' attention to the present time, as a labor practice it also operates within horizons of futurity that are always uncertain. The threat of a yoga teaching career coming to an end is a specter raised in web dramas like *Om City*. Working for studios, Grace teaches for a pittance and is continually under pressure due to newer instructors seeking to make their own place within the teaching economy. The overproduction of yoga teachers is hinted at in an episode where at a meeting of teachers, the studio owner Mitchell adoringly introduces their newest hire. The existing teachers look uncomfortably at this new presence, knowing that she is there to "sub" for them when they cannot teach a class, but that this convenience comes at a price: it reminds them of their own dispensability, the instructor as factory-produced commodity of which there is a seemingly endless supply. The glowing new sub marks the beginning of the current teachers' end.

This seemingly endless supply is not a historical accident. It testifies to the economic precarity of yoga's place within a rent economy in ways that integrate the precarities of holding space and keeping time. At the turn of the millennium, economic pressures on Western yoga studios led many to heavily market teacher trainings, which were often more lucrative than studio classes. This practice offered studios financial security to survive another year. Establishing time-based 200-hour and 500-hour trainings, in contrast to more open-ended practices of study and apprenticeship, transformed paying students into potential teachers. Trainees could understand spending money on yoga training as a capital investment in themselves that would qualify them to earn money in the future. Some large yoga corporations preyed on students' aspirations, recruiting them into expensive teacher trainings even when jobs were unlikely to materialize.[30] Unlike workers taking yoga classes to increase their productivity, which veils economic transactions through layers of psychological management, teacher trainings operate in a more direct financial logic. The homogenous time of the preprogrammed 200-hour or 500-hour training, in contrast to an open-ended experiential process, creates the conditions for production of commodifiable yoga instructors.

The potentially exploitative monetized time of the teacher training industry emerges in Suzanne Morrison's American memoir *Yoga Bitch* (2011), which charts her journey from student to teacher in a context where she is both captivated by and skeptical of yoga's transformative power. Her memoir reveals diverse forms of monetary exploitation, including her own: Morrison participates in a small ring of students who seek to take more classes than they have paid for. As a white female student, she benefits from broader social assumptions around who can be trusted. But she is most critical of what she comes to see as the financial and psychological exploitation within the American-led teacher training she attends in Bali. Teacher trainings, as presented in the memoir, offer an enclosed space and time where a teacher seeks to consolidate her authority over trainees. One student, well versed already in anatomy, resists paying a separate fee to take a required anatomy class. "Here's what's weird," writes Morrison. "[The head teacher] told [the student] that she has attachment issues with money, and that paying for the anatomy class will help her to overcome those issues."[31] Manipulating her own financial gain into a recommendation for the student's psychological growth, the teacher seeks to turn resistance to her authority into evidence that more, not less, yoga is needed. The intensity of this desire exposes an extractive logic at play. A few pages later, the same teacher invites her students to pay her for Balinese wood carvings of herself holding particular yoga poses. "Most of my yogamates got up and offered her thirty, forty dollars for their statues," writes Morrison. "I didn't. . . . I just couldn't do it."[32] The dissonant specter of a Western teacher promoting her own image and profiting from the craft of Balinese workers discredits claims to lofty ideals. As a narrative about faith and eventual disillusionment with structures of authority in the world of yoga, Morrison's memoir invites study on the paradox of teacher training. Although trainees believe they are growing their own authority through the time they invest in themselves, they are expected to depend more deeply on the institution's structures. Through the enclosed time of a teacher training, they provide the capital upon which the future of the studios rests, though their own futures as teachers remain uncertain.

Yoga requires taking charge of time. Teaching demands exquisite attention to the passing of seconds, knowing that the difference between dullness and agony is only a matter of moments. Managing time is the problem of modern life. I come to yoga class to lose my sense of time, to ask someone else to keep it for me. Time is unexpectedly heavy, like space; smooth, like a stone in a creek; and jagged, like a rock in a mountain. We never have enough of it, yet we need someone else to manage it for us. Teachers become shepherds of time that is not their own, protecting their students' present moment while haunted by the precarities of the future. How does a teacher steer time, guard it, stretch it, compress it, order it, sell it?

People say they have no time, and my teacher says, calmly, "That is a lie."

SHOPPING FOR BODIES

Where might Indian bodies fit into this U.S. landscape? If bodies of yoga teachers are often asked to conceal their own hard work, other working bodies also labor in the shadows of the practice. This happens in a cultural context informed by the rise of technology, especially the digital devices that capture attention, command fingers, and mediate everyday life. In this context, the flexible bodies of yoga assume new forms. Representations of yoga crystallize and conceal tensions within emerging ideas of flexible Indian labor since the turn of the millennium.

Indian spiritual experience has long been seen as a form of technological advancement. I suggest that this imaginative work operates in dialogue with a very different source of Indian labor: the work of information technology professionals. Since 1990, they have been able to migrate from India to the United States through the H-1B visa program, which created opportunities for college-educated workers in specialty professions. By the twenty-first century, these two Indian exports—yoga and information technology work—had begun to play uncannily linked roles in the United States. Both the Indian yogi and the Indian H-1B technology migrant can be read as U.S. technology workers: a labor source that has become important both to the U.S. body politic and to the Indian state.

Taken together, these two forms of migrant Indian labor uphold a shared cultural logic that serves the needs of U.S. corporate capitalism and the nationalist aspirations of a rising India. By investigating how symbolic and material worlds are woven together, we can appreciate how the United States has not only turned to fantasies of Indian culture to alleviate its anxieties about technology but also, with distinct political and cultural ambivalence, relied on the labor of Indian bodies. While yoga has been advertised by Indian yogis (and others) as a practice that enables one to enjoy the benefits of technology without falling prey to anomie and alienation, such optimistic visions are symbolically shadowed by a darker narrative of Indian migrants who live and work in a gray legal economy of global traffic in technology labor. Both visions install fantasies of Indianness within the inequalities of capitalist globalization.

These fantasies draw attention to some of the contradictions, complexities, and even abuses that structure a logic in which the United States strives to perfect its cultural relationship to technology through strategic uses of Indianness. On the one hand, technology implies the artificial creations of machine or digital culture. On the other hand, technology implies broader ideas of cultivation captured in the utopian concept of "technê" as craftsmanship or in the Foucauldian technology of the self, where individuals alter themselves in the search for "happiness, purity, wisdom, perfection, or immortality."[33] Embodied and imaginative labor from India has helped to make these two meanings of "technology" converge, but at a price.

The U.S. search for an ideal cultural relationship with technology has long relied on ideas from Asia. In *The Buddha in the Machine* (2014), R. John Williams argues for what he calls "*Asia-as-technê*: a compelling fantasy that would posit Eastern aesthetics as both the antidote to and the perfection of machine culture."[34] Technê, in the sense Williams attributes to Heidegger, refers to ideals of creation through craftsmanship.[35] It conjures a metaphysics of organic wholeness that counterpoints "techno," or industrial ideals of machine culture that rely upon metaphysical divisions between self and machine. Technê offers the allure of a beautiful and unified human spirit, while techno threatens the tyranny of dehumanization. Williams argues that Asian aesthetics are used to invoke technê to allay fears of new technologies.

Yoga has historically integrated ideas of human flourishing with machine and digital culture. Srinivas Aravamudan shows how Indian discourses of spiritual experience, including yoga, offer a vision of a sup-posedly ancient indigenous technê that can support and give meaning to an industrial and colonial techno. This integration of spirit with sci-ence often reflected dialogue with U.S., British, and European move-ments, such as Theosophy and New Thought.[36] It also served the inter-ests of Indian and Hindu nationalists as a way to counter colonial stereotypes of Indian inadequacy. Early twentieth-century Indian writ-ers often presented Indian mysticism as the powerful equal of Western technology while promoting new military technologies, such as nuclear weapons, through what Aravamudan calls a " 'Hindu sublime' enabled by Guru English."[37] Placing yoga within Western scientific frameworks was a prominent project in India's mid-century.[38] In turn, Western sci-entific thinkers, such as Nikolai Tesla, were captivated by yogic concepts such as *prāṇa* (energy) and *ākāśa* (ether).[39] The merger of scientific rhetoric with Indian mysticism eventually flourished within consumer capitalism, as seen in the late twentieth- and twenty-first-century spiri-tual empires of such figures as the Maharishi Mahesh Yogi, Deepak Chopra, and Baba Ramdev.[40] In these discourses, constructing a yogic self has sometimes seemed like making a piece of technology.

A key text that helped to shape this idea emerged from the work of Paramahansa Yogananda, an Indian guru who became an influential proponent of the practice in the early and mid-twentieth century in the United States. *Autobiography of a Yogi* (1946), which influenced West-ern readers for decades, was published in a period of distinct U.S. ambiv-alence about ideas and bodies from India. Yogananda arrived in the United States at a transitional moment when a craze for things Indian that emerged in the 1880s was giving way to tighter restrictions on migra-tion from the subcontinent.[41] Contesting ideas of Indian weakness, technological prowess becomes a defining feature of yogic selfhood in Yogananda's account. His narrative draws attention to yogic *siddhis*, or occult powers, which he presents as advanced forms of technology that surpass Western science.[42] The telepathy of a guru, for example, is under-stood through the language of information technology: "My guru was a perfect human radio."[43] This vision of yoga as a redemptive technê unites machine culture with self-care, aligning spiritual development with

capitalist production. Secret techniques of yoga operate like technological trade secrets, legitimating both the myth of the ancient Indian
renunciate and the spread of yoga into a capitalist United States.[44] These
ideas provide the precursor to the cultural logics that connect yoga,
technology, and capitalist making since the turn of the millennium.

In the simplest alliance between yoga and technology in the twenty-
first century, yoga is therapeutic. For practitioners who understand
themselves as organic bodies surrounded by metal machines, yoga promises to help in coping with the stresses of too many devices. Since the
first years of the new millennium, it has become routine for mainstream
U.S. publications to offer advice columns such as "The Best Yoga Sequence
to Do After Work," where "work" is assumed to be a desk job in front of
a computer and "yoga" is presumed to make this work sustainable.[45] Yoga
is often understood to make practitioners physically flexible, by loosen-
ing muscles stiff from screen time, as well as mentally flexible, by promoting habits of dispassionate observation. In some forms, yoga can
serve as a conduit for fantasies of an imagined ancient India that refresh
the device-dependent practitioner. The sensory and visual language of
U.S. studios that hang images of Indian deities, burn incense, or present
English in fonts inspired by the Devanagari script, for instance, seek to
offer relief from mainstream U.S. office environments where computers, smartphones, wearables, and tablets rule.

The more penetrating aspect of Yogananda's vision that informs
twenty-first-century U.S. culture invites individuals to conceptualize
themselves as devices. In Yogananda's autobiography, the human body
has the capacity to resemble an advanced technological object. Spiritual
development thus becomes remarkably compatible with emergent processes of capitalist product development. Yogananda's vision of the technologized yogic body, which helped to produce new forms of authority
for Indian gurus in a Western context, has infiltrated the discourse available to practitioners in the United States. As described by the influential U.S. yoga center Kripalu, in language that Yogananda (and Foucault)
would have appreciated, yoga represents a "technology for life transformation."[46] The twenty-first-century Indian guru and business consultant Jaggi Vasudev puts the matter starkly: "The human body is the

greatest gadget."[47] Yoga has been embraced by so many corporations because it promises to alleviate the stress of technocentric corporate life while simultaneously encouraging practitioners to treat themselves as products that can be developed and improved.

It is thus not surprising that U.S. tech companies have been at the vanguard of corporate yoga. Google's Chief Evangelist of Brand Marketing, Gopi Kallayil, has argued to business-oriented audiences that the most important "technology" people have is their bodies and brains, and disciplines like yoga (a practice he helped popularize at Google) "optimize this technology."[48] This rhetoric connects Google's digital technology to a humanist wellspring so that its products seem to emerge as new and natural forms of self-development, even as they reflect the values and social hierarchies of global capitalism and U.S. popular culture. Yogananda's heirs thus are not only in yoga studios. They are also in the heart of corporate capital.[49] The language of yoga, as a technology of the self, lends a halo effect to the increasing digitization of modern life.

Such rhetoric since the turn of the millennium implies that, through Indian legacies of yoga, U.S. practitioners can have it all. They can counter the ills of too much machine and digital culture by turning to an Indian export that provides a break from devices through postural practice but also affirms technology's underlying logic of incessant product development. But what about the labor that supports this U.S. thirst for an unending series of technological gadgets and services? Increasingly, this labor is also an Indian export, of information technology professionals.

At just the moment in the 1990s when yoga was becoming more mainstream in the U.S., this parallel movement brought a new wave of Indian migrants who represent the cultural obverse of yoga, via the H-1B visa program. The visa was not created specifically with technology, or India, in mind, but the growth of the computer industry in the 1990s transformed it into a pathway for Indian information technology workers to come to the United States. By 2012, 64 percent of all H-1B visas were granted to Indians.[50] The definition of skilled professional used for the H-1B has favored fields such as computing, not yoga.[51] At the same time that this visa category encouraged mobility of Indian labor, the expansion of U.S. yoga training programs shifted the teaching demographic away from the once iconic Indian male body toward individuals who were more likely to identify as white.[52] The 1990s and beyond thus mark a moment of transformation in the kind of Indian labor desired by U.S. technological structures.

The popularity of the H-1B visa continues a twentieth-century history in which U.S.-centric technological skill has often been seen as integral to modern independent India. Jawarhalal Nehru was famously enthusiastic about science and technology, and connections to the United States were historically vital to the growth and prestige of information technology skills in India. A U.S.-oriented Indian elite promoted computing within the country.[53] The symbolic pressure to keep up with U.S. technology in urban India propelled the success of Rajkumar Hirani's popular Bollywood film *3 Idiots* (2009), based on the first bestselling Indian novel in English, Chetan Bhagat's *Five Point Someone—What Not to Do at IIT* (2004). This story critiques a widespread Indian tendency to measure success as becoming an engineer, especially in the United States. The social status of engineering and computing has inspired thousands of Indian technology workers to migrate through the H-1B program, which promises a job in technology and a life in the United States.

Yet the H-1B visa actually pulls many participants into a distinctly different kind of work and life: one defined by a capitalist search for a flexible workforce that leads to a vulnerable social position. The H-1B visa is highly controversial in the United States. It has been the subject of protracted political battles that have pitted high-tech capital against organized labor, anti-immigration groups, and conservative elements of U.S. politics.[54] Mainstream media discourse has focused on companies that replace expensive older domestic workers with young Indian migrants who work for lower wages.[55] In 1995, *The Washington Post* ran a front-page story titled "White-Collar Visas: Back Door for Cheap Labor?" U.S. companies, it reported, laid off workers to hire programmers on H-1B visas.[56] Twenty years later, a *New York Times* headline revealed the persistence of this phenomenon: "Pink Slips at Disney. But First, Training Foreign Replacements."[57] Critics of the program have testified before Congress that the H-1B unfairly disadvantages domestic workers.[58] While the social status of those who gain such visas may be high in India, their standing in the United States is more uncertain. At its best, the H-1B program places workers in situations where they are likely to be publicly perceived as the cause of STEM job loss in the United States.

At its worst, the H-1B system imprisons Indian tech workers in a globalized gray zone of economic and legal exploitation. Advocates of expanding the program argue that bringing in skilled foreign workers encourages entrepreneurialism, but the great majority of workers on H-1B visas are not in positions to begin exciting ventures. A 2014 expose published by *Reveal*, in association with *The Guardian* and NBC Bay Area, noted that "critics have sounded alarms about immigrant tech workers being treated as indentured servants."[59] The article exposed widespread exploitation in the system: "From 2000 through 2013, at least $29.7 million was illegally withheld from about 4,400 tech workers here on H-1B visas, U.S. Department of Labor documents show."[60] Even enthusiastic defenders of the global circulation of technology professionals have acknowledged the "deleterious effects" of the program.[61] Climates of fear, intimidation, uncertainty, and dependency pervade the world of the H-1B.

This middle-class indenture is most visible in what are, chillingly, called "body shops": Indian-owned subsidiaries that bring Indian technology workers to the United States and contract them out to U.S. corporations. These Indian labor brokers are some of the biggest users of the H-1B visa program. Migrants come to the United States to wait, often without full pay, until an appropriate job is available. If they seek a job on their own, they face expensive penalties. This material flexibility requires workers to wait indefinitely without pay and to move to cities according to the availability of technology work.[62] Such employment conditions might be understood as demanding a grim variant of the physical and mental flexibility cultivated through yoga. U.S. dependence on technologized cultural norms appears to require worker flexibility from H-1B migrants to produce it, and consumer flexibility from yoga to survive it.

To produce a flexible workforce that bends to the changing shape of tech work, body shops circumvent labor protections. While information technology workers may work for a U.S. company, they are technically managed by the body shop, which means that they enjoy few of the labor protections that the company would be required to provide regular employees.[63] An intermediary like a body shop supplies U.S. companies with the most flexible workforce possible, a labor source that can be turned on and off. As a practice in which Indians manage the labor of other Indians, this exploitation is not simple white-against-Indian racism. But it colludes with larger patterns in which nonwhite technology labor in the United States has often struggled for power and recognition.[64]

The metaphor of the body shop is not an accident of language. This is a rhetoric of dehumanization and even dismemberment. Bodies, rhetorically bereft of cognition and culture, become commodities to be ordered, reorganized, and sold. In the connotation drawn from the automotive industry, Indian workers are envisioned as objects and as fundamentally interchangeable exports. While the technology sector frequently invokes the language of innovation and entrepreneurship, arguing that the visa program allows the United States to attract and nurture "foreign talent" or the "best and the brightest," the rhetoric of the body shop forcefully reasserts Fordist images of automated, repetitive, and alienated labor. This positions information technology workers as objectified bodies to be rented for their labor and conjures a form of employment in which they become twenty-first-century factory automatons. Belying the highly skilled mental capacities that these workers are supposed to represent, the phrase "body shop" becomes the professional analogue to the working-class "sweat shop."[65] Information technology workers are portrayed as objectified technology being traded and supposedly robotic makers of digital culture: a dystopian union between the human body and technology production.

The bodies of the H-1B workers thus represent the inverted mirror of that other form of Indian bodily cultivation, yoga. Here we find the obverse of the idealized unity of process and product that yoga, in Yogananda's style, connotes. The workers represent the inverted shadow fantasy of the guru as technê, in which Indian yogic powers of technology represent mastery, control, and autonomy. Skilled Indian professionals are effectively sold, traded, and rented in a gray market to support ongoing U.S. desires for ever cheaper and ever more advanced technological life. Yet they are also critiqued within the U.S. body politic because they are seen to displace more expensive and less flexible domestic labor. Against the benevolent, powerful, and unique Indian body figured by yoga, U.S. media present a faceless and nameless set of Indian workers who are not uncommonly reduced to acronyms, known only bureaucratically as "H-1Bs."

Unlike the gurus of the early and mid-twentieth century, who found some sympathetic audiences in the United States, Indian migrants on the visa program have few friends. Their most visible support has come from Indian Americans but has been limited in its impact. Ronil Hira, an Indian American critic of the H-1B visa program, has testified before Congress about recipients' susceptibility to exploitation.[66] The most systematic political advocacy has come from a group called the Immigrant Support Network, founded in 1998 and backed by Indian entrepreneurs in the United States, which was successful in pushing for limited reforms in 2000.[67] But this network was no longer active a decade later.[68] Workers also encountered obstacles to their own organizing capacity.[69] Indeed, H-1B workers face concerted suspicion in a U.S. public sphere from both liberal and conservative factions that Indian American groups have not been able to counter.

H-1B workers do not find strong support from the state of India either. When India began its economic liberalization in the 1980s, Rajiv Gandhi moved away from nationalist attempts to hold on to Indian workers and instead encouraged their mobility worldwide. He argued that mobility could create a "brain bank" of Indians that could be tapped by the state.[70] Indeed, while the temporary nature of the renewable three-year visa makes workers' lives more uncertain, it benefits such a circulatory system. Inheriting this logic, Prime Minister Modi in September 2015 urged Indian workers in Silicon Valley to contemplate returning to India, exhorting them to consider how the country's "brain drain" could become its "brain gain."[71] The Indian government has historically lobbied for the expansion of the H-1B visa program because it benefits the Indian body shops (officials have equated it with outsourcing).[72] With its capacity to produce and manage fully flexible labor, the program as it exists suits the aspirations of the Indian state, increasingly invested in its international branding as "Digital India."[73]

Unlike Yogananda, who became the leader of an emerging spiritual empire, many information technology migrants labor in the shadows. Twenty-first-century yoga is thought to reshape bodies to make them more fit for the physical and mental tolls of a technology-driven life, developing the self as a product that is both aligned with and designed to ameliorate global capitalism. Yet it is Indian migrants who are forced to become the ultimate flexible citizens of capital and technology. Controversies over migration reflect distinctly ambivalent desires about Indian bodies in the United States. They affirm the logic in which cultural practices from India like yoga can be absorbed and celebrated, but people from India remain vulnerable to xenophobia and legal mistreatment.

Such cultural fantasies simultaneously rely on, yet threaten to erase, ideas of Indian labor. Yogananda's vision of yogic technological futurity offered power and prestige to Indian bodies, but the seamless absorption of his logic into U.S. capitalist product development has spread authority over yoga well beyond those of Indian descent. When members of the Indian diaspora take a class in the United States, they probably study with white teachers. Demographic data on yoga teacher training programs suggest that graduates, like U.S. yoga practitioners more generally, are likely to be both white and female.[74] These statistics correspond to the increasing dominance of white female bodies as authority figures and beauty ideals in the magazine covers, advertisements, and lifestyle periodicals that visually frame yoga in the late twentieth and early twenty-first centuries.[75] Many of these white female teachers experience significant precarity in the economic landscape, but they also collectively claim a secure place within an American idealized vision of yoga. The technê once associated with brown male bodies has effectively transferred to a range of racial and ethnic bodies, particularly white ones. At the same time, U.S. cultures of technologized life rely on the racialized work of Indian H-1B migrants to provide an undervalued source of repetitive labor in the shadows. Brown male bodies are now more likely to be linked to the "techno" of information technology labor, the industrial side that is at once needed and feared. It can seem to members of the diaspora that prestigious forms of authority available to Indians are diminishing, while undervalued sources of flexible labor are on the rise.

THE COST OF LAUGHING FREELY

In the dust of a public park, they wander with no apparent goal. Mothers, grandfathers, middle-aged men; factory workers, barbers, chefs. They attract little notice until one among them calls for their attention. On cue, the park breaks into laughter. At that point, bystanders on the street, on balconies, in taxis, turn and stare.

Laughter yoga is often credited to the work of Madan Kataria, a doctor from the Indian village of Mohrewala, who in 1995 introduced a series of laughter practices designed to promote health and healing. Kataria's model involved bringing together groups of people to form "laughter clubs," where participants would force themselves to laugh in the company of others. The brain benefits, Kataria argued, whether the laughter is genuine or artificial. From a small gathering in Mumbai, laughter clubs spread in subsequent decades to thousands around the world. The practice is from its very origins shot through with ambivalence about the price of laughter; the status of the practice as "yoga" conceals tensions that perpetuate this uncertainty.

Why is this practice considered a form of yoga, given how different it appears from other traditions of postural, devotional, and philosophical practice? The answer lies in laughter as a way of manipulating the energies of breath. In *Laugh for No Reason* (1999), Kataria argues that "laughter yoga combines unconditional laughter with yogic breathing (Pranayama)."[76] As laughter yoga has become increasingly codified, its self-presentation as "yoga" has been developed in multiple dimensions. By the 2020s, Kataria was styled as a guru on his website, where laughter is framed as a spiritual pursuit.[77]

Despite these connections, the genealogy of laughter yoga may be found less in Indian traditions of *prāṇāyāma* than in Kataria's interest in American philosophies of positive thinking. He took particular inspiration from essays on laughter as medicine that appeared in middlebrow American sources such as *Reader's Digest*, along with autobiographical writings about the power of the mind to cure the body, exemplified by Norman Cousins's *Anatomy of an Illness as Perceived by the Patient* (1979), which argued for the agency of the sick in shaping their recovery. Such cultural texts respond to and in some ways replicate cultural logics associated with life under capitalist conditions.

Before Kataria hit upon the idea of laughter yoga, he struggled to establish a medical practice in a world of fierce competition and corruption. He invested family resources in ideas that could not be fully realized.[78] In short, laughter yoga was produced through the crucible of Kataria's own struggle to survive in an India undergoing economic transformation in the 1990s. "Life in Mumbai was stressful," he wrote. "People hardly laughed. A huge population of about 15 million people were forever rushed and hassled to meet their needs and fulfill their dreams."[79] This sober condition, Kataria argues, stems from the competitive structures exemplified through capitalist economies. "All perils of modern living have resulted from competition," he suggests. "While healthy competition is necessary for growth and development, it seems that today's competition is unlimited. It makes us feel like losers even if we are winners."[80] Like the other cultural elaborations of yoga that appeared in force in the first decades of the twenty-first century, laughter yoga reflects and responds to the mix of entrepreneurialism, inequality, and precarity that accompanied late twentieth-century economic reforms.

At one level, the practice rejects capitalist norms around health and medicine in a quest for a new kind of freedom. In *Laugh for No Reason*, Kataria describes his journey as a shift from capitalist anxiety to postcapitalist joy. "Life was tough and it was not easy to make money without any business experience. I was stressed and miserable," he writes. "I embarked on a new search—and this time it was not for money."[81] In his promotion of laughter clubs, Kataria argued that they should be free.[82]

In a documentary made by the Indian American director Mira Nair, *The Laughing Club of India* (2002), Kataria tells the camera, "Right from the beginning, I never liked the idea of charging money for the medical services. And I feel that doctor-patient relation should . . . should not be a business transaction."[83] For those who laugh in the parks with him, laughter is powerful because it is not a commodity to be bought and sold. "So there is nothing like product which somebody is packaging nicely and selling it, you know," says one interviewee.[84] Throughout the documentary, viewers are invited to yoke the concept of free, in a monetary sense, to the concept of freedom. The filmmaking is gentle, sympathetic, and direct, production values muted, perhaps in an attempt to capture a resistance to corporate ideology and aspirational branding. By the end of the documentary, portraits of people laughing grow gradually transcendent. The credits roll over the image of a woman standing on a rooftop, pink sari and long braid whipping around her, rising and bending to the "ha ha ho" of her laughter practice that allows her to unite with the city skyline in the background. Laughter yoga, Nair's *The Laughing Club of India* suggests, liberates.

Yet this rejection of capitalist norms is ironically shaped by modes of thinking intimately connected to capitalist aspirations. In addition to traditions of American positive thinking, Kataria was inspired by American entrepreneurial classics like the writings of Dale Carnegie, whose *How to Win Friends and Influence People* (1936) is often seen as an exemplary self-help text for people living under capitalist conditions.[85] Based on the premise that upward mobility is largely in the control of individuals unhampered by systematic inequalities, Carnegie's book has taken on increased appeal since the turn of the millennium in places like India. Self-help books about how to succeed in business have filled the tables of formal and informal booksellers in urban centers, forming a key part of what Ulka Anjaria identifies as one of India's emergent discourses in the new millennium.[86] These entrepreneurial narratives offer new definitions of what it means to be Indian, even if the narratives are imported from other parts of the world.

Laughter yoga trains practitioners to laugh at money, giving them a tool to mock the oppressiveness that often drives them to the practice.

Nair's documentary includes an interview with an Indian man in the prime of life, surrounded by multiple generations of his family, who suggests that he came to laughter yoga because of the pressures to survive in a changing economic climate. "I was going through ups and downs with my business," he tells the camera, "and my brothers had went to the stock market and doing data processing for the banks for the public issues and dividend WERN. It used to feel that even twenty-four hours in the day were not enough [sic]."[87] Regaining a sense of control over this totalizing force draws him to the liberations experienced through laughter yoga. This situation came to inform the discourse highlighted within the practice. As described in a profile for *The New Yorker* in 2010, Kataria's exercises eventually included "There is No Money Laughter, a pose in which initiates pretend that their pockets are empty, and then laugh; and Visa Bill Laughter, in which they point to an imaginary Visa bill in their palm, and laugh."[88] Impoverishment and debt—two crippling specters—became momentary objects of satire, affording the laughers the illusion of a moment's control. In this kind of exercise, participants are asked to perform a fragment of theater that may, for many, be all too close to reality. Even in its conspicuous absence, money is always close to the heart of laughter yoga.

The specter of the desire for control over and through money thus haunts and informs the practice of laughter yoga. Although laughter clubs are meant to be free, the full range of the phenomenon is enmeshed in economic energies. Laughter teacher trainings with Kataria, costing hundreds of dollars, are not free. By 2021, his organization's website offered, in addition to free services, commodities designed to spread its teaching tools. Gibberish Kits for $15USD, E-learning Kits for $29USD, and a Jumbo pack of training videos for $99USD all suggest the possibilities of monetizing the practice. More subtly, employers value laughter yoga as a capitalist practice that forges a more resilient and compliant workforce. In Nair's documentary, against shots of workers handmaking commodities and forging metal objects before open flames, an authority figure says, "But when you do this kind of exercise, all your tension is relieved. The moment that happens, [the workers are] able to concentrate more on their work and there are less rejections, and productivity is increased. They do more amount of work, because they're now relaxed."[89] Under the sign of "free," economic activity can increase. This situation marks the ongoing tension that the flexibilities of laughter yoga promote.

Like many spiritual practices, laughter yoga can expand capitalist logics by absorbing political critique within neoliberal care of the self.[90] Nair's *The Laughing Club of India* explores the driving purpose of many of the early adherents of laughter yoga who came to the practice to cope with the losses, constraints, and injustices of their lives. One man gestures to a photo of his son, who was killed in a mill workers' protest. A woman speaks of how, engaged at nine and married at sixteen, she has spent thirty-six years in a house that laughter now allows her, momentarily, to escape. These poignant stories point to some of the ways laughter yoga allows practitioners to manage political sites of injustice. The practice can be seen as a double-edged sword, both a necessary route to a freedom unavailable elsewhere and potentially a neoliberal deflection of political critique concerning economic and gendered exploitations.[91]

As laughter yoga aims to alleviate Indian anxieties about economic change, the signifier of "Indianness" takes on new meanings for transnational audiences in ways that animate colonial and Orientalist logics of extraction. Such a narrative emerges in works of fiction like those of Sarah-Kate Lynch, a travel editor for the magazine *Women's Day* in New Zealand, who used a Western woman encountering a laughter club in Mumbai as the conceit of her novel *Heavenly Hirani's School of Laughing Yoga* (2014). Annie, a white American woman adrift after her children have left home and her mother has moved to a dementia ward, is encouraged to accompany her husband on a trip to India. In the style made popular by Elisabeth Gilbert's *Eat Pray Love* (2006), Annie finds herself revived and healed by her trip, particularly through the friendships she makes in a laughing yoga club.

Reflecting the expectations set in motion for international tourists through India's national branding campaigns and Western guidebooks, Lynch describes the events that led her to write the novel. Like Annie, she accompanied her husband on a work trip to Mumbai. "I started writing *Heavenly Hirani's School of Laughing Yoga* the next day from my hotel room, Room 1802, at the Taj Land's End. I had read about laughing yoga in Fiona Caulfield's wonderful guidebook, *Love Mumbai*, and eventually found my way to Chowpatty Beach to join Kishore Kuvavala and his smiling gang of welcoming laughers for their early morning sessions."[92] She then goes on to note the shock she received at the end of her travel: "Kishore wasn't quite the inspiration that Heavenly is (on my last day he told me I owed him a thousand rupees per visit, which somewhat wiped the smile off my face)."[93] One can sympathize, given the sum involved and Kataria's stated norm of making laughter clubs free. In the novel, Lynch corrects this less than happy (for her) ending to instead give Annie the pleasurable feeling of being cared for in community, the kind of escape, relief, and connection described in Mira Nair's documentary by local Mumbai participants.

However, a troubling broader cultural logic is at work in *Heavenly Hirani's School of Laughing Yoga*: the expectation that many things in India should be free, or that the prices should be set by Westerners. Indians of all sorts, from Heavenly of the title to Pinto the taxi driver, are all too willing to care for a vulnerable international tourist. The taxi driver, for instance, refuses to name his price, instead allowing Annie to offer him a sum. Under his guidance, Annie pushes beyond the comforts of her hotel room to explore the world more fully and recover her own sense of self in the process. These patterns reiterate the narrative of wounded innocent whiteness seeking healing and redemption in India.[94] The potential of this logic to sustain colonial and Orientalist tropes becomes evident in the corrective fantasies of the novel, in which the uncomfortable elements of Lynch's autobiographical experience are rewritten into a story where Indians are always happy to help, a new myth of grateful colonial subjects.

In many respects, this cultural logic reflects the end point of the Indian state's insistence that yoga is a gift to the world. Although this phrase is meant to authorize visitors to come as consumers to spend money in India, it also invites Westerners to take it literally. This creates racialized divisions of labor in which India appears as a perpetual service economy for an affluent West. In some respects, the monetary exchanges in the novel disguise and extend capitalist and Orientalist formations for new generations. In the process, these formations grow more resilient. Looking at the imaginative work within *Laugh for No Reason*, *The Laughing Club of India*, and *Heavenly Hirani's School for Laughing Yoga*, we might inquire into the true price of laughing freely. Is it the reinscription into neoliberal norms of entrepreneurialism, the abandonment of political protest in favor of self-perfection, or the resumption of colonial norms of Indian servitude?

Precarity and flexibility are thus intimately yoked. Precarity suggests conditions beyond one's control, while flexibility hints at an individual's ability to gain power in response to those increased demands. States, as they withdraw public goods, have therefore often praised practices that make people more flexible. Such is the promise latent within postural and mental disciplines of yoga. Yet flexibility extends precarity as much as it remedies it. For the teachers holding space and keeping time for the benefit of others, their labor is endlessly uncertain. Within the exchanges that shape yoga in the twenty-first century, changing ideas of Indianness reflect these underlying contradictions. India can be seen as a space of the free in both economic and spiritual terms, yet the costs of being free are paid through hierarchies of servitude, gray labor markets, and colonial and Orientalist logics of extraction. These dangerous forms of work create the illusions, through yoga, that we seek to buy. Imaginative visions reflect and refract these dangers, inviting readers to participate in a practice of *svādhyāya* about the larger forces that free and constrain in a capitalist world.

CONCLUSION

It was required: I had to go to Safety in the Field. I spent three hours in an uncomfortable chair learning about my university's positive legal obligation to care for my health and safety. That loving concern compelled me to distinguish between risks and hazards while I calculated how much the morning cost me in child care. We learned how to use risk meters, discussed the hazards of Spring Festival train travel in China, and drank abysmal coffee.

Many people in the room were headed to remote places like the desert terrain of Australia's outback or the lonely highways of Papua New Guinea. They carried devices that could send an SOS if you pressed a red button. When we were asked to list the main risks associated with our upcoming travel, I thought about the dangers I might encounter. "Concern #1," I wrote. "A Lululemon salesgirl will talk me into really expensive yoga pants."

After the workshop I walked into a Lululemon one wintry August morning. "You must walk the ground," my history professor at university had told us long ago. Lululemon: ground zero for the capitalist yoga industrial complex in the West. Home of expensive clothing sold only to people of a certain size. Lululemon could leave many wondering why the benefits of yoga's global popularity could make a white Canadian man a billionaire, while employees—who would never become rich—spent their lives folding spandex under the spell of relentlessly positive thoughts.

The store was bright. Natural light from skylights was exaggerated by a landscape of mirrors. A hand-lettered chalkboard alerted me to yoga retreats on Australia's south coast and in the Himalayas. Yellow walls popped into my field of vision, as if I had stumbled into a field of daisies. Behind the register, yoga how-tos nestled side by side with a biography of Jack Welsh and Ayn Rand's *Atlas Shrugged*.

I was prepared to be as critical as could be. This was the height of yoga as the thin white fashionable body, the place where consumption disguises itself as spiritual attainment, where an American employee had felt the urge to murder her coworker. (Wouldn't we all, I thought, if *Atlas Shrugged* were on the counter.) As it turned out, I wasn't prepared enough.

The walls of rolled mats, concentric circles of black enlivened by jewel tones of fuchsia, turquoise, and periwinkle, were gorgeous in their symmetry. I touched one. It didn't feel anything like the blue yoga mat I kept in my office, the one I'd had for almost fifteen years since graduate school. It didn't feel anything like the two-for-one sporting goods store mats I had bought for my house. It was spongy and soft and otherworldly.

The wall of yoga pants scared me. They were boxed in open cubbies behind their own shining white counter where a friendly salesgirl stood guard. The young woman working there had long curly hair and an energetic smile. Looking at her, I couldn't help thinking about a *Salon* essay written by a disheartened Lululemon employee who found the company's focus on continuous affirmation to be the ultimate soul killer. This young woman didn't look like her soul was being killed. She seemed, well, happy. When she was away from the counter, I secretly felt the pants and took a look at the price tag. Sensing risk (or was it hazard?), I walked away.

But I walked right into the wall of hoodies. Without thinking too much, I reached out to touch one of the fleecy turquoise jackets. I was surprised at how solid, how heavy, how *good* it felt. At home, I wore a black L.L. Bean fleece hoodie that I'd bought in desperation the year before. I had wanted a hoodie that would elevate my life, something that would free my spirit in the hours wrestling a toddler into clean diapers or flipping blueberry pancakes or Skyping with my family overseas before I had the time to shower. I'd had to settle for a hoodie that reflected the quiet desperation of new parents.

I looked at the hoodie again. I wandered back to the fitting area, where I taught the cheerful salesgirl how to spell my name on the whiteboard outside my dressing room. *It's research*, I told myself.

The fitting room was a miniature work of art: bright, yellow, and mirrored, with chunky circular pegs in a geometric grid in the middle. In my peripheral vision I caught a glimpse of big red tulips reflected in the mirror. There were no crumbs on the floor, no dirty dishes, no buckets of soaking laundry. I wondered if I could stay in this fitting room all day.

I pulled on the hoodie. I looked in the mirror. The jacket was turquoise, brighter than the wall of blacks and grays in my closet, and yet it didn't seem out of place on dark-haired me. It was more architectural than my frumpy forest green fleece from L.L. Bean, the one that I would have given away years ago except that it was what I was wearing when my partner asked me to marry him. We liked to joke that this was how

I knew he loved me no matter what. The turquoise jacket was cozy and solid, form-fitting, with accented stripes running up and down the sides. The sleeves had thumbholes. Wearing it was like putting on a surprisingly comfortable neck brace. All my most fragile parts felt contained.

I looked at the tag. According to the label, this jacket would be perfect for a trip up a mountain or to yoga class. Even discounted, it wasn't cheap. And it was a final sale. But I loved it. It was going to help me do it all.

Maybe it was the broken night's sleep that made me love the Lululemon jacket against my will. It had been my turn that night. I'd slept on an air mattress in my children's room to tend to my sick two-year-old son. He woke me up every few hours, sometimes every thirty minutes, to demand a trip downstairs into our freezing dark kitchen for milk or crackers or medicine. When I put him back in his bed, he wanted me to sit up with him. "Mummy stay," he would plead, though the air mattress was only two feet away. In a hysterical voice, he would cry, "Mummy no sleep!" By the middle of the night, parts of myself I don't like to think exist were starting to take over. Delirious with exhaustion, I would tell my little boy sharply that we all needed to sleep, and only too late catch myself, and stroke his head and tickle his tummy.

Somehow the promise of that turquoise yoga jacket was the unreal, ridiculous, yet vital promise that I would never again have to sleep in my black L.L. Bean hoodie and wake up with crazy hair and hiss at my sick two-year-old son while imagining that he was my CIA torturer. I knew it was a fantasy, all of it. But that didn't mean its power went away.

When my daughter saw me, she said, "Mummy, I love that jumper!"

When my partner saw me, he said, "I wish I had proposed to you in *that* jacket."

Years later, I sleep better. I'm more likely to be woken by my own restless thoughts than by my children. Some days the jacket feels too tight on my midriff. It's hard to laugh in it. Some days I long for the frumpy and forgiving, something like the black L.L. Bean hoodie that I eventually lost on a plane. But this one remains the jacket that stretches to hold things in place. It pushes me to dive for a tennis ball with my son or to take him on a late afternoon bike ride around the sparkling lake. It lets me chase my daughter, now faster than I'll ever be, on endless green lawns. Although I am too embarrassed to wear it to my yoga studio, which puts philosophy before yoga pants, it keeps me warm on chilly May mornings as I write.

The jacket itself has changed with time. Holes have begun to pop at my elbows, little cracks where my skin peeks through. The wrists are fraying into tiny caterpillar threads. Its myth of perfection is mellower.

It is a risk: to be captured by your subject. I cannot pretend that I am outside or above or beyond the corporate fantasies that circulate across oceans and light. In the form-fitting compression of the jacket, my body feels these ambivalent pressures. The forces that I want to speak against are also those which compose me, hold me together, form me into someone able to speak at all. Even if I'd never bought it that sleep-deprived August day, I'd still be wearing this jacket.

6

FRAMING NEW PARTS

Yoga Through Diasporic Critique

When I'm working from home, I sometimes put on a digital yoga class from an app on my iPad. The classes are beautiful, minimalist, spare. Each time, no matter what sequence I choose, the same calming voice greets me. I pretend I'm listening to National Public Radio, the reassuring voice of order I heard in the warm twilight from the back seat of my parents' Camry. Each time, the same yoga model appears on my touch screen. She is young, slender, flexible, and white. She practices in empty space against a white background. There is no actual room; the camera follows only one angle, from the front. The model looks like a real person who's accidentally lost her third dimension. The blue of her top matches the blue in the studio icon at the bottom of my device. It's a perfect alignment of human body and glistening screen. The whole visual space is clean, flat, depthless. It allows me to ignore that I'm practicing next to my unmade bed, my son's puzzle pieces, and my daughter's paper clippings. She loves to cut things out—princesses, fairies, crowns—and make castles. All over our house, little flecks of white paper trail in her wake. It's like practicing in a sea of confetti.

The model is the perfect yogic body. There is no untamed facial hair, no smell of sweat. This body is like the newest model iPhone, glossy and unbroken. My body feels more like the mobile left on my gate the night of a driving thunderstorm. It works, but behind the screen, strange lights pulse with anxiety. The model is a cipher, a subtle map, like the abstract bodies I find in my books on the art of yoga, all symmetry and ease. When I look at her, I think that yoga is perhaps best done by graphic designers. Let's just remove the human body from it all. It is only an inconvenience.

The app is calming. We practice in unison, she and I. As I move my arms to the sky and glimpse the glowing mountains through the window, I forget for a moment about my untended Facebook page, my unwritten tweets, my unread emails. My neglected selves fall from me like invisible leaves scattering to the ground. I become a cleared screen.

But surrounding this world is always my cluttered bedroom. I've come to like the Himalayan snowflakes of paper cuttings that my daughter leaves on the floor. I watch her cutting and twisting and folding, always resizing, always in search of that perfect crown or castle, always in search of the perfect shape.

———— ∞ ————

In this chapter, I explore the cuts and twists and folds of yoga's writers and artists who seek to make something new in the face of the white screens, literal and metaphorical, that shape a globalized capitalist modernity. These experimental voices and visions, from Indians, the Indian diaspora, and those not of Indian background, take shape within twenty-first-century worlds of intense commodification, technological perfectionism, racial hierarchies, and violence of varying speeds.

Protesting this architecture of power from within yogic worlds may appear doomed from the beginning. Andrea Jain makes the compelling argument that"*gestural subversion*, subverting dominant power structures through gestures, is a key area of spirituality's valuation. . . . Although [forms of neoliberal spirituality, such as conscious capitalism] gesture toward wanting to resolve the real devastating social and environmental conditions that neoliberal capitalist structures create and perpetuate, they put the burden for resolving those conditions on individual consumers, as opposed to supporting collective dissent and radical policy changes."[1] When we look at the gestures offered through consumer culture, Jain is right. Yet my lifetime spent with the pages of books also whispers that gestures can matter, as long as we ask of them something they can give.

Imaginative life on its own will not replace collective dissent. It will not overturn cruelties, enact justice, or make the world more equal. Despite what we might hear in the public sphere, it will not automatically make anyone a better person. As Suzanne Keen has shown, developing empathy for a character in a book does not necessarily lead to action for three-dimensional people after the last page is read.[2] Sometimes empathy toward imagined characters displaces empathy toward real people, diffuses a reader's feeling of responsibility, or allows the specifics of one life to screen out the role of systematic injustice. So I do not claim that complex imaginative works, on their own, automatically bolster political projects of justice and equality. But, to make a more modest claim, imaginative forms may reframe the vocabularies people can use to understand their lives and their places within broader systems. They may expose how one person's comfortable life is made possible by someone else's profound discomfort. They may turn an invisible enemy into one that can be seen or offer new insight into unnoticed allies. They may provide dignity within demeaning force fields of subordination. To realize such potential, Keen argues, we must do more than simply read or view these works. We must frame them within critical questions and conversations.[3]

Remixed genealogies of yoga can provide the framework in which to read twenty-first-century representations of the practice. To conduct such a hopeful reading, I turn to imaginative practices found in visual art, literature, and new media. None of these works is outside consumer culture or immune from invisible hierarchies of neoliberal and racialized capitalist logic. But, through their artistic modulation of form and image, they offer a more robust set of critical tools to frame yoga as a resistant practice of deep inquiry.

Such artistic visions of yoga can support political ends oriented to justice of many different kinds. The art of the Indian American artist Chiraag Bhakta in his installation *#WhitePeopleDoingYoga* invites us to consider anew the significance of cultural appropriation, a concept that has grown in power and energy in the twenty-first century in the wake of failed promises of millennial globalization. Bhakta's work makes provocative use of resistant form, where ideas of framing, accumulating, and juxtaposing take center stage. I then turn to the Indian American poet Reetika Vazirani to find evidence of hidden histories of practice and its deeper meaning for the diaspora. Finally, I explore the political possibilities of satire in collaborations between Western groups without Indian backgrounds and the Indian diaspora. Drawing upon my work in *Fiction Across Borders*, I argue that indie media productions like the Canadian mockumentary or mock documentary *Yoga Town* use the instabilities of satire and irony to critique limited ways of envisioning India. Calling direct attention to quests for Indianness, these popular media shape yoga into a way of thinking about the invisible social layers that inform ideas of India. Considering these refractive and reflective visions as practices of a remixed *svādhyāya*, I amplify the voices of those who are keen to use imaginative interpretations of yoga to frame portraits of Indianness in a globalizing world.

The iconic virtue of flexibility afforded through yoga—its ability to conceal points of tension and thus to render those contradictions more resilient—might be seen as the ultimate metaphor for India's diaspora. From labor practices to cultural identity to family structure to political vision, flexibility has long been demanded of India's migrants. Working through and within the circuits of colonialism and capitalism, India's diasporas have often found themselves in distinctly ambivalent positions. They have been embraced as laborers within extractive colonial systems and plantation economies of the nineteenth and twentieth centuries, yet also evicted in the rise of postcolonial nationalisms around the world. Dramatic expulsions from places like Uganda or Myanmar, nationalist coups in places like Fiji, and slow pressures in places like Hong Kong have led to ongoing diasporic journeys across countries and continents.[4] The state of India has viewed its diaspora with a selective eye, most detached from those who travel as indentured laborers or impoverished migrants and most keen to claim kinship with upwardly mobile professionals bearing capital. Layering upon and intersecting with these histories, the millennial surge that sent millions to build cities in the Gulf deserts and to run computer systems in the West has brought intensified demands and desires. Within these complex histories, as Purnima Mankekar argues, Indianness is deeply unsettled.

What makes this unsettlement bankable, I argue, is its recoding as a form of flexibility. Flexibility is diaspora's key asset in neoliberal capitalist conditions, a monetizable quality demanded both by India and by the states to which migrants have traveled.[5] Yet it also, as the condition that renders the ambivalence of states and the precariousness of peoples more resilient, potentially forms the diaspora's prison.

In this chapter, I trace diasporic ambivalence toward ideas of India that emerge under and through yoga as the ultimate metaphor for flexible resilience. Imaginative work from the diaspora has often been critical of the flexibilities demanded of it, presenting them as assets that most benefit non-Indian corporations or individuals. Yet this critique can recuperate flexibility for more politically resistant, imaginatively hopeful ends. I contend that by critiquing the sign of yoga most associated with flexibility—postural practice—and engaging alternative histories of what yoga might mean, diasporic artists and writers call into being a flexibility that works toward their own needs, not simply to benefit the capitalist expansions or racial hierarchies that structure their everyday lives.

#WHITEPEOPLEDOINGYOGA

First one, then another. Then another. Then another. The flat squares and rectangles tower up the first floor of the Asian Art Museum in San Francisco. Magazine spreads. Book jackets. Record covers. Advertisements. White people in saris, white people in leotards, white people in fishnets, white people in nothing much. White gurus and white garbage pail kids. A lot of white people, all doing yoga.

In 2014, the Indian American artist Chiraag Bhakta, who goes by the artist's name *Pardon My Hindi, was invited by the Asian Art Museum to create an installation for the show *Yoga: The Art of Transformation*, co-organized with the Smithsonian's Arthur M. Sackler Gallery. Bhakta chose to collect a range of ephemera depicting yoga in Western popular culture, titling it #WhitePeopleDoingYoga. His artist's statement asserted that the piece was a critique of the appropriation of South Asian cultural signifiers in a Western capitalist context: "Brands like Lulu Lemon [sic] and Nike have started appropriating and trade-marking phrases, moves and clothing—aligning and embedding themselves in our understanding of yoga, while the South Asian face and voice is relegated to an exotic caricature—cartoons, adoption of South Asian names by white Westerners, mystical creatures, Hindu gods."[6] For Bhakta, the remediation of a South Asian legacy through capitalist contexts and racial hierarchies marks a shift from yoga to "YOGA™."

How should we best understand the concept of cultural appropriation at stake here, most simply, the taking of culture from a lifeworld not considered one's own? Theories that circulate in scholarly and popular culture offer diverse possible meanings when this term gains energy. In some conversations, cultural appropriation is simply glossed as cross-cultural exchange: the act of incorporating something from one cultural tradition or location into another. This definition is immediately vulnerable to dismissal as a form of political critique because most, if not all cultures can be shown to exchange with other parts of the world (through trade, ritual, gift, theft, or force). It is unhelpful, I suggest, because it allows no attention to be paid to larger power relations. It thus presumes similitude between a minority group member accessing the cultural repertoire of a more dominant culture and a majority group member doing the reverse, even though the power dynamics of these actions may be very different. I therefore take as a starting point the claim made through the very title of Borrowed Power, that "the important questions about cultural appropriation are the political ones."[7]

A second approach to cultural appropriation focuses on norms of cultural correctness. In this understanding, which is sometimes taken by Hindu right-wing groups who protest uses of Hindu imagery in forms they find offensive in international contexts (for example, deities painted on polluted sites such as toilet covers), the problem is not the invocation of culture by outsiders but the fact that the invocations are incorrect.[8]

Dimensions of this critique matter, as I explore later. But this view is problematic because it relies on unexamined social hierarchies that produce the ideas about what is correct as a respectful form of culture. Such ideas are often used not only to discipline outsiders into specific social behavior but also to repress critique *within* cultural communities. In other words, while the push for correctness appears as a dialogue between those imagined as insiders and as outsiders, it simultaneously marks a hidden dialogue between different kinds of insiders in the context of social hierarchy. Groups assert their power over other community members by projecting their ideas of correctness onto outsiders. This approach is often found in proximity to, and sanctioned by, right-wing politics. It is frequently compatible with state projects of soft power.

A more helpful way of defining cultural appropriation focuses on its commodification of culture, labor, and dissent. This lens takes capitalism as its key explanation, arguing that capitalist practices make culture into commodities and reduce their value to simply what they command on the market. Ownership of artifacts passes completely into new hands through commercial transactions, severing possession from contexts of origin (such as ritual or sacral meanings). This perspective further invites us to consider how these processes rely on the commodification of labor. As William Crane puts it, "appropriation of culture is fundamentally the capitalist appropriation of human labour and lives."[9] This definition acknowledges the transformative role of capitalist power dynamics in the shaping of cultural exchange, removing the need to rely on essentialist ideas of culture or identity. Appropriation of yoga can be understood as a capitalist containment of dissent against structures of power that can include self-commodification as well as the commodification of exotic difference.[10] Yet not all acts of commodification inspire public critique. It may thus be useful to complement attention to capitalism's important role with additional perspectives to explain why some practices are perceived as problematic.

One such complementary approach focuses on negative effects. Drawing on the work of Charles Taylor, Dianne Lalonde argues that cultural appropriation is politically problematic because it can lead to a spectrum of harms that include "nonrecognition, misrecognition, and exploitation."[11] Nonrecognition, when a community lacks political voice or multidimensional representation, constrains the social status and justice claims of members. Such nonrecognition makes what does appear in public discourse more likely to fall into the category of misrecognition, or limiting stereotypes that negatively shape the self-images of groups so represented. Misrecognition might also be experienced by people appropriating the cultures of others. As Véronique Altglas describes in ethnographic work on yoga, those who do not see yoga as their cultural heritage tend to avoid reflection on how their identities are shaped within structures of power, even though their experiences of discomfort hint at these structures.[12] Exploitation, as a third form of harm, indicates that the material benefits of appropriating culture bypass communities of those cultures. This way of thinking connects the seemingly peaceful and consensual side of capitalism to the foundational imperial violence that makes it possible.[13] Appropriation is thus defined by some, as Liz Bucar does in religious studies, as a form of borrowing that causes harm.[14] These perspectives offer a crucial lens that connects cultural signs to political injury.

Cutting elements from these perspectives and reassembling them into a different frame, I suggest that cultural appropriation can be best understood as a constellation of emotional energies that signal dissonance when cultural practices appear to be more valued and valuable than people from those cultures. This way of thinking sits at the intersection of recognition and redistribution projects, suggesting that the problem signaled by "cultural appropriation" is not always nonrecognition, misrecognition, or even the perception of injury, but an excess of recognition in certain areas coupled with a deficit in redistribution. The benefits and costs of those practices are thus unevenly spread: when particular cultural practices are considered uncool, people associated with those parts of the world pay the costs. They face othering, discrimination, and even sometimes outright violence. Yet when particular cultural practices gain social capital, the benefits often seem to bypass those communities of origin.[15]

While I draw upon the layer of political thought that works precisely and rationally to identify exactly what may be wrong when the charge "cultural appropriation" is brought, I also want to look at the term differently: as a term that not only makes its audience think but also makes it *feel*. The phrase carries a bolt of energy. Philosophers tend to conceptualize "cultural appropriation" as a category of wrong, but I take it instead as the kind of speech act that J. L. Austin calls a performative. Performatives, in Austin's sense, are neither true nor false statements. They are social actions.[16] When the phrase "cultural appropriation" appears in public discourses, such as the media, it is not only a description of events that can be judged true or false. In addition, it is a phrase that *does*: it performs an accusation. This signals an energy release on the part of the speaker, who often propels, intensifies, and modulates energies in those accused, as well as in those who witness these encounters. Accusations are by nature hot.

For this reason, rational philosophical analyses of cultural appropriation can miss the mark. Take, for instance, a passage from the work of James Young and Susan Haley. Young is known for the philosophical argument that cultural appropriation, most of the time, causes limited harm.[17] The problem is not simply in what this passage says, though I disagree with many of its foundational assumptions, but is exemplified by the writing style. "Insiders bear the primary responsibility for the perpetuation of their culture. They can be expected to take reasonable precautions to ensure that their cultures are protected. Insiders are able (and probably easily able) to avoid being harmed by any artworks produced by outsiders."[18] Through the signature icy cool of philosophy, roles are clearly defined, responsibilities laid out, and a frictionless environment assumed. Insiders should not be angry, the passage implies, because they should simply take (or have taken) reasonable precautions to protect their cultures. But in evicting emotional energy so vividly, the essay refuses to engage with the real charge posed by cultural appropriation: not a philosophical but an electric one.

Instead of trying (in vain) to rationalize away the energy charge of cultural appropriation, like this Western philosophical style does, we might lean into it. Histories of yoga offer some powerful ways to work with heat. To observe energy circuits and complex emotions is to treat this heat as a *kośa*, or layer, of human experience. For those raising the charge, "cultural appropriation" offers access to a certain kind of empowerment, a making visible of invisibility, a claim to matter in the public sphere. For those being charged, it can raise guilt, betrayal, shock, and shame. Those emotions are unpleasant and may often be covered over by anger. Why does it wound people so badly to be accused of cultural appropriation? Because it is a reminder that they benefit from histories of violence and injustice. This feeling jars against many people's core beliefs in their own goodness and diminishes their sense of individual accomplishment, pushing into the background the obstacles and sacrifices they see so clearly while bringing into the foreground the social norms that ease their path. To resolve this cognitive dissonance, some people diminish themselves in guilt and shame. Others construct defenses—through reason or through emotion—that explain why their actions cannot possibly have caused anyone else harm.

In this world of energetic feeling, a remixed *svādhyāya* is called for: a perspective of inquiry that integrates individual emotions, social scripts, and broader structures of power. Such inquiry observes the energy release of cultural appropriation rather than blindly reacting to its force. This practice can help reveal the workings of broader social injustices, which were not set in motion by the people involved in any given controversy but can maintain momentum through their actions. For those accused of cultural appropriation, seeing this script for perhaps the first time invites them to read their world in a new way.

This invitation serves a key purpose of *#WhitePeopleDoingYoga*, which uses repetitive form to reveal the force fields of power through which the idea of cultural appropriation gains energy. Extending far higher than human height, the rectangular images tower over viewers.[19] Like a wall of bricks, the assemblage dominates the human bodies who come to view it. The ephemera largely feature white bodies within Indian-inspired cultural signifiers. The form of the installation suggests a metaphor of one experience of being Indian American: moving through a world where random pieces of culture, seemingly disconnected, replicate until they form a totalizing story of exclusion through capitalist commodification and racial hierarchies. Using the power of repetition so crucial to *svādhyāya*, Bhakta's art exposes the architectural

186 FRAMING NEW PARTS

connections between what look like isolated acts. By framing yoga in Western popular culture as a set of cultural images that appear separate yet reveal broader patterns of power, the installation testifies to the yogic practice of repetition as a revelatory method. For viewers of color, the exhibit offers a validation, a making visible, of the images that weave through capitalist practices, infecting the heart of commodities, securing their power through ever more intimate technologies of everyday life. Bhakta's installation places the body of the viewer in a position of subordination: the wall of faces is everywhere, rising up, stretching out, so that viewers feel the weight and height. The piece uses sensory experience to bring to light an invisible world of white-ordered centrality that minority subjects negotiate every day.

The installation seeks to make whiteness step out from the wall. In having its white viewers confront an often unacknowledged intimacy with a racial category, the installation asks them to consider how, and why, they engage cultural practices associated with Indianness as part of that intimacy. The power of the title, *#WhitePeopleDoingYoga*, made itself felt from its very inception. In an account of his collaboration with the Asian Art Museum, Bhakta described the reluctance of the white-majority curatorial team to accept it. "They wanted something innocuous like *#PeopleDoingYoga*, without the word 'white,' because the term 'white people' could be 'offensive' to museumgoers, donors, and staff," he wrote.[20] This account was confirmed by museum representatives, who responded to a fact-checking inquiry from the left-wing publication *Mother Jones* with the following:

> According to a museum spokesperson, Bhakta was told that the phrase "white people" could be "offensive or puzzling" to some. As examples, the spokesperson pointed to "Anglo practitioners of yoga unfamiliar with the concepts of cultural appropriation/appreciation, and K-12 students who haven't had the proper exposure to understand the statement implied in 'White People Doing Yoga.'"[21]

An account of the debates from a museum educator involved at the time notes that

Museum staff was divided, and even the exhibition's co-curators were in disagreement. . . . Some curators, educators, and public relations staff claimed the installation title was "reverse racism," inflammatory, and would anger white yoga practitioners. Other curators, educators, and public relations staff vehemently disagreed, arguing that it was important to have a South Asian perspective that differed from the curatorial voice and addressed the missing narrative of cultural appropriation.[22]

"White" is not usually considered a racial slur; it is a category on the U.S. Census. Yet it discomfits. It reminds viewers who are used to thinking of themselves as unmarked, as simply "people," that racial categories have created the social norms and material comforts that surround them like an invisible aura. It reminds this imagined audience that in an American context, they are raced—not only visible minorities "have" race. To see themselves as others might see them is potentially to confront the ways they benefit from structures developed within histories of dispossession and violence. The comforts afforded to particular groups through racial similitude suddenly become uncomfortable when they are named.

The anxieties of the museum spokesperson who used the term "Anglo" as a veil for white are not unfamiliar. When I think of part of my makeup as "white," a great nothingness coexists with a totalizing vision of the American world in which I grew up. What is the meaning of whiteness? It offers everything and nothing. Its comforts cannot be abandoned without material cost, yet constantly seem inadequate, in need of supplementation from a mythical past. They require nourishment from a word like "Anglo," designed to conjure the cultural particularity of "Englishness" even though its actual usage in the United States far exceeds people descended from England. In the post–civil rights era of the 1970s, Matthew Jacobson argues, groups that had entered the category of whiteness began to search for new forms of ethnic differentiation. Ethnic roots, no longer seen as quite so dangerous, could be revived in ways that conjured political deniability around the structural privileges of whiteness.[23] It may be this perception of a cultural or even spiritual absence, as Shreena Gandhi and Lillie Wolff argue, that sub-consciously draws white subjects into the orbit of yoga.[24] This promise of cultural depth, as Amanda Lucia and Rumya Putcha have shown, can help to explain why spaces like transformational festivals and muse-ums prominently feature yoga as a practice where Indianness is ori-ented toward white subjects seeking self-perfection.[25]

The resistance of the museum to the phrase #WhitePeopleDoingYoga exemplifies the condition of white fragility, defined by Robin DiAngelo as "a state in which even a minimum amount of racial stress becomes intolerable, triggering a range of defensive moves."[26] It did not appear to have troubled the museum officials that a change in title would have meant using the word "people" when so little diversity was present, again normalizing the status of whiteness as unmarked and universal. This suggests the equation at the heart of how racial hierarchies conceal their own exclusions: the very concept of "people" could be adequately expressed through the selective representation of *some* people—in this case, those who could be perceived as white. It did not appear to have occurred to them that people of color might have found such a univer-salizing yet exclusive label offensive or puzzling. The controversy gen-erated through Bhakta's artistic engagement—the irony, he pointed out, of "white elites exerting power over Brown critique that was explicitly about white elites exerting power over Brown culture"[27] signals the power of thinking about yoga in this way.

In the squares and grids that the photo of the installation renders seemingly endless, much like the tessellating mats captured on camera on the International Day of Yoga, is an image in search of recognition. The installation gestures toward two interconnected dynamics. The first is the pressing need to be seen. The hashtag of social media signals the broader state in which thoughts and practices must be constantly broad-cast, replicated, and echoed to be considered real. The second, in con-trast, is a pressing need to remain unmarked. The category of whiteness wants to be seen, but not to be recognized as white. The installation invites viewers who occupy some aspect of the category of whiteness to experience emotional and cognitive discomfort as they confront this seemingly endless array of visual evidence. Both ephemeral and enduring, never enough and too much, the images bespeak a need for endless yet edited recognition on the part of a dominant racial category in the twenty-first-century United States.

What was not shown—because cut by the museum—reveals the power of the provocation. Bhakta was asked to remove a shrine in which two white people were presented as gurus. Although such a shrine shows the logical endpoint to which the ephemera collectively point—the elevation of white positionalities through and over Indian cultural forms—it was considered potentially offensive to Indian viewers. In a way, the museum's concern speaks to the rise of the policing of Hindu cultural forms, often in ways compatible with soft Hindutva hierarchies,[28] within right-wing elements of the Indian diaspora. This particular approach, which the museum appeared more keen to accommodate than Bhakta's critique, focuses on disciplining particular groups into using Indian cultural signifiers in ways that tend to benefit internal hierarchies, such as upper-caste practices. Those practices are then normalized as exemplary forms of being "Indian" or "Hindu" in Western spheres. In privileging correctness over critique, the museum played a part in potentially replicating Indian hierarchies while maintaining Western ones.

Prominent on the first floor of the Asian Art Museum, the show perhaps was so unsettling to the staff because it threatened to prompt reflection on the very foundational dynamics of the museum itself: a place of spectatorship built and run by white elites, where Asian art could be experienced via a safely contained form of cultural appreciation. The officials, worried about an audience not familiar with "the concepts of cultural appropriation/appreciation," reveal their own investments in a problematic approach to cross-cultural engagement. Appropriation is perceived as bad, while appreciation (the foundational value of the art museum) is perceived as good. Yet both are shaped by the same architecture of power, in which the person doing the appropriating—or the appreciating—does so from a position of security or even dominance. Appreciation is the conferral of value through the gaze: it implies that one has value to confer. Instead, a more powerful and political form of cross-cultural engagement—a truer realization of the potential of *svādhyāya*—emerges through the provocative critique made by Bhakta's piece. For white viewers to look at white people doing yoga—not on their own terms, but through the lens of minoritization that Bhakta creates for them—is an opportunity to reflect on a reality they may not always see, which shapes their ability to move through the world.

Cultural appropriation is often considered a kind of cut—a severing of a cultural practice from its traditional lifeworld, juxtaposing cultural practices or images in new ways, moving them from one system of value into another. And it might be considered a practice of capitalist accumulation, in which socially dominant positions seek new levels of differentiation to make themselves stand out in a competitive environment. Bhakta's use of cuts, juxtapositions, and accumulation in *#White-PeopleDoingYoga* thrusts that logic back upon a dominant American racial category. Moving these pieces of ephemera out of their original context and juxtaposing them with new objects, his work resituates them within a different value chain that is both an exemplar and a critique of the logic of accumulation. Calling attention to these layers of experience—the intersection among individual, social, and political histories—invites viewers to participate in a new form of *svādhyāya*. *#WhitePeopleDoingYoga* turns to the illuminations of repetition to show that individual, even heartfelt and genuine, engagements with yoga can nonetheless become part of larger patterns that benefit the groups who may need it the least.

The final cut that shapes the significance of the show lies in the heart of its own capitalist formation. Bhakta describes the reluctance of the museum marketing officials to use the phrase #WhitePeopleDoingYoga in advertising in San Francisco publications. He narrates how he took the money the museum had paid him to create the installation—$1,500—and purchased his own advertisement, which amplified the hashtag and overlaid large red block letters of the title upon the images of white practitioners.[29]

As the monetary metamorphosis of the exhibit itself—the fee turns into an advertisement that turns into a work of protest art—the political work of Bhakta's ad is by no means outside the exchanges of capitalism. From one perspective, his real work of art is, in fact, the artist-paid advertisement. Yet the ironic need to purchase his own voice with the fruits of his labor shows the power of political critique. This form of *svādhyāya* looks very, very far from the recitation of texts in isolation of its origin. But it prompts a form of self-study—an inquiry conducted through, about, and within the practice of yoga—of the need to make visible the overpowering assemblages that frame life as a minority. Thinking critically about what repeats itself through yoga is still a pressing political concern.

In critiquing the transformation of yoga into YOGA™, Bhakta's work does not so much ask for recognition for South Asian subjectivities and histories from the dominant public sphere. Indeed, we might read an important politics in what we do not see, a refusal of the simple logic that minority communities wish to render themselves more visible in mainstream space.[30] Instead, Bhakta critiques the dominant public sphere's incessant need for its own mirroring by, ironically, refracting it through his own gaze. The installation does not ask white people to stop doing yoga. It asks only that they look at themselves within larger force fields of power. Although the collected ephemera were all produced to be seen, something unbearable, as witnessed in the museum's ambivalent response, emerges through the act of assembling them together. Inspiring this uncomfortable emotional layer—and asking viewers, as said in so many yoga studios, to sit with it—clarifies a world that many may not have realized they inhabit. Such a perception of energy, one might argue, is the kind of yoga needed in a fraught multiethnic world.

Looking back at the squares and rectangles on the wall of the installation, I am struck by their formal, inflexible structure. The human figures, the groovy waves, and the circular spirals show the flexibility of Indianness to bend to the needs of whomever wants it. But the boxes covering the white wall also signal a secret diasporic resistance. Those straight edges do not bend.

THE SPIROMETRIC ARTS

In childhood I worked hard to forget my breath. When I noticed it, the sensation bothered me. As quickly as possible, I would leap into something to take my mind off it. A book. A song. Breath would recede to the background, where I felt it belonged. Involuntary, unobtrusive, submissive.

By the middle of the road of life, breath began to make demands. Coughs chased me from winter into spring. The labyrinths of my lungs narrowed, my chest tightened. Breathing could no longer be so involuntary, so unobtrusive, so submissive. Without full breaths, the body loses vital force. I began to need the asthmatic's kit of inhalers and spacers and spirometers to make space for air. Through the clarity that only loss can bring, I have begun to learn how breath is energy.

After years of studying postures, I took my first class in *prāṇāyāma*, the art of breathing. The maze through which air becomes part of oneself came to light, like a paper written in invisible ink held over a flame. Unlike the white dust in my asthma inhaler, which could make my head rush and my heart pound, the yogic breathing took me into darker energies. Air stopped at my throat, held like water in a jug, expanding through secret rooms I had not realized I contained.

In breathing, energy moves: tidal, circular, topographic. History and poetry flow through its subtle pulse. Reading, in childhood, regulated my breath. The slowing into a stream of storytelling, the enigmatic holding demanded in a poem. Commas, colons, and full stops tell me when to inhale, hold, and exhale. With oxygen circulates health, memory, power.

In these hidden arts, so difficult to photograph and collect, imaginative life takes shape. To explore such energy, I turn to writings by the Indian American poet and essayist Reetika Vazirani, who delves into the practice of yoga to illuminate the energy currents that shape the Indian diaspora. In reading her work, I build on scholarly insistence that breathing has history and race.[31] Though humans from birth to death all breathe, the energies that circulate through their breath reflect political and historical points of difference. While Chiraag Bhakta's work makes the diaspora visible through its acerbic gaze, it refuses to offer an alternative to the omnipresent spectacles of white people doing yoga. Vazirani's gaze takes us in those new directions. In her essay "The Art of Breathing" and her poem "From Patanjali," both published in the literary magazine *Prairie Schooner* in 2001, Vazirani reflects on her practice of yoga in the context of her complex family history of migration to a United States in the midst of a civil rights racial reckoning. Rejecting the postural practice that had become mainstream by the turn of the twenty-first century, Vazirani instead explores the political potential of *prāṇāyāma*. Breathing takes her on a journey through complex energy circuits that link the body of her person to the body politic of inequitable history.

The essay is haunted by past and future violence. Although yoga offers an emblem for many forms of freedom, it saves no one. The essay tells of how her father, from whom she learned the art of yogic breathing, committed suicide when she was a child. According to one of the thirty-three tiny black journals she hid before she died, Vazirani practiced yoga right up until the day of her own life-ending violence toward herself and her young son.[32] These ghosts, past and yet to come, shadow her essay and poem with unanswered questions and unspeakable pain. To find a path forward from the words of those who found no ultimate comfort in them is a vexed but vital task.

I read Vazirani's life writing to ask how diasporic perspectives on yoga might offer insights into broader forms of *svādhyāya*. Though poetry is not a direct window into the reality of Vazirani's experience, the paired autobiographical essay and poem illuminate how the practice of yoga—in particular, the turn to the breathing—negotiates the social pressures of history in a world of racialized capitalism. As Jahan Ramazani argues, "race-alert writers mine poetry's deep connection to memory. . . . Poetry's mnemonic duration also lends itself to figurations of intergenerational memory."[33] Vazirani's writing, and my reading of her work, resonates with key trends in Asian American poetry in the first decade of the new millennium, when, as Timothy Yu suggests, postconfessional autobiography coexisted with "a desire to make the first person speak within a broader context—of spirituality, philosophy, or politics."[34] Listening to that first-person voice is my practice in these pages.

Vazirani was known for, as Ali Kazim puts it, "splintering poetic form, fracturing the line, abandoning syntax."[35] "The Art of Breathing" fragments the frame of a traditional essay, moving from personal journeys into family narratives and ethnographic observation of American racial and capitalist landscapes. In a study of her own yoga practice, the gaze of Vazirani's speaking self moves across layers of memory. It takes her into her body's interior and the possibilities offered through pregnancy, and into the architectural analogue for her pregnant body, her father's puja closet. Beyond these enclosed spaces, living in the United States for minority subjects requires protective barriers, exemplified by the extra wax Vazirani's father deliberately leaves on the surface of his car. These hidden spaces and obstructive residues, unseen and sometimes unsee-able in a racially complex nation, constitute counterhistories of yoga that might be set against the highly visible projections of whiteness that form the basis for *#WhitePeopleDoingYoga*. Commodified products tell little of the story of Indian diaspora. It is only in the glimpses offered through imaginative work that the presence of counterhistory makes itself felt. Yoga here is not a technology of perfection but a practice charged with the hope of survival.

Vazirani's search to re-represent her history through yoga might be understood through the critique offered by Glen Sean Coulthard, whose work on indigenous perspectives contends that paradigms of recogniz-ing cultural diversity already concede too much to dominant cultures. Such paradigms place minority and especially dispossessed groups in the subordinated position of seeking recognition in ways that are legi-ble within the norms of the dominant culture. Instead, Coulthard argues, what is needed is self-recognition that empowers communities in the work of decolonization.[36] This self-recognition is most compelling for Coulthard because it speaks to larger issues of sovereignty. From a perspective that does not recognize the dominant state as legitimate, seeking approval from that state is a lost cause. In the case of the Indian diaspora in the United States, such strong sovereignty claims cannot be made. Yet it is worth posing Coulthard's key question:Should minority communities accept the idea that they need to be recognized by domi-nant states and popular cultures? Or instead, is self-recognition—even self-study— called for?

Vazirani's essay "The Art of Breathing" begins with a frustrated search for outside recognition: the narrator's quest to hear her name pro-nounced by others as she would pronounce it. The symbolic weight of this ordinary moment speaks to a broader desire to be named, to be visible, and to have one's full background make claims upon American public space. These quests make their way through broad spectrums of public life, ranging all the way from what individuals are called up to the classifications they are offered on the census. "Calling me for my ultrasound, the receptionist leans toward the glass window, Retinka Varzeenee. How can this be? I have been here once a month for seven months and have corrected her four times."[37] In her yoga class, Vazirani's "I" finds herself renamed anew through the pronunciation of Sanskrit words: "When the class mispronounces surya namaskara, sun salutation, I feel a murmur of discomfort, the way I feel today in my obstetrician's office when my own name is mangled."[38] Observing the flexibilities demanded of diasporic subjects, Vazirani feels compelled to respond to a name that is mispronounced, that is almost but not her own, yet is laid like a screen over her sense of self. As a member of the diaspora, she becomes a person who cannot be seen directly or in full.

Yoga, studied through the prism of white America, fails on its own to offer Vazirani's speaking self a path to meaningful recognition. She writes, "learning yoga from white people is, for me, like copying down the ingredients of a vegan lentil dal burger from a Whole Foods deli sticker. I feel there are things I should know, that might have been handed down to me but were not."[39] In the learning is an absence, a gap not in the circulation of commodities or the supply of ingredients but in the people available to mediate and pass down knowledge. This palpable absence takes us into the condition of cultural appropriation, the valuing of cultural practices over people.

Vazirani is able to shift her approach by rethinking yoga as the art of breathing. Like Bhakta, she critiques the capitalist commodification of the seemingly perfectible body through yoga, reading into mainstream U.S. postural practice a cipher for the individualist competition of capitalist society writ large. Living without attention to breath, Luce Irigaray speculates, locks the self within the prison of history. "We remain passive at the level of breathing, bathing in a sort of socio-cultural placenta that passes on to us an already exhaled, already used, not truly pure air," she writes.[40] Cultivating breathing enables Vazirani's speaker to become conscious of that "socio-cultural placenta" that exists in parallel with the biological placenta through which her body breathes for her unborn child. *Prāṇāyāma* takes her into the unseeable parts of her own body that are not yet extractable as a capitalist resource. Pregnant with her son in the essay, the speaking self uses *prāṇāyāma* to explore what is below and beyond the skin: "The heat in my body leads me to spaces within myself, as if to rooms in a house I had never let myself fully inhabit. . . . The heat generated by my audible breathing leads me underground and overseas."[41] Understood as a form of remixed *svādhyāya*, this journey of breath expands physical selfhood like a work of poetry in which the inside is as expansive as the outside. No longer seeking validation from the pronunciation of Sanskrit words in the classroom, instead exploring her own inner generative capacity, the speaker turns to the art of breathing to animate self-recognition for a person caught within competing currents of energy.

The art of breathing invokes the powers of genealogy and lineage. While many explorations of the body modifications possible through *prāṇāyāma* focus on physiology,[42] for Vazirani *prāṇāyāma* is political. Air is politically shaped, whether we are thinking about the invisible pollutants that circulate within it, the inequitable access to respiratory care in the global pandemic, or the legacies of racial injustice that continue to haunt who can breathe freely in American space.[43] Vazirani traces her encounter with the practice back to her father, who taught her how to control her breath through his own practice before he died. This genealogy is precisely what makes breathing powerful, yet fraught. Yogic breathing is a failure, it cannot save her father, and for many years afterward she rejects it. And yet the art of breathing becomes his legacy to Vazirani's speaking self that she hopes to pass on to her unborn child. In such a context, what matters in the practice of yoga is the relationship it calls her into. This relationship encompasses the most intimate bonds of a father to his daughter, the broader histories of devotion to his gurus that he brings into American space, the histories of complex race relations that interconnect Indian, white, and black experiences in Vazirani's childhood, and the mystifications of American capitalism that conceals its own predatory impulses. In the section entitled "Oamkar,"

Vazirani's choice of transliteration moves away from the "om" readily found in mainstream American studios toward the genealogy of "*Omkāra*" of the *Ā 'īn-i Akbarī*, a more hopeful legacy of cross-cultural engagement. In this sense, although breathing draws away from the outward and visible, human histories are at the heart of the art of breathing.

Self-recognition, at its most powerful, inspires a new form of belonging for a diasporic subject. Such recognition is not necessarily in a fixed place or a specific name but in a flow of inhalation, holding, and exhalation, a circular rhythm that makes space for the competing demands placed on people in a state of diasporic difference. This mobility, by the end of the essay, makes room for an altered relationship with racial differences from which it begins. If, in the beginning passage, white Americans are placed under the kind of critical eye that years later shapes *#WhitePeopleDoingYoga,* the ending passages of the essay highlight how the struggles for political racial justice in the United States—exemplified by the civil rights movement that informed Vazirani's childhood—suggest alternative relations. "My teacher is a white woman in Virginia. . . . Somebody like her might have helped my father, who turned to pharmaceuticals, who in the end stopped breathing."[44] Breath, unlike medicines in jars, is not yet extractable. It offers the possibility—though never the certainty—of new human connections that challenge racial inequalities and capitalist commodification.

Vazirani creates new frames of possibility through such a genealogy of self-recognition in the poem that accompanies "The Art of Breathing." "From Patanjali" places the speaking self in a lineage that anchors itself in the systematizer Patañjali, for whom—as "The Art of Breathing" points out—postural practice meant relatively little. Through poetry, Vazirani explores the potential of yogic practice to become a kind of *svādhyāya* that connects cellular interiority to politics and history. In the poem, the speaking self enters into a meditation that draws attention to one point of repetition: the words "or else," repeated ten times in a one-page poem, always as either the first or last foot of the line. This sense of an unspoken, perhaps unspeakable alternative that does not always make syntactic sense haunts the poem. The meditative state transformed into words is both present and absent, observable and elusive. Within the lines of the poems are gaps, visual spaces of blankness that hint at changes in consciousness and the pacing of breath. The meditation focuses on the speaker's unborn son, her son's father, and the histories of racial perceptions, inequalities, and injustices that shape the bodies of all three held together in the emotional layer created by the poem. In the middle, the speaker turns into a body composed of breath:

> I open my fingers and feel their breath
> or else centuries pouring into out of
> people yes we judge them light and dark
> or else height and hair
> and whose god made gold
> rise above aleph let me go from that
> gnawing at straw houses[45]

Vazirani's syntax often leaves it unclear whether the lines are end-stopped or enjambed, offering alternative possibilities—the "or else" that echoes again and again—as part of the reading experience. Poetry modulates breath, so the alternatives change the way breath is held or released, as do the blank spaces that work as a *kumbhaka*, or breath retention, within a practice of *prāṇāyāma*. In the passage quoted here, the fragment "into out of" places the holding of breath after an inhalation and before an exhalation, mirroring a common structure in *prāṇāyāma* in which breath is contained before the diaphragm releases.

As fingers take on the ability to breathe, new layers open up to the weight and travel of history. Centuries pour into and out of people, circulating through their bodies. Breath is not only about the intake of air or even the search for poetic inspiration (the literal breathing in of the divine), but also about the ways histories move through and within human bodies, how perceptions of skin color, height, hair, or wealth are brought into an interior layer. Resonating with Fanon's classic argument that minoritized subjects internalize their own oppression, the poem reveals how such subjects might become aware of this: how they might observe its comings and goings as these ideas circulate within their minds and bodies. In observing the makings of judgment around racial-ized and capitalist perceptions of value, the poem turns to meditative practice to clarify how broader social structures shape the way different people breathe in and out in the world.

A racial longing becomes palpable throughout "The Art of Breathing" and "From Patanjali," for the powers of blackness and the political clarity afforded by that position within American culture. If one strand of anxiety in Vazirani's writings notes the white American and Indian histories of privileging lightness over darkness and the need to defend her own skin coloration from those who wish her lighter, another strand seeks to embed herself more closely within the glamour, power, and passion that the writings link to African American histories. The poem meditates from her unborn son to an image of

> his father on a green bed Virginia
> plantation back to the first
> four generations of stress

If we read this as an autobiographical reference to the father of Vazirani's child, the African American poet Yusef Komunyakaa, the poem enfolds these histories that the father brings to their son, evoking through enjambment plantation slavery and multigenerational forms of oppression. This historical makeup, again through the sliding, wrapping force of the lines, then becomes part of the mother's body:

> my own skin I am in
> you in your rest and
> above everything I wish you well

If read end-stopped, the line reads as a mode of self-recognition, a sense of completeness within the narrator's skin and its ambivalent, ambiguous positioning in a transnational racial landscape: sometimes too dark, sometimes too light. If read enjambed, however, it rests that sense of self-recognition in dependence on the unborn child and its multiracial histories that claim black as well as Indian ancestry.

The longing to integrate with African America, to share in the clarity that such positionality can offer, is echoed in "The Art of Breathing": "The university where my father teaches is African American. . . . I notice they seem very rich and stylish, and in them resides a certain power, a glamour I am not a part of. . . . I am intoxicated and full of admiration for a drama I do not understand."[46] In becoming the mother to a multiracial child, the speaker writes her way into a form of American belonging. Genealogy is reversed, it works backward, not simply something she passes on to her son but something that she inherits from him. In understanding inheritance to work in this way, as a circular rather than unidirectional process, Vazirani's poem recodes cultural identities to resemble the circuits of breathing. In breathing for and through her son, she reminds herself that no one fully breathes alone.

Published at the historical moment in the fall of 2001 when the twin towers of Manhattan were demolished in a terrorist attack, Vazirani's words offer fragile hope in light of intensified personal and national violence. They show how for a woman in the Indian diaspora, yoga provides a crucial set of potential insights into how she might negotiate the flexibilities demanded of her. The art of breathing, as she comes to conclude, reminds her of writing a poem. This is how I feel too in a yoga studio, arms extended, foot turned in, breathing out. Journeys of *svādhyāya* within the body are also journeys into family, community, history, into ways of being human in an often inhuman world. Moving on different feet, they offer interwoven transformations.

Yoga is imagined in these pages as a practice of survival for the Indian diaspora. In history, none of the practitioners of yoga in Vazirani's essay—father, narrative self, and unborn son—survive. All we are left with is fragments of their practice, breathing made word, aligned in new frames of possibility, hidden within the "or else."

MOCKING MASTERY

In my *prāṇāyāma* class, I learn to pull in my intercostal muscles smoothly for long, gliding breaths. When those muscles contract sharply, they change my breathing. I laugh.

What use might this alternative form of breathing offer? How can breath itself be cut and framed to illuminate new ends? To explore this question, I turn to a director's cut: the Canadian *Yoga Town*, released as an indie web series in 2013. Written and produced by Jill Hope Johnson and Ashwin Sood, *Yoga Town* satirizes the ethnic politics of yoga by leaning into, rather than away from, essentialist stereotypes in order to access a new point of view through comedy. At some points, it leans so hard into stereotype that its images almost explode. The flexibilities of Indianness—the question of how far this category can stretch, how far people of different backgrounds can stretch within it, and what all this resilience might conceal—are revealed through the lens of satire.

As I have argued in my earlier work on cross-cultural engagement, stereotypes can create paradoxically fruitful terrain for an ethics of comic border crossing.[47] As Homi Bhabha has suggested, within their seeming fixedness lies an anxious instability of meaning that must be repeated in order to exist. Satire both relies on and exposes this instability. The possibilities latent within these seemingly rigid emblems of discursive domination find further theoretical articulation in the work of Mrinalini Chakravorty, who argues that "stereotypes about South Asia that we encounter in global narratives force us to define ourselves as consumers of these texts. That is, even as stereotypes provoke us to imagine South Asia's remarkable differences, they also reveal ourselves to us, and at times remake us."[48] The stereotype is not something that simply exists; it is called into being through a dynamic relationship between text and audience. This intimacy brings with it political and ethical possibility: "Seeing the stereotype as something that involves us intimately in it means recognising its ethical force."[49] Compelling audiences to reflect on their own complicity thus is a key part of a stereotype's potentially productive work, and what satires like *Yoga Town* can do.

As a collaboration among writers, actors, and production teams that include both members of the Indian diaspora and people not of Indian background, *Yoga Town* turns to the instabilities of irony and satire to mock many of the specters of capitalist commodification and ethnic essentialism through a classic contest: Who owns the soul of yoga? The story tells of the struggle of Willow, a white hippie protagonist whose yoga studio seeks to offer "real yoga" but is brought to the brink of ruin by a new competitor, Elijah. Dressed in colorful, Indian-inspired clothes,

which render him ethnically ambiguous—is he Indian or not?—Elijah
in his "Go Yoga" mobile van seduces away Willow's dwindling clientele,
including her daughter. *Yoga Town* plays with these dynamic dimensions
of stereotype through comic invitations to audience reflection. Made as
a mockumentary, the series was released in twelve short episodes that
combine dramatic action with faux-confessional modes where characters address the camera directly. The form of the mock documentary
questions the premise of truth that the documentary genre is thought
to seek, yet also pursues its own revelations. Under the guise of speaking to an audience, the camera allows characters to overhear themselves.
The direct address to the camera creates a state in which characters know
and do not know themselves at the same time.

To save her studio, Willow enlists the help of Neela, the Indian Canadian owner of a consultancy called Tandoori Loving Care. "I come into
your business, I spice it up with a little ethnic chic, and badda bing, you
feel better, I make a buck or two," she tells the camera in a Canadian
accent. "From nine to five," she shifts to an Indian accent, "I talk like
this." Shifting back to a Canadian accent, "And from five to nine I talk
like this." "Turn it on" (in a Canadian accent); "turn it off" (in an Indian
one). "No—turn it off—turn it on—" (in an Indian accent)—she then
looks very confused—"Turn it off" (in a Canadian accent). She looks
helplessly at the camera. "You know what I mean."[50] Played by Veena
Sood, an improvisational comedy actor, Neela satirically embodies the
flexibilities she seeks to monetize and dramatizes the impossibilities of
living in this world of ethnic commodification. The one "real" experience portrayed through the satire is confusion: the toll taken on the diaspora, always asking who others around them need them to be.

As a professional maker of stereotype, Neela exposes Indianness as a
sign always under renovation, composed through the commodity chains
of other countries and through the perceptions of ethnic difference that
operate in Canada. Her direct address to the camera, in the style beloved
of mockumentaries, invites the viewer to consider how their presence
is implicated within such fantasy. Neela's job evokes the self-exoticizing
strategies of the Indian state, where the diaspora is celebrated for its ability to sell a spiritual otherness in global markets. "Neela, it says it's

made in China," Willow says anxiously, looking at the bottom of a Buddha head that Neela has brought as studio décor. "Yeah," says Neela, looking unfazed. "I got it at the dollar store."[51] The series thus illuminates how the ethnic "touch" seen to be so valuable within white-oriented spaces is a market-oriented production of difference—an imagined essence that is actually a combination of performance and consumption. The cuts of the camera frame, which move between action scenes and direct confessions, use the formal devices of juxtaposition and fragmentation to push forward the satire, both of the character and of the audience's complicity with mythmakings of Indianness.

The cinematic cuts and juxtapositions of *Yoga Town* mock mastery over ideas of Indianness by diasporic and nondiasporic subjects. For most of the characters featured, Indianness is cast within the shadow of fraudulence and ambiguity. The satire sheds light on the flexibilities demanded by and through the differently raced characters. The quest for Indianness is figured in *Yoga Town* as destructive. The ambiguously presented Elijah steals Willow's business, then offers to "help" her with an offer of sex. The "good Indian" whom Neela imports to enliven Willow's studio, the Indian Canadian celebrity chef Vikram Vij, is rerouted in a wave of enthusiasm to Elijah's van. Neela, after the collapse of Willow's business, returns as a steely-eyed villain to demand payment for service. All the productions meant to benefit Willow's studio now flow to Elijah and his "Go Yoga" alternative. Turned into a commodity, Indianness moves with waves of social capital, eluding firm control. *Svādhyāya* as a practice invites us to expand from an observation of content to a broader awareness of the framing and cutting powers of the camera. As those formal techniques expose failings, fraudulence, and even dangers within desperate and exploitative pursuits, satire is the *svādhyāya*: the place of comic disconnect where an idea is cut open and juxtaposed with its internal contradictions to expose hierarchical structures of power.

In many ways, *Yoga Town* remains ensnared within limited frames that reinforce racialized cultural scripts. Even as it mocks these images, it relies on the trope of the innocent white woman who turns to a Hinducentric vision of India to heal her wounds.[52] This vision relies on the erasure of two important systems of power: an understanding of whiteness that does not recognize how that category benefits from long-standing systems of colonial exploitation and racialized capitalism, and an understanding of Hindu-centric India that cannot admit how that configuration has also repressed its own minorities.[53] Dressed initially in earth-toned, billowing clothes so iconic of hippiedom that audience members can almost smell the patchouli through the screen, Willow gradually shifts to bright and more ornate Indian fabrics that contrast with the norms of yoga wear both in Western studios and in twentieth-century Indian postural manuals. The frame of *Yoga Town*, which begins with Willow's distress and ends with her potential self-immolation, centers sympathy on the problem of a white woman who copes with her own suffering by draping herself—literally and figuratively—in signs of Indianness.

Yet this healing power is itself subject to a critical look. In the final scene of the web series, a distraught Willow pours kerosene in a circle around her yoga mats and Indian-inspired cushions, then lights a match. Resonating with subcontinental histories of female self-immolation as well as Sita's trial by fire in the *Rāmāyaṇa*, this final—and distinctly noncomic—ending suggests that a search for the heart of yoga, conducted under the sign of Indianness, will quite literally burn down the house. An unexpectedly confronting moment for a comic series, the jarring finale portrays Indianness as most authentic when it destroys its own object. The idea of India masters, but cannot be fully mastered.

CONCLUSION

Ideas of Indianness work within, through, and upon the diverse white screens of popular culture. While the obvious and visible images of India turn such ideas into commodities, often for the benefit of white corporations but also for ethnic self-commodification, more resistant—and sometimes dangerous—ideas of Indianness emerge in the cuts, juxtapositions, and frames of these imaginative forms. In the art installation, the essay and poem, and the video series, reflecting on the power of form—rather than remaining fixed on content—leads to the most critical reflective gestures. If the art of breathing teaches one how to move energy, form directs where the energy goes, how it flows, where it is held, and how it is released. Though these gestures will not overturn systems of power, they can introduce important notes of friction. In this sense, representations of yoga—read through a remixed and remediated vision of *svādhyāya*—can offer a counterpoint to the endless sculpting of the perfect working body to suit the needs of neoliberal states. As a metaphor for the flexibilities desired by and often demanded of India's diaspora, yoga offers a space to reflect on what it means to become a more flexible subject. Critical pieces, like *#WhitePeopleDoingYoga*, suggest that for a diaspora, sometimes insisting on rigidity is important.

From this perspective, contesting cultural appropriation is not about getting culture correct or avoiding offense, but about engaging—politically, socially, and materially—with the perspectives of people intimately connected to those cultures who may be both amplified and erased in an act of cultural exchange. The first danger of focusing only on nonrecognition and misrecognition is that we may be asking too much of culture, demanding that it fix legacies of injustice, dispossession, and other political harms. The second danger, of focusing only on exploitation, is that we may ask too little of culture, assuming that until material debts and inequalities are settled, cultural engagement remains all sound and fury, signifying nothing. Instead, we might ask how debates over and within imaginative life are invitations to consider the energy channels of history, justice, and memory that shape diverse lifeworlds. Like Liz Bucar, who ends her critique of religious appropriation in Western yoga with a call to think critically about how practitioners amplify, erase, or perform elements of Indian culture, I suggest that an effective response to the structural harms of appropriation requires practitioners to deepen their understanding not only of yoga's complexity but also of the broader political dynamics shaping ideas of flexible Indianness.[54]

Such form directs energy. Like the "Mobius strip" of breath,[55] the inverted figure of eight that intertwines inhalation and exhalation, art circulates forces of life with a twist. Words come to look more and more like breath, the life force needed to survive a changing world. They bespeak what Achille Mbembe has called "the universal right to breathe," the struggle against "everything that, in the long reign of capitalism, has constrained entire segments of the world population, entire races, to a difficult, panting breath and life of oppression."[56] India's diaspora has aligned new parts to tell a new story through yoga, creating bricolage out of mainstream culture, excavating hidden histories in the art of breathing, and offering satiric frames for the flexibilities demanded of the diaspora in so many of its dimensions.

In Bombay in 1986, my parents bought a quilt. It was large enough to cover their king-sized bed, the bed that was big enough for me to snuggle in at the edge when I woke up in the night from dreams of snakes and lions. The quilt was covered with hand-embroidered flowers and vines on a creamy background. My parents loved it. You couldn't buy anything like it from the shiny parquet displays in the windowless Belk's department store at home.

The people who sold my parents the quilt wrapped it up tightly, making it small enough to fit into our floppy brown vinyl suitcase with duct tape on the corners. My mother pushed and pulled our clothes around its contours when it came time to pack for our flight back to South Carolina. The suitcase bulged in improbable ways. My job was to sit on the top so that the bag would flatten long enough for my mother to coax the nearly broken zipper around the perimeter. No one checked baggage weights in 1986. If you could force something into your suitcase, you could take it home.

Back in our ranch house on a suburban street, my parents unfurled the quilt. The greens of the vines mirrored the forest green of their bedroom wall. It was glorious. But it was also strange. The quilt was padded with a foam so stiff that it stuck straight out from the sides of the bed. It didn't bend. It didn't drape.

My mother blinked at the Indian quilt. We so often blinked at the textiles we brought back from Bombay. Ochres, reds, oranges the color of the sun setting over the Indian Ocean. They all looked captivating in my aunt and uncle's flat. In American light, those colors changed. They challenged. They dared. They did not quite fit. It always seemed so much safer to pull out something from L.L. Bean. But my parents loved the flowers and vines. They didn't want to fold the quilt up and put it into the guest room drawer where my mother kept her out-of-date saris. So they began to unquilt it.

That January, the quilt made itself at home in a basket by the fireplace my parents never lit. It sat next to the piles of library books that covered the flagstone hearth. When my mother had a moment, she sat down in our bucket chair, pulled out my grandmother's orange-handled sharp sewing scissors, and began to cut the threads that bound the top of the quilt to the industrial-strength inner foam. When my father had a minute, he did a bit too. Soon I would sit on Saturday mornings, curled in the chair in the house by the cold fireplace, and snip away at the threads myself.

I remember this as a cozy time. Cutting, pulling, unthreading. Each stitch came out at the pace of my breath. Slowly, the scraps of stiff foam began to vanish. In their place appeared a strong, supple, flexible bedspread. When my parents and I looked at the emerging quilt, we felt a sense of shared pride. The three of us, unquilting, had made something we could use.

Now, decades later, I look back and wonder. What would it have been like to live under a stiff Indian quilt?

7

LYING OUT

Spectral Yoga

Stories and spectacles, circulating within and upon the practice of yoga, tell of the promise and peril of a flexible India in the twenty-first-century world. Transforming tension into harmony, the "culture peace" offered through yoga ironically can prevent the injuries of political and economic life from gaining a chance to heal.

Visions of yoga give the illusion of order. They allow practitioners to document and quantify progress toward ideal bodies. In its modern form, the practice provides a way to regulate time and create oases in modern lives that are increasingly irregular and always "on." Yoga can promise the perfection of discipline in an era when so much seems to be beyond our control. If measurement, counting, and incessant data collection were once the utopian dreams of states, international organizations, and scholarly disciplines, today these projects have entered into the heart of middle-class personhood in many parts of the world. Devices record our steps, apps count our hours of sleep, "likes" record our popularity. For many people, these projects of quantification are not simply physical. Scales measure moral worth, screens record success and failure, social media statistics calculate personal and economic value. Numbers are rarely morally neutral.

Yet pushing us to grasp what we cannot ordinarily measure is one of yoga's historical goals. Stories and spectacles of yoga can also present remixed approaches to *svādhyāya*, self-studies that teach readers to see the world from complex critical positions that dive into the depths of often inequitable histories. In different ways, yoga has invited its practitioners to look beyond the visible and quantifiable world to apprehend something bigger and deeper. Today, we might take up some of that promise as part of the practice. We might become curious about what is left out of the frame, what is not counted, what eludes our quantified and bounded selves.

Who's there?

My Indian family is dying. Ghosts are invading my townhouse in Australia. On the wall above the steep staircase, amid snapshots of my children running by the Tasman Sea, are black-and-white images of faces who have crossed over. My grandfather, always the tallest man in the photo, looks out from a line of young men behind the fabric counter of Kaymally's in Hong Kong. "Who's there?" my children ask, pointing to the wall.

In other shots on our wall my grandfather sits next to his wife, his eyes framed by the elegant sunglasses that became his signature. My grandmother, whose picture haunted my childhood, shoots the disapproving stare I have gradually learned to live with. Gone before I was born, my grandmother was the one who took up yoga in our family. It was recommended for her diabetes, my mother said, in the 1960s. My uncle took up headstands in the 1980s for his health. My aunt practiced mudras during chemotherapy for the breast cancer that eventually took her life.

In many of the memoirs I read, yoga prepares the self for death. Ending in *śavāsana*, or corpse pose, yoga can be a place to rethink the meaning of dying. Most of the time I spend in *śavāsana*, I watch my thoughts write emails. But, every once in a while, a radiant darkness spreads over my body.

Diasporas watch this radiant darkness claim their living ties to India. I watch my cousins, all of whom married people without Indian descent, and our beautiful tousle-haired children whose skin tones run all the way from freckled rose to olive glow to burnt sienna. We circulate and recirculate through changing ideas of India, passing into spaces shaped by loss as much as by the warmth of human hands. The idea of India changes with each generation. My children, with one Indian grandparent, ask if they are Indian. Sometimes I fill up their Yumboxes with dosa and their bookshelves with Indian freedom fighter comics and make them listen to audiobooks of the *Ramayana* in the car, but I'm not sure whom I'm forming.

The first moment I asked myself if I were Indian was at Stanford in 1999. Alone, I went to a screening of the film *Earth*, about the agonies of Partition. It was a story of division I had never heard before. My PhD studies in literature had recently begun. After several quarters of reading modernist poems and Shakespeare and structuralist theory, I had become increasingly unsure that I should devote my hours to the minute details of Virginia Woolf's novels.

The theater was filled almost entirely with people of South Asian descent. This was the world of Silicon Valley, and Indian tech money was paying for us to watch the film. I had never been in a room with this many Indians outside of India in my life. As if I were fifteen again, I became convinced that everyone was looking at me. I would be thrown out of the screening for my inability to list India's emperors or for having received an insufficient number of racist comments in my childhood.

Pain legitimates. We know who we are by how we have been hurt. My mother left behind so much of India in her journey because her world had the ability to wound. She protected me from pain. To this day, my aunts and uncles are continually surprised by how little I know of their past. A great-uncle confined like an animal to a madhouse in Pune. A cousin murdered by the Mumbai mafia for property. A family, half racing to Pakistan, half staying put in India. An uncle, wandering the streets of Hong Kong with a suitcase filled with cash for the end of the world. My generation was protected from pain through the stories not told, the gatherings not attended, the relatives never phoned, the cuts not performed.

My looks have protected me from pain. I don't look like what people expect from Indians, even multiracial ones. A worn, folded piece of paper kept in my wallet in my early twenties listed guesses I had received about my ethnicity. Latina, Greek, Mediterranean, Iranian, Uyghur. Australian officials look at me and tick "white" on their form without asking. Because as a child I thought about Indianness so little, I almost never interpreted cruel comments, prank calls, noninvitations to parties, or occasional unfriending as signs of its presence. I was quiet, nerdy, and bookish, a sufficient explanation for not fitting into a world of cheerleaders and duck hunters.

If this pain is missing for multiethnic minorities, who are we? Pleasure does not seem to work. New Age selfhoods define themselves through the experience of pleasure, which is why we distrust them. Madonna wearing *mehndi* has simply not experienced enough Indian pain. If one grows fed up with a cultural practice, one can leave it without cost. No departure tax, no exit fee.

One part of me feels that there is something true about this cultural logic. When I can read my losses as losses, they bring to life an Indianness I did not always know I had. The fact that I am so unsettled when I can't speak Hindi in India marks me as a child of the diaspora. In Mexico or Indonesia or Japan, I can simply not know. In India, my not-knowing is shot through with wrongness and guilt. Over time, I've come to embrace anxiety as the best proof of belonging. If we're anxious, we own it.

I now ask my family ghosts to guide me. Through their spirits, absence takes on meaning and form. I think of Derek Parfit writing on death: "My death will break the more direct relations between my present experiences and future experiences, but it will not break various other relations. . . . Now that I have seen this, my death seems to me less bad."[1] The last time I saw my aunt alive, she blessed me on my journey home. Her hands upon me, on the threshold before the carved wooden door; her words in a language I could not understand. By the end of that year, she was the one who made the grander journey. This book is my way of sending blessings in return.

In *śavāsana* at the end of a practice, I try to keep myself open to the ghosts. Who's there? If the sayings are right, that I am practicing for death, and if Parfit is right, that the dead are not fully gone, then yoga turns bodies and minds into a new threshold of possibility. If I take yoga seriously as a way of knowing the world, I find some comfort in its ability to haunt. In a way, in *śavāsana* I am most alone. No one speaks. After class, we avoid each other's eyes. And yet in *śavāsana* I am not alone at all. The ghosts help me with the anxious, stylized repetition of claims to something—what?—from India. I don't look Indian. I don't sound Indian. I don't live in India. I don't carry a card. Indianness is a never-ending series of losses.

At the same time, I find myself loath to accept that the only path to belonging is through pain. For those who have not experienced enough pain, or the right kinds of pain, or the visible and accepted forms of pain, what is left to legitimate who we are? Yoga offers another answer: practice.

EPILOGUE

The Moon

I wake early in India. When I open my eyes, it feels like they are still closed. Darkness and silence fill the space. I have no idea what time it is until I feel for my phone. Five a.m. A good time to rise.

It is peaceful. Time seems long and limitless without the framing grid of school trips and afternoon pickups and child bedtimes to shape my day. I pull out my yoga mat and push aside the drapes.

In the blackness, a full golden moon shines over the Arabian Sea.

It is the closest to perfect moon I have ever seen. Its reflection streams down over the invisible water in a column of light. Just beneath I can see the dark pillar of my image in the mirror.

I am immediately gripped by two desires: to open the window to see the moon without glass between us, and to take a photograph to preserve it forever. The tension between these two desires doesn't reach me right away. My fingers search on the window frame for the latch. I pull and pull, but the window will not budge. Even though I opened it the day before, today it is sealed shut.

There's nothing to do but look through the glass that divides me from the moon. If I shift my balance just so, standing on my mat, I can move the moon into a small clear space on the glass where rivulets of water have made a path through the speckled dust. I see the moon, warm and gold as if it were the sun. I see the glass. I see the dust just at the edges of my vision. It is as if I watch the moon through a small clear keyhole. A small space through which the moon can also see me.

Without thinking about it too much, I raise my arms and begin my sun salutations. I know that it is unlikely that ancient yogis did these sequences at dawn, but that does not really matter. It is a good way to greet the day. Yesterday the quality of my limbs was so heavy that I could barely move. A sluggish, slothful practice, one filled with sadness. Today my limbs seem different. My arms rise up without my realizing it as I look steadily at the moon. I watch the trifold column, the moon at the top, its long streaming reflection across the dark water, my shadowy self stacked at the bottom. Some of what I am seeing is glass, some is water, some is sky, but for a moment all seems like moon.

My limbs begin to move effortlessly through the sequence. I let the pattern carry me, floating through the forms like a leaf floating downstream. In my head, I hear the voices of many teachers. Yoga is an experience. Yoga is an experiential science. Yoga is an art. Even when I'm crouched low to the ground, I can still see the moon in its fullness, as if it is following me rising and falling.

When I stand and look straight through the clear rivulet, the moon is lighter. The column of tessellated light has thinned. I practice and watch. I can tell what will come, the beginning of the end. The column vanishes first. The globular moon hovers in the darkness. Then it too thins and vanishes. I have no photograph to remember it by.

Blackness surrounds. Even in the daytime, it's often hard here to tell the sea from the sky. In this absence of light it is impossible to know what is water, what is air, what is rock. Other ways of knowing must be called upon.

Then, a sparkle of light where the moon once was. Perhaps a star, perhaps a pinprick—a hint of something beyond the black curtain of sky.

This window is the window my grandfather looked out of until he died. The room I am staying in is what I still think of as his room, which I remember from my childhood as filled with medical equipment and the sound of Koranic chanting on a scratchy tape deck. My grandfather, white-bearded and banging his cane against the building lift in impatience. We were said to look a little bit alike, to share the same oval face, the same skin tone the color of tea with too much milk, and the same habit of fingers in perpetual motion.

This flat where I look out the window is the one place I can still stand as I did as a child. My parents sold my childhood home. My other aunts and uncles moved from place to place, island to island. I live ten thousand miles from where I was born. The invisible absences, the world that is passing, the world that is gone. Absences surround the borders of what I think of as my self.

I keep practicing in the loss of the moon. Slowly the rocks at the water's edge appear, and then the moving sea comes into view, and finally the sky brightens with morning sun. I can see the apartment tower on the left and the slum homes down at the tideline. A recognizable world takes form.

A gift has been offered. Of that I am sure. An experience and a frame, solar and lunar, dark and light. The moon and the glass and the ghosts, all part of yoga's flexible form.

NOTES

1. SETTING UP

1. David Gordon White, ed., *Yoga in Practice* (Princeton, NJ: Princeton University Press, 2011), 2.

2. Because my focus is on ideas of Indianness, I do not largely address practices of yoga that claim genealogies from other parts of the world, such as Kemetic yoga. I do include forms that reflect complex entanglements between South Asian and non-South Asian influences.

3. White, *Yoga in Practice*, 2–4.

4. See, among others, Geoffrey Samuel, *The Origins of Yoga and Tantra: Indic Religions to the Thirteenth Century* (Cambridge: Cambridge University Press, 2008); Gavin Flood, *The Ascetic Self: Subjectivity, Memory and Tradition* (Cambridge: Cambridge University Press, 2004); David Gordon White, *The Yoga Sutra of Patanjali: A Biography* (Princeton, NJ, and Oxford: Princeton University Press, 2014); Satya Prakash Singh, ed., *History of Yoga* (New Delhi: Munshiram Manoharlal Publishers, 2010); Andrew J. Nicholson, *Unifying Hinduism: Philosophy and Identity in Indian Intellectual History* (New York: Columbia University Press, 2010); James Mallinson and Mark Singleton, trans., *Roots of Yoga* (London: Penguin, 2017); Karl Baier, Philipp A. Maas, and Karin Preisendanz, eds., *Yoga in Transformation: Historical and Contemporary Perspectives* (Gottingen: V&R Unipress, 2018); Suzanne Newcombe and Karen O'Brien-Kop, eds., *Routledge Handbook of Yoga and Meditation Studies* (Abingdon, UK: Routledge, 2021); Karen O'Brien-Kop, *Rethinking "Classical Yoga" and Buddhism: Meditation, Metaphors and Materiality* (London: Bloomsbury, 2022).

5. Barbara A. Holdrege, *Bhakti and Embodiment: Fashioning Divine Bodies and Devotional Bodies in Kṛṣṇa Bhakti* (Abingdon, UK: Routledge, 2015); Patton E. Burchett,

A Genealogy of Devotion: Bhakti, Tantra, Yoga, and Sufism in North India (New York: Columbia University Press, 2019).

6. William R. Pinch, *Warrior Ascetics and Indian Empires* (Cambridge: Cambridge University Press, 2006); David Gordon White, *Sinister Yogis* (Chicago: University of Chicago Press, 2009); Hugh B. Urban, *Tantra: Sex, Secrecy, Politics and Power in the Study of Religions* (Berkeley: University of California Press, 2003); Knut A. Jacobsen, ed., *Yoga Powers: Extraordinary Capacities Attained Through Meditation and Concentration* (Leiden: Brill, 2012).

7. Elizabeth De Michelis, *A History of Modern Yoga: Patanjali and Western Esotericism* (London and New York: Continuum, 2004); Joseph S. Alter, *Yoga in Modern India: The Body Between Science and Philosophy* (Princeton, NJ, and Oxford: Princeton University Press, 2004); Sarah Strauss, *Positioning Yoga: Balancing Acts Across Cultures* (Oxford: Berg, 2005); Mark Singleton and Jean Byrne, eds., *Yoga in the Modern World: Contemporary Perspectives* (London and New York: Routledge, 2008); Mark Singleton, *Yoga Body: The Origins of Modern Posture Practice* (New York: Oxford University Press, 2010); Andrea R. Jain, *Selling Yoga: From Counterculture to Pop Culture* (New York: Oxford University Press, 2014); Beth Berila, Melanie Klein, and Chelsea Jackson Roberts, eds., *Yoga, the Body, and Embodied Social Change: An Intersectional Feminist Analysis* (Lanham, MD: Lexington Books, 2016); Andrea R. Jain, *Peace Love Yoga: The Politics of Global Spirituality* (New York: Oxford University Press, 2020); Suzanne Newcombe, *Yoga in Britain: Stretching Spirituality and Educating Yogis* (Sheffield, UK: Equinox, 2019); Stephanie Y. Evans, *Black Women's Yoga History: Memoirs of Inner Peace* (Albany: State University of New York Press, 2021); Laurah E. Klepinger, *Transnational Yoga at Work: Spiritual Tourism and Its Blind Spots* (Lanham, MD: Lexington Books, 2022); Farah Godrej, *Freedom Inside? Yoga and Meditation in the Carceral State* (New York: Oxford University Press, 2022); Amanda J. Lucia, *White Utopias: The Religious Exoticism of Transformational Festivals* (Oakland: University of California Press, 2020); Cara Hagan, ed., *Practicing Yoga as Resistance: Voices of Color in Search of Freedom* (London: Routledge, 2021); Anya Foxen and Christa Kuberry, *Is This Yoga? Concepts, Histories, and the Complexities of Modern Practice* (London: Routledge, 2021).

8. Singleton, *Yoga Body*; Anya P. Foxen, *Inhaling Spirit: Harmonialism, Orientalism, and the Western Roots of Modern Yoga* (New York: Oxford University Press, 2020); Evans, *Black Women's Yoga History*; Theodora Wildcroft, *Post-Lineage Yoga: From Guru to #MeToo* (Sheffield, UK: Equinox Ebooks Publishing, 2020).

9. Mallinson and Singleton, *Roots of Yoga*, xii.

10. Agi Wittich, "Iyengar Yoga for Women: A Practising Tradition in the Making," *Religions of South Asia* 11, no. 2–3 (August 1, 2018): 231–53, https://doi.org/10.1558/rosa.37025; Newcombe, *Yoga in Britain*; Evans, *Black Women's Yoga History*; Emanuela Mangiarotti, "The Politics of Tending to the Body: Women Doing Yoga in Genoa (Italy)," *European Journal of Women's Studies*, October 27, 2022, 135050682211290, https://doi.org/10.1177/13505068221129063; Barbara Humberstone and Carol Cutler-Riddick, "Older Women, Embodiment and Yoga Practice," *Ageing & Society* 35, no. 6

(July 2015): 1221–41; Narin Hassan, "Travelers, Translators, and Spiritual Mothers: Yoga, Gender, and Colonial Histories," *Race and Yoga* 5, no. 1 (2020): 24–41, https://doi.org/10.5070/R351046982; Foxen, *Inhaling Spirit*.

11. Jain, *Peace Love Yoga*; Shameem Black, "Yoga, Sexual Violation and Discourse: Reconfigured Hegemonies and Feminist Voices," *Australian Feminist Studies* 35, no. 105 (2020): 277–92; Karen-Anne Wong, "Inclusive Identities: The Lens of Critical Theory," in *Routledge Handbook of Yoga and Meditation Studies*, ed. Suzanne Newcombe and Karen O'Brien-Kop (Abingdon, UK: Routledge, 2021), 481–83; Diana York Blaine, "Mainstream Representations of Yoga: Capitalism, Consumerism, and Control of the Female Body," in *Yoga, the Body, and Embodied Social Change*, ed. Beth Berila, Melanie Klein, and Chelsea Jackson Roberts (Lanham, MD: Lexington Books, 2016), 129–40.

12. Christine E. Spadola et al., "Enhancing Yoga Participation: A Qualitative Investigation of Barriers and Facilitators to Yoga among Predominantly Racial/Ethnic Minority, Low-Income Adults," *Complementary Therapies in Clinical Practice* 29 (November 2017): 97–104, https://doi.org/10.1016/j.ctcp.2017.09.001; Sandi M. Tenfelde, Lena Hatchett, and Karen L. Saban, " 'Maybe Black Girls Do Yoga': A Focus Group Study with Predominantly Low-Income African-American Women," *Complementary Therapies in Medicine* 40 (October 2018): 230–35, https://doi.org/10.1016/j.ctim.2017.11.017; Sabrina Smith and Matthew Atencio, " 'Yoga Is Yoga. Yoga Is Everywhere. You Either Practice or You Don't': A Qualitative Examination of Yoga Social Dynamics," *Sport in Society* 20, no. 9 (2017): 1167–84, https://doi-org.virtual.anu.edu.au/10.1080/17430437.2016.1269082.

13. Godrej, *Freedom Inside?*

14. One historical formation that links yoga to egalitarian social politics is the *bhakti* (devotional) Sant tradition from the fifteenth century to the present. See Daniel Gold, "The Hindi Sants' Two Yogic Paths to the Formless Lord," in *Meditation and Culture: The Interplay of Practice and Context*, ed. Halvor Eifring (London: Bloomsbury, 2015), 131–46.

15. Jain, *Peace Love Yoga*, 8.

16. Lee Siegel, *Trance-Migrations: Stories of India, Tales of Hypnosis* (Chicago: University of Chicago Press, 2014).

17. On yoga's potential for critique, see Hagan, *Practicing Yoga as Resistance*.

18. For a fascinating approach that also attends to language, see Matylda Ciolkosz, "The Quasi-Linguistic Structure of Iyengar Yoga Asana Practice: An Analysis from the Perspective of Cognitive Grammar," *Studia Religiologica* 47, no. 4 (2014): 263–73.

19. See, among others, Alter, *Yoga in Modern India*; Strauss, *Positioning Yoga*; Pinch, *Warrior Ascetics and Indian Empires*; Singleton, *Yoga Body*; De Michelis, *A History of Modern Yoga*; White, *Sinister Yogis*; White, *The Yoga Sutra of Patanjali*; Jain, *Selling Yoga*; Jain, *Peace Love Yoga*; Anya P. Foxen, *Biography of a Yogi: Paramahansa Yogananda and the Origins of Modern Yoga* (New Delhi: Oxford University Press, 2017); Newcombe, *Yoga in Britain*; Foxen, *Inhaling Spirit*.

20. For a diversity of texts, see White, *Yoga in Practice*; Mallinson and Singleton, *Roots of Yoga*.

21. For example, see Knut Jacobsen's analysis of allegorical narrative fictions that were used to teach yoga in early twentieth-century Bengal. Knut A. Jacobsen, *Yoga in Modern Hinduism: Hariharānanda Āraṇya and Sāṃkhyayoga* (Abingdon, UK: Routledge, 2018).

22. Singleton, *Yoga Body*, Kindle Loc 261.

23. Strauss, *Positioning Yoga*, 15–16; Srinivas Aravamudan, *Guru English: South Asian Religion in a Cosmopolitan Language* (Princeton, NJ: Princeton University Press, 2006).

24. On the history of this literary tradition, see Ulka Anjaria, ed., *A History of the Indian Novel in English* (New York: Cambridge University Press, 2015). As essays in the collection show, English has never developed in isolation from India's other languages. For an exploration of this dynamic, see Rashmi Sadana, *English Heart, Hindi Heartland: The Political Life of Literature in India* (Berkeley and Los Angeles: University of California Press, 2012).

25. Significant sociological work has been done to analyze dominant patterns that shape the mainstream representation of yoga in periodical culture and social media, especially in Western contexts. See Kristen C. Blinne, *Pop Culture Yoga: A Communication Remix* (Lanham, MD: Lexington Books, 2020); Angela Hinz et al., "Practice or Performance? A Content Analysis of Yoga-Related Videos on Instagram," *Body Image* 39 (December 2021): 175–83, https://doi.org/10.1016/j.bodyim.2021 .08.002; Angela Hinz et al., "Is This What a Female Yogi Looks Like? A Content Analysis of Yoga Images on Instagram," *Body Image* 36 (March 2021): 117–26, https://doi.org/10.1016/j.bodyim.2020.11.003; K. Alysse Bailey et al., "Is #YogaForEveryone? The Idealised Flexible Bodymind in Instagram Yoga Posts," *Qualitative Research in Sport, Exercise and Health* 14, no. 5 (2022): 827–42, https://doi.org /10.1080/2159676X.2021.2002394; Nandini Bhalla and David Moscowitz, "Yoga and Female Objectification: Commodity and Exclusionary Identity in U.S. Women's Magazines," *Journal of Communication Inquiry* 44, no. 1 (January 2020): 90–108, https://doi.org/10.1177/0196859919830357; Agi Wittich and Patrick McCartney, "Changing Face of the Yoga Industry, Its Dharmic Roots and Its Message to Women: An Analysis of *Yoga Journal* Magazine Covers, 1975–2020," *Journal of Dharma Studies* 3 (2020): 31–44, https://doi.org/10.1007/s42240-020-00071-1; Nandini Bhalla, Jane O'Boyle, and Leigh Moscowitz, "Selling Yoga 'Off the Mat': A 10-Year Analysis of Lifestyle Advertorials in *Yoga Journal* Magazine," *Journal of Communication Inquiry*, September 15, 2022, 019685992211186, https://doi.org/10 .1177/01968599221118646; Mary Grace Antony, "That's a Stretch: Reconstructing, Rearticulating, and Commodifying Yoga," *Frontiers in Communication* 3, no. 47 (October 23, 2018), https://doi.org/10.3389/fcomm.2018.00047.

26. Tessa Morris-Suzuki, "Liquid Area Studies," *positions: asia critique* 27, no. 1 (February 1, 2019): 209–39, https://doi.org/10.1215/10679847-7251897. See also Zygmunt Bauman, *Liquid Modernity* (Cambridge: Polity Press, 2000).

27. See, for instance, Sunil Khilnani, *The Idea of India* (New York: Farrar, Straus and Giroux, 1997); Ravinder Kaur, "Nation's Two Bodies: Rethinking the Idea of 'New' India and Its Other," *Third World Quarterly* 33, no. 4 (2012): 603–21; Jelle J.P. Wouters and Tanka B. Subba, "The 'Indian Face,' India's Northeast, and 'The Idea of India,'" *Asian Anthropology* 12, no. 2 (December 2013): 126–40, https://doi.org/10.1080/1683478X.2013.849484.

28. See, among others, Edward Anderson and Arkotong Longkumer, "'Neo-Hindutva': Evolving Forms, Spaces, and Expressions of Hindu Nationalism," *Contemporary South Asia* 26, no. 4 (2018): 371–77, https://doi.org/10.1080/09584935.2018.1548576; Priya Chacko, "Marketizing Hindutva: The State, Society, and Markets in Hindu Nationalism," *Modern Asian Studies* 53, no. 2 (March 2019): 377–410, https://doi.org/10.1017/S0026749X17000051; Christophe Jaffrelot, "India's Democracy at 70: Toward a Hindu State?," *Journal of Democracy* 28, no. 3 (July 2017): 52–63; Jain, *Peace Love Yoga*; Arkotong Longkumer, *The Greater India Experiment: Hindutva and the Northeast* (Stanford, CA: Stanford University Press, 2020).

29. Rumya Sree Putcha, "After *Eat, Pray, Love*: Tourism, Orientalism, and Cartographies of Salvation," *Tourist Studies* 20, no. 4 (2020): 461, https://doi.org/10.1177/1468797620946808. For demographic studies on the centrality of white women within U.S. yoga, see Crystal L. Park, Tosca Braun, and Tamar Siegel, "Who Practices Yoga? A Systematic Review of Demographic, Health-Related, and Psychosocial Factors Associated with Yoga Practice," *Journal of Behavioral Medicine* 38, no. 3 (June 2015): 460–71; Holger Cramer et al., "Prevalence, Patterns, and Predictors of Yoga Use," *American Journal of Preventive Medicine* 50, no. 2 (February 2016): 230–35, https://doi.org/10.1016/j.amepre.2015.07.037.

30. Lucia, *White Utopias*.

31. The journal *Race and Yoga* most directly addresses these questions, along with Berila, Klein, and Roberts, *Yoga, the Body, and Embodied Social Change*.

32. Jain, *Selling Yoga*; Sarah Sharma, *In the Meantime: Temporality and Cultural Politics* (Durham, NC: Duke University Press, 2014); Jain, *Peace Love Yoga*; Klepinger, *Transnational Yoga at Work*.

33. Frederick Errington, Tatsuro Fujikura, and Deborah Gewertz, *The Noodle Narratives: The Global Rise of an Industrial Food into the Twenty-First Century* (Berkeley: University of California Press, 2013), 14.

34. Satya P. Mohanty, *Literary Theory and the Claims of History: Postmodernism, Objectivity, Multicultural Politics* (Ithaca, NY: Cornell University Press, 1997), 122.

35. On the diverse approaches taken by scholar-practitioners, see Mark Singleton and Borayin Larios, "The Scholar-Practitioner of Yoga in the Western Academy," in *Routledge Handbook of Yoga and Meditation Studies*, ed. Suzanne Newcombe and Karen O'Brien-Kop (Abingdon, UK: Routledge, 2021), 37–50.

36. See Nancy Miller, *But Enough About Me: Why We Read Other People's Lives* (New York: Columbia University Press, 2002); Saidiya Hartman, *Lose Your Mother: A Journey Along the Atlantic Slave Route* (New York: Farrar, Straus and Giroux, 2008); Ann Cvetkovich, *Depression: A Public Feeling* (Durham, NC: Duke University Press, 2012);

Carrie J. Preston, *Learning to Kneel: Noh, Modernism, and Journeys in Teaching* (New York: Columbia University Press, 2016).

37. Sara Suleri, *Meatless Days* (Chicago: University of Chicago Press, 1989); Amitava Kumar, *Passport Photos* (Berkeley: University of California Press, 2000); Kirin Narayan, *My Family and Other Saints* (Chicago: University of Chicago Press, 2007); Kirin Narayan, *Everyday Creativity: Singing Goddesses in the Himalayan Foothills* (Chicago: University of Chicago Press, 2016); Siegel, *Trance-Migrations*.

38. Kirin Narayan, "Statement," in *Living in America: Poetry and Fiction by South Asian American Writers*, ed. Roshni Rustomji-Kerns (New York: Routledge, 1995), 155.

39. Siegel, *Trance-Migrations*.

40. Catherine Malabou, *The Future of Hegel: Plasticity, Temporality and Dialectic*, trans. Lisabeth During (Abingdon, UK: Routledge, 2005), 9.

41. Malabou, *The Future of Hegel*, 12.

42. Aihwa Ong, *Flexible Citizenship: The Cultural Logics of Transnationality* (Durham, NC: Duke University Press, 1999), 6.

43. Aihwa Ong, "(Re)Articulations of Citizenship," *PS: Political Science and Politics* 38, no. 4 (October 2005): 697.

44. Bauman, *Liquid Modernity*.

45. Ravinder Kaur, *Brand New Nation: Capitalist Dreams and Nationalist Designs in Twenty-First-Century India* (Stanford, CA: Stanford University Press, 2020), 8.

46. Dhooleka Sarhadi Raj, "The Overseas Citizen of India and Emigrant Infrastructure: Tracing the Deterritorializations of Diaspora Strategies," *Geoforum* 59 (February 2015): 159–68, https://doi.org/10.1016/j.geoforum.2014.11.015. On the broader complexities raised through identity documents in a South Asian context, see Vasudha Chhotray and Fiona McConnell, "Certifications of Citizenship: The History, Politics and Materiality of Identity Documents in South Asian States and Diasporas," *Contemporary South Asia* 26, no. 2 (2018): 111–26, https://doi.org/10.1080/09584935.2018.1471042.

47. Purnima Mankekar, *Unsettling India: Affect, Temporality, Transnationality* (Durham, NC: Duke University Press, 2015), 18.

48. Mankekar, *Unsettling India*, 5.

49. Amit S. Rai, *Jugaad Time: Ecologies of Everyday Hacking in India* (Durham, NC: Duke University Press, 2019), 2.

50. Navi Radjou et al., *Jugaad Innovation: Think Frugal, Be Flexible, Generate Breakthrough Growth* (Hoboken: Wiley, 2012), 4, 86.

51. Marta Rohatynskyj, "Empowering the Dividual," *Anthropological Theory* 15, no. 3 (September 2015): 317–37, https://doi.org/10.1177/1463499615570919.

52. Assa Doron, "Mobile Persons: Cell Phones, Gender and the Self in North India," *The Asia Pacific Journal of Anthropology* 13, no. 5 (2012): 417.

53. See, for instance, Udeni M. H. Appuhamilage, "A Fluid Ambiguity: Individual, Dividual and Personhood," *The Asia Pacific Journal of Anthropology* 18, no. 1 (January 1, 2017): 1–17, https://doi.org/10.1080/14442213.2016.1249020; Nayanika Mookherjee, "Introduction: Self in South Asia," *Journal of Historical Sociology* 26, no. 1 (March 2013): 1–18, https://doi.org/10.1111/johs.12008.

54. "Review: Memoir of the Late Major Antony Bumble, of the Bengal Army. By John William Braye. London: 1867," *The Pioneer*, May 10, 1867, 3.

55. "Tamar Indien," *The Pioneer*, November 12, 1877, 10.

56. Alter, *Yoga in Modern India*; Singleton, *Yoga Body*; Suzanne Newcombe, "Stretching for Health and Well-Being: Yoga and Women in Britain, 1960–1980," *Asian Medicine* 3, no. 1 (October 16, 2007): 37–63, https://doi.org/10.1163/157342107X207209; Alison Shaw and Esra S. Kaytaz, "Yoga Bodies, Yoga Minds: Contextualising the Health Discourses and Practices of Modern Postural Yoga," *Anthropology & Medicine* 28, no. 3 (2021): 279–96, https://doi.org/10.1080/13648470.2021.1949943; Foxen, *Inhaling Spirit*.

57. Singleton, *Yoga Body*, Kindle Loc 3085.

58. "Live on the Floor," *The Leader*, August 25, 1921, 11.

59. Shari L. Dworkin and Faye Linda Wachs, *Body Panic: Gender, Health and the Selling of Fitness* (New York: New York University Press, 2009), 109.

60. Christiane Brosius, *India's Middle Class: New Forms of Urban Leisure, Consumption and Prosperity* (Abingdon, UK: Routledge, 2010), 307.

61. "PM Narendra Modi Launches 'Fit India Movement,'" *Money Control*, August 29, 2019, https://www.moneycontrol.com/news/india/pm-narendra-modi-to-launch-fit-india-movement-at-10-am-where-to-watch-live-4383891.html.

62. For a more detailed account of *svādhyāya* as a remixed approach to yogic style, see Shameem Black, "Yogic Style in Motion: Experiments in Power and Knowledge," *Textual Practice* 36, no. 4 (2022): 605–25.

63. Ichiyo Muto, "Asia, Inter-Asia, and Movement: Decolonization into the Future," *Inter-Asia Cultural Studies* 11, no. 2 (2010): 179.

64. Dipesh Chakrabarty, *Provincializing Europe: Postcolonial Thought and Historical Difference* (Princeton, NJ: Princeton University Press, 2000).

65. On the complex nature of categories used to articulate indigenous rights and identities in India, see Bengt G. Karlsson, "The Social Life of Categories," *Focaal-Journal of Global and Historical Anthropology* 65 (2013): 33–41, https://doi.org/10.3167/fcl.2013.650104.

66. IP Singh and Siddhartha Sarma, "'Ravana's Airports,' 'Modi Waves' Leave Science Congress Stunned,'" *The Times of India*, January 6, 2019, https://timesofindia.indiatimes.com/india/ravanas-airports-modi-waves-leave-science-congress-stunned/articleshow/67402208.cms.

67. Suhas Palshikar, "The BJP and Hindu Nationalism: Centrist Politics and Majoritarian Impulses," *South Asia: Journal of South Asian Studies* 38, no. 4 (2015): 719, https://doi.org/10.1080/00856401.2015.1089460.

68. Daniel Heifetz, "Religion, Science, and the Middle Class in the All World Gayatri Pariwar," *International Journal of Hindu Studies* 23, no. 1 (April 2019): 32, https://doi.org/10.1007/s11407-019-09249-0.

69. Bhuvi Gupta and Jacob Copeman, "Awakening Hindu Nationalism through Yoga: Swami Ramdev and the Bharat Swabhiman Movement," *Contemporary South Asia* 27, no. 3 (2019): 313–29, https://doi.org/10.1080/09584935.2019.1587386; Arkotong Longkumer, "'Nagas Can't Sit Lotus Style': Baba Ramdev, Patanjali, and Neo-Hindutva,"

Contemporary South Asia 26, no. 4 (2018): 400–20, https://doi.org/10.1080/09584935 .2018.1545008; Jain, *Peace Love Yoga.*

70. On this direction, see Shameem Black, "Decolonising Yoga," in *Routledge Handbook of Yoga and Meditation Studies*, ed. Suzanne Newcombe and Karen O'Brien-Kop (Abingdon, UK: Routledge, 2021), 13–21.

71. Patrick McCartney, "Jhirī: A 'Sanskrit-Speaking' Village in Madhya Pradesh," *Journal of South Asian Languages and Linguistics* 4, no. 2 (2017): 167–209.

72. Prachi Patankar, "Ghosts of Yogas Past and Present," *Jadaliyya*, February 26, 2014, http://www.jadaliyya.com/Details/30281/Ghosts-of-Yogas-Past-and-Present.

73. Longkumer, *The Greater India Experiment*, 54.

74. "Whose Yoga Is It Anyway?," *Tehelka*, June 21, 2016.

75. Bharatiya Janata Party, *Toward Ram Rajya* (New Delhi: Bharatiya Janata Party, 1991).

76. Amish, *The Immortals of Meluha* (Chennai: Westland Publications, 2008), 35.

77. Gold, "The Hindi Sants' Two Yogic Paths to the Formless Lord," 131–32.

78. Veena Howard, "Divine Light and Melodies Lead the Way: The Santmat Tradition of Bihar," *Religions* 10, no. 4 (2019): 230, https://doi.org/10.3390/rel10040230.

79. "The awareness that these Sants brought to a society struggling against superstition and suppression," Sthanewshwar Timalsina argues, "demonstrates the wider social application of Yoga, with language as an important tool in individual and social transformation. . . . Most significantly, the instruction that liberation cannot dawn in the absence of social justice is a principle [they] observe in their personal lives." Sthaneshwar Timalsina, "Songs of Transformation: Vernacular Josmani Literature and the Yoga of Cosmic Awareness," *International Journal of Hindu Studies* 14, no. 2–3 (December 2010): 218, 219, https://doi.org/10.1007/s11407-011-9091-x.

80. Peter Friedlander, "Reassessing Religion and Politics in the Life of Jagjivan Rām," *Religions* 11, no. 5 (May 1, 2020): 224, https://doi.org/10.3390/rel11050224.

81. Borayin Larios, "The Vedamūrti: Embodying the Veda in Contemporary Maharashtra," *International Journal of Hindu Studies* 17, no. 3 (December 2013): 291, https://doi .org/10.1007/s11407-014-9141-2.

82. Dermot Killingly, "Svādhyāya: An Ancient Way of Using the Veda," *Religions of South Asia* 8, no. 1 (August 22, 2014): 112, https://doi.org/10.1558/rosa.v8i1.109.

83. Philipp A. Maas, " 'Sthirasukham Āsanam': Posture and Performance in Classical Yoga and Beyond," in *Yoga in Transformation: Historical and Contemporary Perspectives*, ed. Karl Baier, Philipp A. Maas, and Karin Preisendanz (Vienna: Vienna University Press, 2018), 52.

84. Mallinson and Singleton, *Roots of Yoga*, xvi, 84.

85. Larios, "The Vedamūrti," 291.

86. *Annual Report of the Mysore Archaeological Department for the Year 1929 with the Government Review Thereon* (Bangalore: Government Press, 1931), 120.

87. Asiya Bibi, "Abul Fazl's Comparative Study of Hindu Culture: An Analysis,'" *Journal of Asian Civilizations* 39, no. 1 (2016): 141, 153.

88. Audrey Truschke, *Culture of Encounters: Sanskrit at the Mughal Court* (New York: Columbia University Press, 2016), 165.

89. On Iyengar's life, see Rashmi Palkhivala, *A Life of Light: The Biography of B.K.S. Iyen-gar* (Noida, Uttar Pradesh: Harper Element, 2017); Julia Pedersen, ed., *Guruji BKS Iyengar and His Institute in the '70s* (London: YogaWords, 2020).

90. De Michelis, *A History of Modern Yoga*, 208–10.

91. Andrea R. Jain, "Branding Yoga: The Cases of Iyengar Yoga, Siddha Yoga and Anu-sara Yoga," *Approaching Religion* 2, no. 2 (December 2012): 3–17.

92. Palkhivala, *A Life of Light*.

93. B.K.S. Iyengar, *Light on Yoga: Yoga Dipika*, rev. ed. (New York: Schocken Books, 1966), 38.

94. On late colonial articulations of "East-West" syncretism in print culture, see Tanya Agathocleous, "'The Coming Clash of East and West': Syncretism, Cosmopolitanism, and Disaffection in the Colonial Public Sphere," *Textual Practice* 31, no. 4 (June 7, 2017): 661–85, https://doi.org/10.1080/0950236X.2016.1189454.

95. Shameem Black, "Yoga by the Book," *Contemporary South Asia* 28, no. 1 (2020): 15–27, https://doi.org/10.1080/09584935.2019.1666091. Gerald Yorke, editor at Allen and Unwin, also played an important role in shaping the English of the volume. Suzanne Newcombe and Philip Deslippe, "Anglophone Yoga and Meditation Outside of India," in *Routledge Handbook of Yoga and Meditation Studies* (Abingdon, UK: Routledge, 2021), 356; Palkhivala, *A Life of Light*.

96. Iyengar, *Light on Yoga*, 39.

97. For a portrait of Vinoba Bhave's movement, see Arthur Koestler, "Last of the Saints," *Commentary*, February 1960.

98. Candace Brunette-Debassige, "From Subjugation to Embodied Self-in-Relation: An Indigenous Pedagogy for Decolonization," in *Sharing Breath: Embodied Learning and Decolonization*, ed. Sheila Batacharya and Yuk-Lin Renita Wong (Edmonton, AB: Athabasca University Press, 2018), 204.

99. Dianne Bondy, "Yoga, Race and Culture," *Yoga International*, n.d., https://yoga international.com/article/view/yoga-race-and-culture.

100. Evelyn B. Tribble and John Sutton, "Minds in and out of Time: Memory, Embodied Skill, Anachronism, and Performance," *Textual Practice* 26, no. 4 (August 2012): 592, https://doi.org/10.1080/0950236X.2012.696485.

101. Benjamin Richard Smith, "Body, Mind and Spirit? Towards an Analysis of the Prac-tice of Yoga," *Body & Society* 13, no. 2 (June 2007): 32, https://doi.org/10.1177/1357 034X07077771.

102. Oren Ergas, "Overcoming the Philosophy/Life, Body/Mind Rift: Demonstrating Yoga as Embodied-Lived-Philosophical-Practice," *Educational Philosophy and Theory* 46, no. 1 (January 2, 2014): 74–86, https://doi.org/10.1111/j.1469-5812.2011.00811.x.

103. Feminist analytical and methodological critiques of depersonalized and disembodied voice claim a long history within scholarship, yet major scholarly conventions con-tinue to make it challenging to incorporate such critique. See, for instance, feminist reflections on embodied experience within new scholarship in Judith Gill et al., "The-sis Writing as a Feminist Project: Negotiating Space for Women's Embodied Selves in New Scholarship," *Australian Feminist Studies* 23, no. 56 (June 2008): 249–61, https://doi.org/10.1080/08164640802068443.

104. Kirin Narayan, "Refractions of the Field at Home: American Representations of Hindu Holy Men in the 19th and 20th Centuries," *Cultural Anthropology* 8, no. 4 (November 1993): 476–509; White, *Sinister Yogis*; David N. Lorenzen and Adrian Munoz, eds., *Yogi Heroes and Poets: Histories and Legends of the Naths* (Albany: State University of New York Press, 2011); Siegel, *Trance-Migrations*.

105. Farah Godrej, "The Neoliberal Yogi and the Politics of Yoga," *Political Theory* 45, no. 6 (2017): 772–800.

106. On this broader world, see Ketaki Pant, "A Poet's Ocean: Merchants and Imagination across Indian Ocean Gujarat," *South Asia: Journal of South Asian Studies* 44, no. 4 (2021): 684–702, https://doi.org/10.1080/00856401.2021.1939104.

107. Peter Morey and Amina Yaqin, *Framing Muslims: Stereotyping and Representation After 9/11* (Cambridge, MA: Harvard University Press, 2011), 22.

108. Elizabeth Kadetsky, *First There Is a Mountain* (Westland, MI: Dzanc Books, 2011), Kindle Loc 1649.

109. Still and video images on social media show idealized bodies that often refract dominant social norms. Hinz et al., "Practice or Performance?"

110. K. S. Joshi, "On the Meaning of Yoga," *Philosophy East and West* 15, no. 1 (January 1965): 53.

2. CONDUCTING MASS PRACTICE

1. In 2003 the Department of Indian Systems of Medicine and Homeopathy was renamed the Department of Ayurveda, Yoga and Naturopathy, Unani, Siddha and Homeopathy.

2. "PM's Remarks at Presentation of Kabir Puraskar and National Communal Harmony Awards," Former Prime Minister of India Dr. Manmohan Singh, May 1, 2006, https://archivepmo.nic.in/drmanmohansingh/speech-details.php?nodeid=318.

3. Akhil Gupta, *Red Tape* (Durham, NC: Duke University Press, 2012), 143. See also Matthew Hull, *Government of Paper: The Materiality of Bureaucracy in Urban Pakistan* (Berkeley and Los Angeles: University of California Press, 2012).

4. Gauri Kartini Shastry, "Human Capital Response to Globalization: Education and Information Technology in India," *Journal of Human Resources* 47, no. 2 (2012): 294. Shastry notes that India's information technology sector, for instance, requires English proficiency.

5. Andrea R. Jain, *Peace Love Yoga: The Politics of Global Spirituality* (New York: Oxford University Press, 2020), 131.

6. David Gordon White's *Sinister Yogis* (Chicago: University of Chicago Press, 2009) shows that practitioners of yoga in folklore across India's many languages were often spies in the pay of kings.

7. William R. Pinch, *Warrior Ascetics and Indian Empires* (Cambridge: Cambridge University Press, 2006).

8. Christophe Jaffrelot, "The Story of Indian Politicians and Tantrics," Carnegie Endowment for International Peace, November 7, 2015, https://carnegieendowment.org /2015/11/07/story-of-indian-politicians-and-tantrics-pub-61928.

9. See, among many others, Elizabeth De Michelis, *A History of Modern Yoga: Patanjali and Western Esotericism* (London and New York: Continuum, 2004); Joseph S. Alter, *Yoga in Modern India: The Body Between Science and Philosophy* (Princeton and Oxford: Princeton University Press, 2004); Mark Singleton, *Yoga Body: The Origins of Modern Posture Practice* (New York: Oxford University Press, 2010).

10. Geoffrey Samuel, *The Origins of Yoga and Tantra: Indic Religions to the Thirteenth Century* (Cambridge: Cambridge University Press, 2008); Patton E. Burchett, *A Genealogy of Devotion: Bhakti, Tantra, Yoga, and Sufism in North India* (New York: Columbia University Press, 2019).

11. Dipesh Chakrabarty and Rochona Majumdar, "Gandhi's Gita and Politics As Such," *Modern Intellectual History* 7, no. 2 (August 2010): 341, https://doi.org/10.1017 /S1479244310000107.

12. Joseph S. Alter, *Gandhi's Body: Sex, Diet, and the Politics of Nationalism* (Philadelphia: University of Pennsylvania Press, 2000), 19.

13. Joseph S. Alter, "Body, Text, Nation: Writing the Physically Fit Body in Post-Colonial India," in *Confronting the Body: The Politics of Physicality in Colonial and Post-Colonial India*, ed. James H. Mills and Satadru Sen (London: Anthem, 2004), 17.

14. Andrew Bingham Kennedy, *The International Ambitions of Mao and Nehru: National Efficacy Beliefs and the Making of Foreign Policy* (New York: Cambridge University Press, 2012), 142.

15. Kadira Pethyagoda argues, for instance, that India's reputation as "non-violent" with a "benign international influence" facilitates material deals, such as Australia's 2014 decision to sell India uranium. Kadira Pethiyagoda, "India's Soft Power Advantage," *Australia India Institute* (blog), November 4, 2014, http://www.aii.unimelb.edu.au /news/blog/india%E2%80%99s-soft-power-advantage. This reputation is presumably not the sole cause of such decisions. Australia-India trade in goods jumped dramatically from almost $11 billion AUD in 2007–08 to almost $18 billion AUD in 2010–11 and $27.5 billion AUD in 2017. However, this reputation allows advocates for India to justify and legitimate India's growing global role.

16. Sarah Strauss, *Positioning Yoga: Balancing Acts Across Cultures* (Oxford: Berg, 2005).

17. Robert Love, *The Great Oom: The Mysterious Origins of America's First Yogi* (New York: Penguin, 2010); Anya P. Foxen, *Biography of a Yogi: Paramahansa Yogananda and the Origins of Modern Yoga* (New Delhi: Oxford University Press, 2017).

18. Suzanne Newcombe, *Yoga in Britain: Stretching Spirituality and Educating Yogis* (Sheffield, UK: Equinox, 2019).

19. Andrea R. Jain, *Selling Yoga: From Counterculture to Pop Culture* (New York: Oxford University Press, 2014), Kindle Loc 778; Singleton, *Yoga Body*.

20. Srinivas Aravamudan, *Guru English: South Asian Religion in a Cosmopolitan Language* (Princeton, NJ: Princeton University Press, 2006), 194, 203; Bhavdeep Kang,

"Indira and the 'Indian Rasputin,'" *The Asian Age*, June 6, 2016, https://www.asianage .com/books/indira-and-indian-rasputin-604; Kirin Narayan, "Refractions of the Field at Home: American Representations of Hindu Holy Men in the 19th and 20th Centuries," *Cultural Anthropology* 8, no. 4 (November 1993): 476–509.

21. Peter van der Veer, "Global Breathing: Religious Utopias in India and China," *Anthropological Theory* 7, no. 3 (September 2007): 324, https://doi.org/10.1177/146 3499607080193.

22. Raphaël Voix, "Hindu Ascetics and the Political in Contemporary India," in *Routledge Handbook of Yoga and Meditation Studies*, ed. Suzanne Newcombe and Karen O'Brien-Kop (Abingdon, UK: Routledge, 2021), 152.

23. Joseph S. Alter, "Pahalwan Baba Ramdev: Wrestling with Yoga and Middle-Class Masculinity in India," *Modern Asian Studies* 55, no. 4 (July 2021): 1360.

24. Chandrima Chakraborty, "The Hindu Ascetic as Fitness Instructor: Reviving Faith in Yoga," *The International Journal of the History of Sport* 24, no. 9 (2007): 1184.

25. Jain, *Peace Love Yoga*.

26. Arkotong Longkumer, "'Nagas Can't Sit Lotus Style': Baba Ramdev, Patanjali, and Neo-Hindutva," *Contemporary South Asia* 26, no. 4 (2018): 401, https://doi.org/10.1080 /09584935.2018.1545008.

27. "Our Five National Movement," Bharat Swabhiman, n.d., http://bharatswabhiman trust.org/ReadMore.aspx?ContentType=Bharat%20Swabhiman%20details&Con tentID=28.

28. Ramdev quoted in Harmony Siganporia, "Who Dreams This Dreaming? Patanjali's Symbolic Usurpation of the Trope of the 'Enslaved' Indian Economy," *Continuum* 32, no. 6 (November 2, 2018): 762, https://doi.org/10.1080/10304312.2018.1525926.

29. Venera R. Khalikova, "The Ayurveda of Baba Ramdev: Biomoral Consumerism, National Duty and the Biopolitics of 'Homegrown' Medicine in India," *South Asia: Journal of South Asian Studies* 40, no. 1 (2017): 109, https://doi.org/10.1080/00856401 .2017.1266987.

30. Jyotirmaya Tripathy, "Consuming Indigeneity: Baba Ramdev, Patanjali Ayurveda and the Swadeshi Project of Development," *Journal of Developing Societies* 35, no. 3 (September 2019): 414, https://doi.org/10.1177/0169796X19873213.

31. Manisha Pande, "BJP Does Shirshasana over Ramdev Remark: Yoga Guru's Distasteful Anti-Dalit Remarks May Harm Party's Cause," *DNA: Daily News and Analysis*, May 3, 2014.

32. Priyanka Rawal, "Indian Monk Who Wants a Billion-Dollar Company: A Yogic Business Revolution," *International Journal of Management Research and Review* 6, no. 9 (September 2016): 1170; Jain, *Peace Love Yoga*, 77–78.

33. Suzanne Newcombe, "Yoga and Meditation as a Health Intervention," in *Routledge Handbook of Yoga and Meditation Studies*, ed. Suzanne Newcombe and Karen O'Brien-Kop (Abingdon, UK: Routledge, 2021), 158.

34. "DRDO Ties up with Ramdev to Market Supplements, Food Products," *The Times of India*, August 23, 2015, http://timesofindia.indiatimes.com/india/DRDO-ties-up-with -Ramdev-to-market-supplements-food-products/articleshow/48643649.cms.

35. Pragati Ratti Sharma, "Yoga: A Multi-Billion Dollar Opportunity Market Poised to Grow," Wellness India.com, November 21, 2016, http://www.franchiseindia.com /wellness/Yoga-A-multi-billion-dollar-opportunity-market-poised-to-grow.8983. In the United States alone, spending in 2016 was estimated at USD$16 billion. Ipsos Public Affairs, "The 2016 Yoga in America Study Conducted by Yoga Journal and Yoga Alliance," January 2016, 4, https://www.yogaalliance.org/2016yogainamericastudy.

36. Susannah Myrtle Lazarus, "Meet Sarvesh Shashi, India's New Millionaire Yogi," *The Hindu*, May 10, 2019, https://www.thehindu.com/society/meet-27-year-old-sarvesh -shashi-indias-new-millionaire-yogi/article27094190.ece.

37. Government of India, "Income-Tax Act, 1961–2016" (2016), http://www.incometaxindia .gov.in/pages/acts/income-tax-act.aspx.

38. Lubna Kablyl, "Ramdev Trust Wins I-T War on Tax-Exempt Tag for Yoga," *The Times of India*, February 18, 2017, http://timesofindia.indiatimes.com/business /india-business/ramdev-trust-wins-i-t-war-on-tax-exempt-tag-for-yoga /articleshow/57215759.cms.

39. Pankaj Jalote, Bijendra Nath Jain, and Sudhir Sopory, "Classification for Research Universities in India," *Higher Education* 79, no. 2 (February 2020): 227, https://doi.org /10.1007/s10734-019-00406-3.

40. Meera Nanda, *The God Market: How Globalization Is Making India More Hindu* (New York: Monthly Review Press, 2009), 119.

41. "Swami Vivekananda Yoga Anusandhana Samsthana—S-VYASA," S-VYASA Swami Vivekandanda Yoga Anusandhana Samsthana, accessed May 16, 2019, https://svyasa .edu.in/#.

42. Nanda, *The God Market*, 126.

43. Puja Pednekar, "Patanjali to Hold Monthly Yoga Sessions in Schools," *Hindustan Times*, August 19, 2016, https://www.hindustantimes.com/cities/patanjali-to-hold -monthly-yoga-sessions-in-schools/story-XQk2gHzWRhKBepB4CNzd2I.html.

44. Central Board of Secondary Education, quoted in Neelam Pandey, "CBSE Students Will Earn Grades in Class 10 by Doing Yoga, Showing Patriotism," *Hindustan Times*, February 1, 2017, https://www.hindustantimes.com/education/cbse-students-will -earn-grades-in-class-10-by-practising-yoga-showing-patriotism/story-990rKCg mqP6X1rtLOx6RQJ.html.

45. Ritika Chopra, "Panel Picks Patanjali, Ramdev Likely to Head First Vedic Board," *The Indian Express* (blog), February 25, 2019, https://indianexpress.com/article /education/baba-ramdev-likely-to-head-first-vedic-board-patanjali-5599448/.

46. In May 2016, the Indian Ministry of Human Resource Development requested that all states make yoga compulsory in schools. "Yoga to Be Made Compulsory in Schools," *DNA: Daily News and Analysis*, May 6, 2016, http://www.dnaindia.com /india/report-yoga-to-be-made-compulsory-in-schools-govt-2209866.

47. Jain, *Selling Yoga*.

48. Susan (Sixue) Jia, "Leisure Motivation and Satisfaction: A Text Mining of Yoga Centres, Yoga Consumers, and Their Interactions," *Sustainability* 10, no. 12 (November 27, 2018): 4458, https://doi.org/10.3390/su10124458.

49. Peter Martin, "Yoga Diplomacy: Narendra Modi's Soft Power Strategy," *Foreign Affairs*, January 25, 2015, http://www.foreignaffairs.com/articles/142812/peter-martin /yoga-diplomacy.

50. Ian Hall, "India's New Public Diplomacy: Soft Power and the Limits of Government Action," *Asian Survey* 52, no. 6 (December 2012): 1107.

51. Ravinder Kaur, "'I Am India Shining': The Investor-Citizen and the Indelible Icon of Good Times," *The Journal of Asian Studies* 75, no. 3 (August 2016): 629, https://doi .org/10.1017/S0021911816000619.

52. Ravinder Kaur, *Brand New Nation: Capitalist Dreams and Nationalist Designs in Twenty-First-Century India* (Stanford, CA: Stanford University Press, 2020), 13.

53. David Geary, "Incredible India in a Global Age: The Cultural Politics of Image Branding in Tourism," *Tourist Studies* 13, no. 1 (2013): 37; Vrushali Patil, "Reproducing-Resisting Race and Gender Difference: Examining India's Online Tourism Campaign from a Transnational Feminist Perspective," *Signs: Journal of Women in Culture and Society* 37, no. 1 (September 2011): 204.

54. "Discover True Wellness with Tailor-Made Yoga Tours in India," *Guided Tours India*, accessed January 2, 2023, http://guidedtoursindia.blogspot.com/2014/12/Discover -True-Wellness-with-Tailor-Made-Yoga-Tours-in-India.html.

55. Interview by the author, November 2018.

56. Interview by the author.

57. "Prathap Suthan, NCD, Cheil India," *Desi Creative* (blog), September 7, 2010, http:// www.desicreative.com/prathap-suthan-ncd-cheil-india/.

58. For images, see Grey Worldwide India, *Ministry of Tourism India—"Yoga 4,"* 2006, https://www.adforum.com/talent/6697276-prathap-suthan/work/6686093; Grey Worldwide India, *Yoga*, 2006, https://www.adforum.com/creative-work/ad/player /6686100/yoga/ministry-of-tourism-india; Grey Worldwide India, *Yoga 2*, 2006, https://www.adforum.com/creative-work/ad/player/6686091/yoga-2/ministry-of -tourism-india.

59. Grey Worldwide India, *Yoga*.

60. Grey Worldwide India, *Yoga Microsite*, 2006, https://www.adforum.com/creative -work/ad/player/6686099/yoga-microsite/ministry-of-tourism-india.

61. Samuel, *The Origins of Yoga and Tantra*, 3–8.

62. Manjari Chatterjee Miller and Kate Sullivan de Estrada, "Pragmatism in Indian Foreign Policy: How Ideas Constrain Modi," *International Affairs* 93, no. 1 (2017): 37.

63. Swati Mathur, "Incredible India 2.0 to Take a Spiritual Bent," *The Times of India*, June 21, 2017, http://timesofindia.indiatimes.com/india/incredible-india-2-0-to -take-a-spiritual-bent/articleshow/59243906.cms.

64. The UN Convention on Biological Diversity includes under Article 8(j) the obligation to "respect, preserve and maintain knowledge, innovations and practices of indigenous and local communities embodying traditional lifestyles relevant for the conservation and sustainable use of biological diversity." United Nations, "Convention on Biological Diversity" (1992), 6, https://treaties.un.org/doc/Treaties/1992/06 /19920605%2008-44%20 p.m./Ch_XXVII_08p.pdf. Placed alongside the respect for

cultural practices established through the 1948 Universal Declaration on Human Rights and the 1966 International Covenant on Economic, Social and Cultural Rights, "traditional knowledge" is understood to contribute to the cultural vitality of its traditional owners. David R. Downes, "How Intellectual Property Could Be a Tool to Protect Traditional Knowledge," *Columbia Journal of Environmental Law* 25 (2000): 254n2; 255n7.

65. Downes, "How Intellectual Property Could Be a Tool to Protect Traditional Knowledge," 278.

66. Jean-Paul Gaudilliere, "An Indian Path to Biocapital? The Traditional Knowledge Digital Library, Drug Patents, and the Reformulation Regime of Contemporary Ayurveda," *East Asian Science, Technology and Society: An International Journal* 8 (2014): 399.

67. Pradip N. Thomas, "Traditional Knowledge and the Traditional Knowledge Digital Library: Digital Quandries and Other Concerns," *The International Communication Gazette* 72, no. 8 (2010): 663.

68. V. K. Gupta, "Protecting India's Traditional Knowledge," *WIPO Magazine*, June 2011, http://www.wipo.int/wipo_magazine/en/2011/03/article_0002.html.

69. Mohd Shoaib Ansari, "Evaluation of Role of Traditional Knowledge Digital Library and Traditional Chinese Medicine Database in Preservation of Traditional Medicinal Knowledge," *DESIDOC Journal of Library and Information Technology* 36, no. 2 (March 2016): 75.

70. Allison Fish, "The Commodification and Exchange of Knowledge in the Case of Transnational Commercial Yoga," *International Journal of Cultural Property* 13, no. 2 (2006): 200.

71. Allison Fish, "Authorizing Yoga: The Pragmatics of Cultural Stewardship in the Digital Era," *East Asian Science, Technology and Society: An International Journal* 8, no. 4 (2014): 457.

72. "Traditional Knowledge and Traditional Medicine," World Trade Organization, n.d., https://www.wto.org/english/tratop_e/trips_e/trilatweb_e/ch2d_trilat_web_13_e.htm.

73. Most prominent among these has been the attempts of Bikram Choudhury to copyright the specific sequence of poses and conditions of practice (rooms heated to specific temperatures) in the United States.

74. "Siddha at a Glance," Traditional Knowledge Digital Library, accessed January 31, 2023, http://www.tkdl.res.in/tkdl/langdefault/Siddha/Sid_Siddha-Glance.asp?GL=Eng.

75. David Gordon White, *The Alchemical Body: Siddha Traditions in Medieval India* (Chicago: University of Chicago Press, 1996), 2–3. On the complex relation between siddha medicine and yoga in the context of health, see Newcombe, "Yoga and Meditation as a Health Intervention," 161.

76. Christèle Barois, Suzanne Newcombe, and Dagmar Wujastyk, "Introduction to The Usman Report (1923): Translations of Regional Submissions," *EJournal of Indian Medicine* Supplement 4 (n.d.): xxi, https://doi.org/10.21827/61e814114457b. Siddha was

sometimes presented in a syncretic relation to Sanskrit traditions of medicine, such as Ayurveda, but it was also, as Richard Weiss shows, used to construct a distinctive Tamil identity in the context of Tamil revivalism. See Richard S. Weiss, *Recipes for Immortality: Healing, Religion, and Community in South India* (New York: Oxford University Press, 2009).

77. White, *The Alchemical Body*, 347.

78. White, 346–47.

79. "United Nations A/Res/69/131" (2014), http://undocs.org/A/RES/69/131.

80. van der Veer, "Global Breathing," 315.

81. For an analysis of this dynamic as it shapes different elements of India's nation branding, see Shameem Black, "State Spectacles of Yoga: Invisible India and India Everywhere," *South Asia: Journal of South Asian Studies* 46, no. 1 (2023): 1–17,https://doi.org /10.1080/00856401.2023.2135847.

82. V. Ravi Kumar, *Yoga: Bharat's Invaluable Gift to the World* (New Delhi: Niyogi Books, 2015).

83. For example, a paragraph on yoga's popularity declaring that "Justice Sandra Day O'Connor and 15 others faithfully take their class each Tuesday morning" is taken without attribution from a 2001 *Time* magazine article. See Richard Corliss, "The Power of Yoga," *Time*, April 15, 2001, http://content.time.com/time/health/article /0,8599,106356,00.html.

84. Kumar, *Yoga*, 173.

85. Author's note, Kumar, 15.

86. Marcel Mauss, *The Gift: Forms and Functions of Exchange in Archaic Societies*, trans. Ian Cunnison (London: Cohen & West Ltd, 1969), 1.

87. Daniele Conversi, "Irresponsible Radicalisation: Diasporas, Globalisation and Long-Distance Nationalism in the Digital Age," *Journal of Ethnic and Migration Studies* 38, no. 9 (2012): 1368–70.

88. Press Information Bureau, Government of India, "Ministry of AYUSH and WHO Working Group Meeting on Benchmarks for Training in Yoga from Today," February 26, 2019, http://pib.nic.in/newsite/PrintRelease.aspx?relid=188950.

89. "BJP Becomes Largest Political Party in the World," *The Times of India*, March 30, 2015, http://timesofindia.indiatimes.com/india/BJP-becomes-largest-political-party -in-the-world/articleshow/46739025.cms.

90. Seetha Lakshmi, "Yoga Must Be Proof-Based to Be Popular: PM Narendra Modi's Guru," *The Times of India*, December 20, 2016, http://timesofindia.indiatimes.com /city/bengaluru/yoga-must-be-proof-based-to-be-popular-pm-narendra-modis -guru/articleshow/56072050.cms; Ellen Barry, "Prime Minister Modi's Yoga Consultant, H.R. Nagendra," *The New York Times*, June 15, 2015, http://www.nytimes.com /2015/06/16/world/asia/prime-minister-modis-yoga-consultant-hr-nagendra.html ?partner=bloomberg.

91. Christophe Jaffrelot, "Narendra Modi between Hindutva and Subnationalism: The Gujarati Asmita of a Hindu Hriday Samrat," *India Review* 15, no. 2 (2016): 196.

92. Celia W. Dugger, "Religious Riots Loom Over Indian Politics," *The New York Times*, July 27, 2002, http://www.nytimes.com/2002/07/27/international/asia/27INDI.html.

93. Ashis Nandy, "Obituary of a Culture," *Seminar*, May 2002, http://www.india-seminar .com/2002/513/513%20ashis%20nandy.htm.

94. Suguna Ramanathan, "Ordeal by Fire," *Seminar*, May 2002, http://www.india-seminar .com/2002/513/513%20suguna%20ramanathan.htm.

95. Outlook Web Desk, "PM Modi Gets Clean Chit From SC In 2002 Gujarat Riots Case: A Timeline Of Events," *Outlook*, June 24, 2022, https://www.outlookindia.com /national/pm-modi-gets-clean-chit-in-2002-gujarat-riots-case-a-timeline-of -events-news-204382.

96. Outlook Web Desk, "'The Modi Question:' India Slams BBC Documentary On PM Modi And 2002 Gujarat Riots, Calls It 'Propaganda Piece,'" *Outlook*, January 19, 2023, https://www.outlookindia.com/national/-a-propaganda-piece-india-slams-bbc -documentary-on-pm-modi-and-2002-gujarat-riots-youtube-takes-down-video -news-255000.

97. Alyssa Ayres, *Our Time Has Come: How India Is Making Its Place in the World* (New York: Oxford University Press, 2018), 123.

98. Asoke Mukerji, "Revealed: The Diplomatic Moves That Delivered Modi His Yoga Day," *The Wire* (blog), June 21, 2016, http://thewire.in/44205/revealed-the-diplomatic -moves-that-delivered-modi-his-yoga-day/.

99. Anusha Lakshmi, "Choreographing Tolerance: Narendra Modi, Hindu Nationalism, and International Yoga Day," *Race and Yoga* 5, no. 1 (2020): 44.

100. Jain, *Peace Love Yoga*, 131–56; Sunila S. Kale and Christian Lee Novetske, "Some Reflections on Yoga as Political Theology," *The Wire*, January 28, 2016, https://thewire .in/culture/some-reflections-on-yoga-as-political-theology. This political work has also had an impact beyond India. See, for example, analyses of mass yoga in Kajal Nisha Patel, "White Womanhood, Hindutva and Spiritual Bypass: Museum Yoga and the Mass-Participation Spectacle," *The Jugaad Project* 5, no. 1 (2023), www.thejugaad project.pub/museum-yoga.

101. Amit Chaturvedi, "On International Yoga Day, PM Modi to Join 35,000 People at Raj-path," NDTV, June 21, 2015, http://www.ndtv.com/cheat-sheet/stage-set-for-inter national-yoga-day-pm-modi-to-join-35-000-people-at-rajpath-773691.

102. See, for instance, "International Day of Yoga," Wikipedia, January 9, 2023, https:// upload.wikimedia.org/wikipedia/commons/e/e8/The_Prime_Minister%2C_Shri _Narendra_Modi_participates_in_the_mass_yoga_demonstration_at_Rajpath _on_the_occasion_of_International_Yoga_Day%2C_in_New_Delhi_on_June _21%2C_2015_(3).jpg.

103. Freya Noble, "That's A LOT of Downward Dogs!," *Daily Mail Australia*, June 21, 2015, http://www.dailymail.co.uk/news/article-3133167/That-s-LOT-downward-dogs -Incredible-photos-millions-people-world-taking-International-Day-Yoga-army -prime-minister-involved.html.

104. Alter, "Body, Text, Nation," 31–32.

105. On the strength of feelings and public affects generated through Bollywood, see Purnima Mankekar, *Unsettling India: Affect, Temporality, Transnationality* (Durham, NC: Duke University Press, 2015); Vijay Mishra, *Bollywood Cinema: Temples of Desire* (New York: Routledge, 2002).

106. Douglas Kellner, "The Media, Democracy, and Spectacle: Some Critical Reflections," *Cultural Politics* 11, no. 1 (2015): 55.

107. Vikas Swarup, ed., *International Day of Yoga* (New Delhi: MaXposture Media Group [1] Pvt Ltd, 2015).

108. Stephanie March, "International Yoga Day: 35,000-Strong New Delhi Crowd Sets World Record for Largest Yoga Session," *ABC News*, June 22, 2015, http://www.abc .net.au/news/2015-06-22/india-sets-new-world-record-for-international-yoga-day /6562300.

109. Swati Sharma, "Here's What Narendra Modi's Fashion Says about His Politics," *The Washington Post*, January 26, 2015, https://www.washingtonpost.com/news/world views/wp/2014/06/06/heres-what-narendra-modis-fashion-says-about-his-politics /?utm_term=.5a9b8d699e80; Zahir Janmohamed, "The Rise of Narendra Modi: The Man Who Doesn't Wear Dark Green," *Boston Review*, June 28, 2013, http://bost onreview.net/world/zahir-janmohamed-narendra-modi-india-gujarat-man-who -refuses-wear-green.

110. Noble, "That's A LOT of Downward Dogs!"

111. Express Web Desk, "10 Quotes from Narendra Modi's Yoga Day Speech: 'Make Yoga a Part of One's Life,'" *The Indian Express*, June 21, 2016, http://indianexpress.com /article/india/india-news-india/ten-quotes-from-narendra-modis-address-on -international-yoga-day-in-chandigarh-2865991/.

112. C. M. Bhandari, "Prime Minister Modi Defies Research Findings," *Devamber Arogya Dham* (blog), August 26, 2015, http://www.bhandariyogayurveda.com/single-post /2015/08/26/Prime-Minister-Modi-defies-Research-Findings.

113. Sarah Sharma, *In the Meantime: Temporality and Cultural Politics* (Durham, NC: Duke University Press, 2014), 100.

114. Karan Singh, "Nets of Maya: Gorakhnath as a Trickster Saint in the Folktale of Raja Bharthari and Gopi Chand," *Marvels & Tales* 32, no. 1 (2018): 15, https://doi.org/10.13110 /marvelstales.32.1.0013.

115. "BJP: Those Opposing Yoga Should Drown in Ocean," *The Muslim News*, June 9, 2015, https://muslimnews.co.uk/news/south-asia/india-those-opposing-yoga-surya -namaskar-should-drown-in-ocean/.

3. ALIGNING BOTH HANDS

1. Sazana Jayadeva offers ethnographic evidence that proficiency in English is used to assert membership in and negotiate the Indian middle class. At the same time, Bollywood films like *Hindi Medium* (2017) satirize the impulse to overvalue English. See Sazana Jayadeva, "'Below English Line': An Ethnographic Exploration of Class

and the English Language in Post-Liberalization India," *Modern Asian Studies* 52, no. 2 (2018): 576–608.

2. Ulka Anjaria, *Reading India Now: Contemporary Formations in Literature and Popular Culture* (Philadelphia: Temple University Press, 2019), 29.

3. Ulka Anjaria argues that a key trend within twenty-first-century fiction in India is a "'realist impulse,'" which takes shape through "gestures such as stories set in the present rather than the past and the trimming of modernist, metaphorical, and metafictional language for a more stripped-down and less ostensibly self-conscious aesthetic. This impulse signals a new political urgency in both nonfiction and fiction writing alike." Ulka Anjaria, "The Realist Impulse and the Future of Postcoloniality," *Novel* 49, no. 2 (August 2016): 278, https://doi.org/10.1215/00295132-3509035. See also Anjaria, *Reading India Now*.

4. E. Dawson Varughese describes a genre of "Bharati fantasy," or this way of reimagining India as a mythically ennobled "Bharat," as a key element of postmillennial Indian fiction. See E. Dawson Varughese, "Celebrate at Home: Post-Millennial Indian Fiction in English and the Reception of 'Bharati Fantasy' in Global and Domestic Literary Markets," *Contemporary South Asia* 22, no. 4 (2014): 350–61, https://doi.org/10.1080/09584935.2014.963513.

5. Maseeh Rahman, "Indian Prime Minister Claims Genetic Science Existed in Ancient Times," *The Guardian*, October 29, 2014, https://www.theguardian.com/world/2014/oct/28/indian-prime-minister-genetic-science-existed-ancient-times. Since then, Indian scientific gatherings, such as the 106th Indian Scientific Congress, have witnessed similar claims. See IP Singh and Siddhartha Sarma, "'Ravana's Airports,' 'Modi Waves' Leave Science Congress Stunned," *The Times of India*, January 6, 2019, https://timesofindia.indiatimes.com/india/ravanas-airports-modi-waves-leave-science-congress-stunned/articleshow/67402208.cms.

6. Srinivas Aravamudan, *Guru English: South Asian Religion in a Cosmopolitan Language* (Princeton, NJ: Princeton University Press, 2006).

7. Stereotypes, of course, are not always rigid containers, and as Homi Bhabha has argued, their repetitive nature is often a sign not of certainty but of anxiety. Homi K. Bhabha, *The Location of Culture* (London: Routledge, 1994), 66. For ways they can lend themselves to more open and surprising readings, see Shameem Black, *Fiction Across Borders: Imagining the Lives of Others in Late Twentieth-Century Novels* (New York: Columbia University Press, 2010), 99–134; Mrinalini Chakravorty, *In Stereotype: South Asia in the Global Literary Imaginary* (New York: Columbia University Press, 2014).

8. See Shameem Black, "Flexible Indian Labor: Yoga, Information Technology Migration, and U.S. Technoculture," *Race and Yoga* 1, no. 1 (2016): 23–41; Shameem Black, "Yoga by the Book," *Contemporary South Asia* 28, no. 1 (2020): 15–27, https://doi.org/10.1080/09584935.2019.1666091; Suzanne Newcombe, *Yoga in Britain: Stretching Spirituality and Educating Yogis* (Sheffield, UK: Equinox, 2019), 12–34.

9. Andrea R. Jain, *Selling Yoga: From Counterculture to Pop Culture* (New York: Oxford University Press, 2014), Kindle Loc 1760–2200.

10.   Purnima Mankekar, *Unsettling India: Affect, Temporality, Transnationality* (Durham, NC: Duke University Press, 2015).

11.   Wendy Doniger, for instance, encourages her readers to "face the violence embedded in the Vedic sacrifice of cattle and horses and situate the ritual violence in the social violence that it expresses, supports, and requires, the theft of other people's cattle and horses." Wendy Doniger, *The Hindus: An Alternative History* (New York: Penguin, 2009), 103.

12.   Patton E. Burchett, *A Genealogy of Devotion: Bhakti, Tantra, Yoga, and Sufism in North India* (New York: Columbia University Press, 2019), 171–72.

13.   On authorizing practices, see Jean Byrne, "'Authorized by Sri K. Pattabhi Jois': The Role of Parampara and Lineage in Ashtanga Vinyasa Yoga," in *Gurus of Modern Yoga*, ed. Mark Singleton and Ellen Goldberg (Oxford: Oxford University Press, 2014), 107–21.

14.   Sushmi Dey, "Yoga Set to Get WHO Stamp of Approval," *The Times of India*, June 21, 2015, https://timesofindia.indiatimes.com/india/Yoga-set-to-get-WHO-stamp-of -approval/articleshow/47752286.cms; Press Information Bureau, Government of India, "Ministry of AYUSH and WHO Working Group Meeting on Benchmarks for Training in Yoga from Today," February 26, 2019, http://pib.nic.in/newsite /PrintRelease.aspx?relid=188950.

15.   Government of India, Ministry of AYUSH, "Guidelines for Organizing of Yoga Fest/ Utsav in States/UTs," n.d., http://ayush.gov.in/sites/default/files/Guidelines%20 for%20organizing%20of%20Yoga%20Fest%20and%20utsav_1.pdf.

16.   Patrick McCartney, "Stretching into the Shadows: Unlikely Alliances, Strategic Syncretism, and De-Post-Colonizing Yogaland's 'Yogatopia(s)," *Asian Ethnology* 78, no. 2 (2019): 375.

17.   "The Author," Mohan Ashtakala, accessed April 9, 2019, https://www.mohanashtakala .com/the-author/.

18.   Ashtakala, "The Author."

19.   Mohan Ashtakala, *The Yoga Zapper* (Calgary: Books We Love, 2015), Kindle Loc 5055.

20.   Ashtakala, "The Author."

21.   Patton Burchett, "Bhakti Rhetoric in the Hagiography of 'Untouchable' Saints: Discerning Bhakti's Ambivalence on Caste and Brahminhood," *International Journal of Hindu Studies* 13, no. 2 (August 2009): 115–17, https://doi.org/10.1007/s11407-009 -9072-5.

22.   Judith G. Martin, "The Pedagogy of Conciliation in the Bhagavata Purana: A 'Sporting' Way of Understanding Jnana-Yoga" (Master's thesis, McMaster University, 1975), 38. Patañjali, whose *Yogasūtras* set out a range of yogic practices in a much earlier historical period, is usually linked to a dualistic classical Sāṃkhyan philosophy that is not necessarily theistic or devotional. On yoga and sacred sound in the *Bhāgavatapurāṇa*, see Guy L. Beck, "Hari Krishna Mahamantra: Gaudiya Vaishnava Practice and the Hindu Tradition of Sacred Sound," in *The Hare Krishna Movement: The Postcharismatic Fate of a Religious Transplant*, ed. Edwin F. Bryant and Maria L. Ekstrand (New York: Columbia University Press, 2004), 40.

23. The *Bhāgavata Māhātmya*, a late sixteenth- or early seventeenth-century Vaiṣṇava text associated with the Gauḍīya tradition of north India that sings the praises of the *Bhāgavatapurāṇa*, makes it clear that reciting the stories over seven days (a "*saptāha*") is far preferable to any other practice: "The *saptāha* is superior to *yoga*, and it is superior to meditation (*dhyāna*) and *jñāna*." Barbara A. Holdrege, *Bhakti and Embodiment: Fashioning Divine Bodies and Devotional Bodies in Kṛṣṇa Bhakti* (Abingdon, UK: Routledge, 2015), 128, 138.

24. Ashtakala, *The Yoga Zapper*, Kindle Loc 5035.

25. McComas Taylor, *Seven Days of Nectar: Contemporary Oral Performance of the Bhāgavatapurāṇa* (New York: Oxford University Press, 2016).

26. McComas Taylor, "'Stories of God': Contemporary Oral Performance of Bhāgavatakathā," *International Journal of Hindu Studies* 17, no. 3 (December 2013): 263, https://doi.org/10.1007/s11407-014-9145-y.

27. Luis González-Reimann, "The *Yugas*: Their Importance in India and Their Use by Western Intellectuals and Esoteric and New Age Writers: The Importance of Yugas," *Religion Compass* 8, no. 12 (December 2014): 357–70, https://doi.org/10.1111/rec3.12139.

28. Patrick McCartney, "Jhirī: A 'Sanskrit-Speaking' Village in Madhya Pradesh,"*Journal of South Asian Languages and Linguistics* 4, no. 2 (2017): 167–209.

29. Ashtakala, *The Yoga Zapper*, Kindle Loc 4972.

30. Ashtakala, Kindle Loc 1239.

31. On the colonial shaping of Indian beauty norms via capitalism, see Mobeen Hussain, "Combining Global Expertise with Local Knowledge in Colonial India: Selling Ideals of Beauty and Health in Commodity Advertising (c. 1900–1949)," *South Asia: Journal of South Asian Studies* 44, no. 5 (2021): 926–47, https://doi.org/10.1080/00856401.2021.1968599.

32. Vanita Reddy, "The Nationalization of the Global Indian Woman: Geographies of Beauty in *Femina*," *South Asian Popular Culture* 4, no. 1 (April 2006): 62, https://doi.org/10.1080/14746680600555691.

33. I use such phrasing because whiteness is often not explicitly marked in U.S. novels and instead rests on readerly assumptions.

34. "W+K's Incredible India! Campaign Puts Spotlight on Die-Hard Indophiles," Campaign India, January 22, 2009, https://www.campaignindia.in/article/wks-incredible-india-campaign-puts-spotlight-on-die-hard-indophiles/409566.

35. Chandra traces the complex ways in which nineteenth-century Indians used sexualized constructions of whiteness to constitute their own difference, not only from white Europeans, but also from other lower caste Indians. See Shefali Chandra, "Whiteness on the Margins of Native Patriarchy: Race, Caste, Sexuality, and the Agenda of Transnational Studies," *Feminist Studies* 37, no. 1 (Spring 2011): 127–53.

36. Ann Morning, "The Racial Self-Identification of South Asians in the United States," *Journal of Ethnic and Migration Studies* 27, no. 1 (January 2001): 61–79, https://doi.org/10.1080/13691830125692.

37. United States v. Bhagat Singh Thind 261 U.S. 204, No. 204 (U.S. Supreme Court 1923).

38. Indians did find other avenues to access some of the benefits associated with white-ness. Most disturbingly, as Vijay Prashad has shown, some members of Indian com-munities aggressively defined themselves against Black Americans. Vijay Prashad, *The Karma of Brown Folk* (Minneapolis: University of Minnesota Press, 2000).

39. For more on the complexities of race, see Sharmila Sen, *Not Quite Not White: Losing and Finding Race in America* (Gurgaon, Haryana: Penguin Viking, 2018).

40. Ashtakala, *The Yoga Zapper*, Kindle Loc 4997.

41. Marcel Mauss, *The Gift: Forms and Functions of Exchange in Archaic Societies*, trans. Ian Cunnison (London: Cohen & West Ltd, 1969). The logic of *The Yoga Zapper* also offers an inverted mirror of patterns traced by Shefali Chandra in her critique of how white American women have sought guidance from Hindu authorities, figuring "India" in Hindu-centric ways and concealing complicities between whiteness and imperialism. See Shefali Chandra, "'India Will Change You Forever': Hinduism, Islam, and Whiteness in the American Empire," *Signs* 40, no. 2 (Winter 2015): 487–512.

42. For an analysis of how this logic informs the Incredible India campaign, see Shameem Black, "State Spectacles of Yoga: Invisible India and India Everywhere," *South Asia: Journal of South Asian Studies* 46, no. 1 (2023): 1–17, https://doi.org/10.1080/00856401 .2023.2135847.

43. Ashtakala, *The Yoga Zapper*, Kindle Loc 4972.

44. Ashtakala, *The Yoga Zapper*, Kindle Loc 4617.

45. Ashtakala, *The Yoga Zapper*, Kindle Loc 3466.

46. Ashtakala, *The Yoga Zapper*, Kindle Loc 376.

47. Aalif Surti, "Annapurna Devi: The Tragedy And Triumph Of Ravi Shankar's First Wife," *Man's World India*, May 2000, https://www.mansworldindia.com/people /annapurna-devi-the-tragedy-and-triumph-of-ravi-shankars-first-wife/.

48. Surti.

49. Atul S. Merchant, *Taskari* (Mumbai: Atul S. Merchant, 2014), acknowledgments.

50. Merchant, 104–5.

51. Craig Harris, "Allauddin Khan | Biography & History," AllMusic, accessed May 10, 2019, https://www.allmusic.com/artist/allauddin-khan-mn0000002677.

52. Anastasia Tsioulcas, "She Was Poised To Be A Star—Instead, She Spent 60 Years In Her Apartment," National Public Radio, October 23, 2018, https://www.npr.org/2018 /10/23/659786993/annapurna-devi-poised-star-surbahar-spent-60-years-her -apartment.

53. Justin Scarimbolo, "Brahmans Beyond Nationalism, Muslims Beyond Dominance: A Hidden History of North Indian Classical Music's Hinduization" (PhD diss., Univer-sity of California, Santa Barbara, 2014); Peter Manuel, "North Indian Sufi Popular Music in the Age of Hindu and Muslim Fundamentalism," *Ethnomusicology* 52, no. 3 (Fall 2008): 379.

54. Max Katz, "Institutional Communalism in North Indian Classical Music," *Ethno-musicology* 56, no. 2 (Spring/Summer 2012): 279–98, https://doi.org/10.5406/ethno musicology.56.2.0279.

55. Merchant, *Taskari*, 167.

56. Merchant, *Taskari*, 106.

57. White, *Sinister Yogis.*

58. Karan Singh, "Nets of Maya."

59. Narayan, "Refractions of the Field at Home;" Aravamudan, *Guru English.*

60. Siegel, *Trance-Migrations.*

61. Raphaël Voix, "Denied Violence, Glorified Fighting: Spiritual Discipline and Controversy in Ananda Marga,'" *Nova Religio* 12, no. 1 (2008): 3–25, https://doi.org/10.1525/nr.2008.12.1.3; Helen Crovetto, "Ananda Marga and the Use of Force," *Nova Religio* 12, no. 1 (2008): 26–56.

62. See, for instance, Love, *The Great Oom*; Stefanie Syman, *The Subtle Body: The Story of Yoga in America* (New York: Farrar, Straus and Giroux, 2010); Jain, *Selling Yoga.*

63. Merchant, *Taskari*, 136.

64. Patrick McCartney, "Spiritual Bypass and Entanglement in Yogaland: How Neoliberalism, Soft Hindutva and Banal Nationalism Facilitate Yoga Fundamentalism," *Politics and Religion Journal* 13, no. 1 (2019): 137–75.

65. Merchant, *Taskari*, 82.

66. "India Destroys Stockpile of Chemical Weapons," *India Today,* May 14, 2009, https://www.indiatoday.in/latest-headlines/story/india-destroys-stockpile-of-chemical-weapons-47447-2009-05-14.

67. Merchant, *Taskari*, 147.

68. Chakrabarty and Majumdar, "Gandhi's Gita and Politics As Such," 341–42.

69. Shringi Diva Vikram, "Mystery, Mythology and Masala," *The Hindu,* June 14, 2017, https://www.thehindu.com/books/books-authors/mystery-mythology-and-masala/article19047862.ece.

70. Bodhisattva Chattopadhyay, "Speculative Utopianism in Kalpavigyan: Mythologerm and Women's Science Fiction," *Foundation* 46, no. 127 (2017): 6–19.

71. David Gordon White, *Sinister Yogis* (Chicago: University of Chicago Press, 2009).

72. Vikram, "Mystery, Mythology and Masala."

73. Sowmya Rajaram, "'Indian Readers Largely Read Realism Fiction,'" *Bangalore Mirror,* July 8, 2018.

74. James Mallinson and Mark Singleton, trans., *Roots of Yoga* (London: Penguin, 2017, 259; Geoffrey Samuel, *The Origins of Yoga and Tantra: Indic Religions to the Thirteenth Century* (Cambridge: Cambridge University Press, 2008).

75. Julian Strube, *Global Tantra: Religion, Science, and Nationalism in Colonial Modernity* (New York: Oxford University Press, 2022), 119–23.

76. Hugh B. Urban, *Tantra: Sex, Secrecy, Politics and Power in the Study of Religions* (Berkeley: University of California Press, 2003), 92.

77. Urban, *Tantra*, 111.

78. Urban argues that the most influential figure in the twentieth-century reworking of Tantra for India and Western imaginaries has been Bhagwan Shree Rajneesh (Osho), who redefined Tantra as a path of "spiritual sex" and enthusiastically linked orgasmic energy to unbridled capitalist individualism.

79. While Osho's brand of Neo-Tantra was pleasure-oriented and not concerned with black magic, it nonetheless unapologetically kept Tantric capacities for violence and advertised itself as politically undemocratic. Hugh B. Urban, *Zorba the Buddha: Sex, Spirituality and Capitalism in the Global Osho Movement* (Oakland: University of California Press, 2015), 98.

80. Shweta Taneja, *The Rakta Queen* (Noida, Uttar Pradesh: HarperCollins Publishers India, 2018), 47.

81. Taneja, 54.

82. Radha Sarkar and Amar Sarkar, "Sacred Slaughter: An Analysis of Historical, Communal, and Constitutional Aspects of Beef Bans in India," *Politics, Religion & Ideology* 17, no. 4 (October 2016): 329–51, https://doi.org/10.1080/21567689.2016.1259108.

83. Dawson Varughese, "Celebrate at Home."

84. Debjani Ganguly, *This Thing Called the World: The Contemporary Novel as Global Form* (Durham, NC: Duke University Press, 2016).

4. ASSUMING CORPSE POSE

1. Peter Morey and Amina Yaqin, *Framing Muslims: Stereotyping and Representation After 9/11* (Cambridge, MA: Harvard University Press, 2011), 22.

2. Karen Leonard, "Historical Constructions of Ethnicity: Research on Punjabi Immigrants in California," *Journal of American Ethnic History* 12, no. 4 (Summer 1993): 3–26; Juan L. Gonzalez, Jr., "Asian Indian Immigration Patterns: The Origins of the Sikh Community in California," *International Migration Review* 20, no. 1 (1986): 40–54.

3. On these early histories of migration, including the application of the Alien Land Law to migrants from India, see Karen Leonard, "Punjabi Farmers and California's Alien Land Law," *Agricultural History* 59, no. 4 (October 1985): 549–62.

4. Paul Hendrickson, "Cesar Chavez's Causa," *The Washington Post*, April 22, 1979.

5. "Muhammad Ahmad Writings, Undated" (Archives Unbound), accessed June 20, 2019, http://go.galegroups.com/gdsc/i.do?&id=GALE%7CSC5103270679&v=2.1&u=ucberkeley&it=r&p=GDSC&sw=w&viewtype=Manuscript.

6. Stephanie Y. Evans, *Black Women's Yoga History: Memoirs of Inner Peace* (Albany: State University of New York Press, 2021); Jana Long, dir., *The Uncommon Yogi: A History of Blacks and Yoga in the U.S.*, 2016, https://www.youtube.com/watch?v=xQqSdB9PD38.

7. Philip Deslippe, "The Swami Circuit: Mapping the Terrain of Early American Yoga," *Journal of Yoga Studies* 1 (May 1, 2018): 10, https://doi.org/10.34000/JoYS.2018.V1.002.

8. Tria Blu Wakpa, "Yoga Brings You Back to Who You Are: A Conversation Featuring Haley Laughter," *Race and Yoga* 3, no. 1 (2018): 1–11; Rachel Panton and Stephanie Evans, eds., "Sassin' Through Sadhana," *Race and Yoga* 2, no. 1 (2017).

9. Evans, *Black Women's Yoga History*, 40.

10. For a range of voices, see Cara Hagan, ed., *Practicing Yoga as Resistance: Voices of Color in Search of Freedom* (London: Routledge, 2021).

11. Jessamyn Stanley, *Yoke: My Yoga of Self-Acceptance* (New York: Workman, 2021), 103.

12. Michelle Goldberg, *The Goddess Pose: The Audacious Life of Indra Devi, the Woman Who Helped Bring Yoga to the West* (New York: Knopf, 2015).

13. Philip Goldberg, *American Veda: From Emerson and the Beatles to Yoga and Meditation—How Indian Spirituality Changed the West* (New York: Harmony Books, 2010).

14. Enoch H. Page, "The Gender, Race, and Class Barriers: Enclosing Yoga as White Public Space," in *Yoga, the Body, and Embodied Social Change: An Intersectional Feminist Analysis*, ed. Beth Berila, Melanie Klein, and Chelsea Jackson Roberts (Lanham, MD: Lexington Books, 2016), 41–65.

15. Anya P. Foxen, *Biography of a Yogi: Paramahansa Yogananda and the Origins of Modern Yoga* (New Delhi: Oxford University Press, 2017).

16. Deslippe, "The Swami Circuit," 10.

17. Reetika Vazirani, "The Art of Breathing," *Prairie Schooner* 75, no. 3 (Fall 2001): 63–74; Roopa Kaushik-Brown, "Toward Yoga as Property," in *Yoga, the Body, and Embodied Social Change: An Intersectional Feminist Analysis*, ed. Beth Berila, Melanie Klein, and Chelsea Jackson Roberts (Lanham, MD: Lexington Books, 2016), 67.

18. Andrea R. Jain, *Selling Yoga: From Counterculture to Pop Culture* (New York: Oxford University Press, 2014).

19. Vijay Prashad, *Uncle Swami: South Asians in America Today* (Noida, Uttar Pradesh: HarperCollins India, 2013); Sunaina Maira, *Missing: Youth, Citizenship, and Empire after 9/11* (Durham, NC: Duke University Press, 2009).

20. Soniya Munshi, "Multiplicities of Violence: Responses to September 11 from South Asian Women's Organizations," *Race/Ethnicity: Multidisciplinary Global Contexts* 4, no. 3 (July 2011): 419–36, https://doi.org/10.2979/racethmulglocon.4.3.419.

21. David Gordon White, *Sinister Yogis* (Chicago: University of Chicago Press, 2009).

22. William R. Pinch, *Warrior Ascetics and Indian Empires* (Cambridge: Cambridge University Press, 2006).

23. Diana Killian, *Corpse Pose* (New York: Berkley Prime Crime, 2008), Kindle Loc 1096.

24. Neal Pollack, *Stretch: The Unlikely Making of a Yoga Dude* (New York: HarperCollins, 2010).

25. Neal Pollack, *Downward-Facing Death* (Las Vegas: Thomas & Mercer, 2013); Neal Pollack, *Open Your Heart* (Las Vegas: Thomas & Mercer, 2013).

26. Pollack, *Downward-Facing Death*, 210.

27. Pollack, *Downward-Facing Death*, 214.

28. Pollack, *Downward-Facing Death*, 219.

29. Eileen Luhr, "Seeker, Surfer, Yogi: The Progressive Religious Imagination and the Cultural Politics of Place in Encinitas, California," *American Quarterly* 67, no. 4 (2015): 1169–93, https://doi.org/doi:10.1353/aq.2015.0072.

30. Jayshree Bajoria and Esther Pan, "The U.S.-India Nuclear Deal," Council on Foreign Relations, November 5, 2010, https://www.cfr.org/backgrounder/us-india-nuclear-deal.

31. Kadira Pethiyagoda, "India's Soft Power Advantage," *Australia India Institute* (blog), November 4, 2014, http://www.aii.unimelb.edu.au/news/blog/india%E2%80%99s-soft-power-advantage.

32. Cynthia Aaron, Sedlock v. Baird, No. D064888 (Court of Appeal, Fourth Appellate District, Division One, State of California, April 3, 2015).

33. Bethany McLean, "Whose Yoga Is It, Anyway?," *Vanity Fair*, March 5, 2012, https://www.vanityfair.com/news/business/2012/04/krishna-pattanbhi-trophy-wife-ashtanga-yoga.

34. Maya Burger, "What Price Salvation? The Exchange of Salvation Goods between India and the West," *Social Compass* 53, no. 1 (March 2006): 87, https://doi.org/10.1177/0037768606061579.

35. Burger, 85–86.

36. McLean, "Whose Yoga Is It, Anyway?"

37. Sedlock v. Baird, No. 37-2013-00035910-CU-MC-CTL (Superior Court of San Diego County, 2013).

38. *Sedlock v. Baird* at 5.

39. *Sedlock v. Baird* at 10.

40. Osho, "Sanskrit Is a Divine Language," *Speaking Tree*, n.d., https://www.speakingtree.in/article/sanskrit-is-a-divine-language#:~:text=The%20Sanskrit%20language%20is%20called%20Devavani%20%E2%80%94%20the,certain%20music%20and%20aroma.%20How%20did%20this%20happen?

41. Patrick McCartney, "Jhirī: A 'Sanskrit-Speaking' Village in Madhya Pradesh," *Journal of South Asian Languages and Linguistics* 4, no. 2 (2017): 167–209.

42. For more on tensions between Christian evangelical culture and yogic practice, see Candy Gunther Brown, "Christian Yoga: Something New Under the Sun/Son?," *Church History* 87, no. 3 (2018): 659–83, https://doi.org/10.1017/S0009640718001555; Candy Gunther Brown, *Debating Yoga and Mindfulness in Public Schools: Reforming Secular Education or Reestablishing Religion?* (Chapel Hill: University of North Carolina Press, 2019).

43. *Sedlock v. Baird* at 9.

44. Malnak v. Yogi (U.S. Court of Appeals, Third Circuit 1979).

45. Sunila S. Kale and Christian Lee Novetske, "Yoga and the Means and Ends of Secularism," *The Wire*, June 21, 2018, https://thewire.in/government/yoga-means-ends-secularism.

46. *Sedlock v. Baird* at 25.

47. "Religious Landscape Study," Pew Research Center, accessed February 9, 2021, https://www.pewforum.org/religious-landscape-study/.

48. Brief of Amicus Curiae Yoga Alliance in Support of Respondents and Affirmance, No. 37-2013-00035910-CU-MC-CTL (n.d.).

49. *Brief of Amicus Curiae*, No. D064888 at 5.

50. Dia Dabby and Amélie Barras, "Bent Out of Shape: Fictions of Yoga and Religion before the Courts," *Religion & Human Rights* 13, no. 3 (2018): 288, https://doi.org/10.1163/18710328-13021142.

51. The amicus curiae brief further uses this vital, but dispensable, South Asian antiquity to legitimize an ahistorical definition of yoga's purpose. "Yoga developed some 5,000 years ago as a comprehensive system for well-being on all levels: physical, mental, emotional and spiritual" (5), it argues. Even putting aside scholarly doubts about this figure, there is relatively little evidence from scholars of South Asian philosophy, history, and religious studies that yoga in early historical periods was meant to further "well-being" as it would be understood in a coastal suburb of twenty-first-century San Diego. Yogis of past centuries strove more for supernatural power, military might, and immortality than for stress relief. This approach to historical origins creates an unsupported fantasy of an assumed Indian past to justify particular visions of U.S.-based postural practice that Yoga Alliance has a financial stake in expanding.

52. Aaron, *Sedlock v. Baird*, at 32.

53. Aaron, *Sedlock v. Baird*, at 25.

54. Gary Warth, "Yoga Funders Offer New Grant to EUSD," *The San Diego Union-Tribune*, July 31, 2013, accessed August 19, 2015, http://www.sandiegouniontribune.com/news/2013/Jul/31/tp-yoga-funders-offer-new-grant-to-eusd/2/#article-copy.

55. A worker at Lululemon, a store for yoga wear and gear, killed a colleague in 2011 in Bethesda, Maryland.

56. Maira, *Missing*.

57. Vijay Prashad, "The Day Our Probation Ended," *Race/Ethnicity: Multidisciplinary Global Contexts* 4, no. 3 (July 2011): 362, https://doi.org/10.2979/racethmulglocon.4.3.361.

58. Shameem Black, "Yoga, Sexual Violation and Discourse: Reconfigured Hegemonies and Feminist Voices," *Australian Feminist Studies* 35, no. 105 (2020): 277–92.

59. Michael Richards, "B. K. S. Iyengar," *Time*, April 26, 2004, http://content.time.com/time/specials/packages/article/0,28804,1970858_1970910_1972051,00.html.

60. Hilary De Vries, "Yoga's Great Teacher Draws Crowds on Final U.S. Tour," *The New York Times*, October 13, 2005, http://www.nytimes.com/2005/10/13/arts/yogas-great-teacher-draws-crowds-on-final-us-tour.html?_r=0.

61. B. K. S. Iyengar, John J. Evans, and Douglas Abrams, *Light on Life: The Yoga Journey to Wholeness, Inner Peace, and Ultimate Freedom* (Emmaus, PA: Rodale, 2005).

62. Debesh Banerjee, "*Eat, Pray, Love* Promotes Tourism to India," *The Indian Express*, August 16, 2010, http://archive.indianexpress.com/news/eat-pray-love-promotes-tourism-to-india/660833/1.

63. Banerjee.

64. Beth J. Harpaz, "'Eat, Pray, Love' Tourism Courted by Travel Industry," *The Huffington Post* (blog), May 8, 2010, http://www.huffingtonpost.com/2010/08/04/eat-pray-love-tourism-cou_n_671130.html?ir=Australia.

65. Saritha Rai, "India's Tourism Banks on 'Eat, Pray, Love,'" *Globalpost* (blog), August 22, 2010, http://www.globalpost.com/dispatch/india/100804/tourism-international-travel-eat-pray-love.

66. Shefali Chandra, "'India Will Change You Forever': Hinduism, Islam, and Whiteness in the American Empire." *Signs* 40, no. 2 (Winter 2015): 488.

67. Chandra, 488.

68. Associated Press in Washington, "Obama Unveils New Curbs on Racial Profiling in US," *The Guardian*, December 9, 2014, http://www.theguardian.com/world/2014 /dec/09/obama-curbs-racial-profiling-us. This phenomenon is not unique to the United States. In Britain, despite national guidelines warning against ethnic profiling, ethnic minorities have been far more likely than whites to be detained under counterterrorism laws. See Vikram Dodd, "Asian People 42 Times More Likely to Be Held under Terror Law," *The Guardian*, May 24, 2011, http://www.theguardian.com /uk/2011/may/23/counter-terror-stop-search-minorities.

69. Charu A. Chandrasekhar, "Flying While Brown: Federal Civil Rights Remedies to Post 9/11 Airline Racial Profiling of South Asians," *Asian Law Journal* 10, no. 2 (2003): 217.

70. Niraj Warikoo, "Ohio Woman Sues FBI, Airline for Racial Profiling," *USA Today*, January 22, 2013, http://www.usatoday.com/story/news/nation/2013/01/22/racial -profiling-lawsuit/1856619/.

71. The Associated Press, "Lawmakers Criticize US Law Enforcement Profiling Guidelines," *The New York Times*, March 11, 2015, http://www.nytimes.com/aponline/2015 /03/11/us/ap-us-racial-profiling-guidelines.html.

72. Sayantani Dasgupta, "The Perils of Flying While Brown," *Salon* (blog), July 4, 2014, http://www.salon.com/2014/07/05/the_perils_of_flying_while_brown_partner/.

73. Nor are these practices limited to people of South Asian ancestry. In 2012, federal officers in a behavioral detection program at Boston's Logan Airport described how the program, rather than being based on observations of suspicious behavior, focused on race and ethnicity. Officers tended to target Middle Easterners, Blacks, Hispanics, and other minorities for searching and questioning. Michael S. Schmidt and Eric Lichtblau, "Racial Profiling Rife at Airport, U.S. Officers Say," *The New York Times*, August 11, 2012, http://www.nytimes.com/2012/08/12/us/racial-profiling-at-boston -airport-officials-say.html?paewanted=all&_r=1.

74. Tariq Ali, "Karl Marx Led to My Arrest as a Terrorist in Germany," *Independent*, October 30, 2001, https://www.independent.co.uk/voices/commentators/tariq-ali-karl -marx-led-my-arrest-terrorist-germany-9194216.html.

75. "State of California Hopes to Boost Trade Ties with India," *The Economic Times*, January 16, 2020, https://economictimes.indiatimes.com/news/economy/foreign -trade/state-of-california-hopes-to-boost-trade-ties-with-india/articleshow /73276995.cms.

5. BENDING OVER BACKWARD

1. Andrea R. Jain, *Selling Yoga: From Counterculture to Pop Culture* (New York: Oxford University Press, 2014); Sarah Sharma, *In the Meantime: Temporality and Cultural Politics* (Durham, NC: Duke University Press, 2014); Verena Schnäbele, *Yoga in Modern Society* (Hamburg: Verlag Dr Kovac, 2010); David Harvey, *A Brief History of Neoliberalism* (Oxford: Oxford University Press USA, 2005).

2. Michael Hardt, "Affective Labor," *boundary 2* 26, no. 2 (Summer 1999): 96.

3. Hardt, "Affective Labor," 100.

4. Capitalist structures, as many theorists have argued, divide the work of "production" from that of "reproduction," even though those two forms of labor rely on each other in complex ways. Joan Acker, "Gender, Capitalism and Globalization," *Critical Sociology* 30, no. 1 (January 2004): 24, https://doi.org/10.1163/156916304322981668.

5. Clara Han, "Precarity, Precariousness, and Vulnerability," *Annual Review of Anthropology* 47 (2018): 332.

6. Department of Economic and Social Affairs, "World Social Report 2020: Inequality in a Rapidly Changing World" (United Nations, 2020), 26.

7. On the diversity of what precarity might entail, see Fran Martin, John Nguyet Erni, and Audrey Yue, "(Im)Mobile Precarity in the Asia-Pacific," *Cultural Studies* 33, no. 6 (November 2, 2019): 895–914, https://doi.org/10.1080/09502386.2019.1660690.

8. See competing interpretations in Amanda J. Lucia, "'Give Me Sevā Overtime': Selfless Service and Humanitarianism in Mata Amritanandamayi's Transnational Guru Movement," *History of Religions* 54, no. 2 (November 2014): 188–207, https://doi.org/10.1086/677812.

9. Shannon Wagner, "Workers Say They Were Manipulated into Free Labor For National Yoga Brand," *Vice*, October 30, 2020.

10. Ravinder Kaur, *Brand New Nation: Capitalist Dreams and Nationalist Designs in Twenty-First-Century India* (Stanford, CA: Stanford University Press, 2020).

11. Helen Avery, "The Importance of Holding Space," *Wanderlust*, n.d., https://wanderlust.com/journal/the-importance-of-holding-space/.

12. Jade Lizzie, "'Holding Space': What It Means for Yoga Teachers and You," *Yogapedia*, January 29, 2016, https://www.yogapedia.com/holding-space-what-does-it-mean/2/7018.

13. Beth Gibbs, "Holding Space in Yoga Class: What the Yoga Sutras Can Teach Us," *YogaUOnline.com*, October 9, 2017.

14. Tracy Weber, *Murder Strikes a Pose* (Woodbury, MN: Midnight Ink, 2013), Kindle Loc 304.

15. Matthew Remski, "Modern Yoga Will Not Form a Real Culture Until Every Studio Can Also Double as Soup Kitchen, and Other Observations from the Threshold between Yoga and Activism," in *21st Century Yoga: Culture, Politics and Practice*, ed. Carol Horton and Roseanne Harvey (Chicago: Kleio Books, 2012), Kindle Loc 2021. Italics in the original.

16. Yuk-hang Ng and Natalie Ornelland Lana Lam, "Seventh Yoga Centre Goes Bust," *South China Morning Post*, June 27, 2011; MS Nawaz, "Almost Half the Yoga Centres in Rishikesh, Regarded as the Yoga Capital of the Country, Forced to Shut as Many Can't Afford Rent," *The Times of India*, August 10, 2020.

17. Rain Mitchell, *Tales from the Yoga Studio* (New York: Penguin, 2011), Kindle Loc 2621, 2633.

18. Mitchell, *Tales from the Yoga Studio*, Kindle Loc 2621.

19. Mitchell, *Tales from the Yoga Studio*, Kindle Loc 2734.

20.   Mitchell, *Tales from the Yoga Studio*, Kindle Loc 2739.

21.   Kathryn A. Cady, "Flexible Labor: A Feminist Response to Late Twentieth-Century Capitalism?," *Feminist Media Studies* 13, no. 3 (July 2013): 403, https://doi.org/10.1080 /14680777.2012.678876.

22.   Cady, "Flexible Labor," 409.

23.   Sarah Jones, "Yoga Teachers Are Unionizing to Heal the Wellness Industry," *New York Magazine*, September 12, 2019, https://www.thecut.com/2019/09/yogaworks-teachers -first-yoga-teacher-union.html.

24.   Sharma, *In the Meantime*, 84.

25.   Sharma, *In the Meantime*, 84.

26.   Melissa Gregg, *Counterproductive: Time Management in the Knowledge Economy* (Durham, NC: Duke University Press, 2018), 105–6.

27.   Weber, *Murder Strikes a Pose*, Kindle Loc 103.

28.   Tom O'Brien, "Episode 5: 'Think Of Others,'" *Om City: The Series*, 2014, http:// omcityseries.com/episodes.

29.   Alexandra Gray, *The Yoga Teacher* (New York: Grove/Atlantic, 2008), Kindle Loc 2566.

30.   Alice Hines, "Inside CorePower Yoga Teacher Training," *The New York Times*, April 6, 2019, https://www.nytimes.com/2019/04/06/style/corepower-yoga-teacher-training .html.

31.   Suzanne Morrison, *Yoga Bitch: One Woman's Quest to Conquer Skepticism, Cynicism and Cigarettes on the Path to Enlightenment* (New York: Three Rivers Press, 2011), Kindle Loc 2986.

32.   Morrison, *Yoga Bitch*, Kindle Loc 3036.

33.   Michel Foucault, "Technologies of the Self," in *Technologies of the Self: A Seminar with Michel Foucault*, ed. Luther H. Martin, Huck Gutman, and Patrick H. Hutton (Amherst: University of Massachusetts Press, 1988), 18.

34.   R. John Williams, *The Buddha in the Machine: Art, Technology, and the Meeting of East and West* (New Haven, CT: Yale University Press, 2014), 1.

35.   Martin Heidegger, *The Question Concerning Technology, and Other Essays* (New York: Harper & Row, 1977), 34.

36.   Srinivas Aravamudan, *Guru English: South Asian Religion in a Cosmopolitan Language* (Princeton, NJ: Princeton University Press, 2006), 105–41; Elizabeth De Michelis, *A History of Modern Yoga: Patanjali and Western Esotericism* (London and New York: Continuum, 2004), 112–19; Philip Goldberg, *American Veda: From Emerson and the Beatles to Yoga and Meditation—How Indian Spirituality Changed the West* (New York: Harmony Books, 2010), Kindle Loc 893–1222; Julian Strube, *Global Tantra: Religion, Science, and Nationalism in Colonial Modernity* (New York: Oxford University Press, 2022).

37.   Aravamudan, *Guru English*, 142.

38.   Joseph S. Alter, *Yoga in Modern India: The Body Between Science and Philosophy* (Princeton, NJ and Oxford: Princeton University Press, 2004).

39.   Anya P. Foxen, *Biography of a Yogi: Paramahansa Yogananda and the Origins of Modern Yoga* (New Delhi: Oxford University Press, 2017), 80.

40. Aravamudan, *Guru English*, 259.

41. Vivek Bald, *Bengali Harlem and the Lost Histories of South Asian America* (Cambridge, MA: Harvard University Press, 2013), 16.

42. For a more extended analysis of how Yogananda engaged with scientific theories of electromagnetism, see Foxen, *Biography of a Yogi*, 84–88.

43. Paramahansa Yogananda, *Autobiography of a Yogi* (Los Angeles: Self Realization Fellowship, 1946), 177.

44. For a more detailed reading of *Autobiography of a Yogi*, see Shameem Black, "Flexible Indian Labor: Yoga, Information Technology Migration, and U.S. Technoculture." *Race and Yoga* 1, no. 1 (2016): 23–41.

45. "The Best Yoga Sequence to Do After Work," *Shape*, July 12, 2003, http://www.shape.com/blogs/working-it-out/best-yoga-sequence-do-after-work.

46. Timothy McCall, "Yoga as a Technology for Life Transformation," Kripalu: Center for Yoga and Health, Fall 2005, http://kripalu.org/article/179.

47. Satish Padmanabhan, "If Yoga Is Hindu, Then Gravity Is Christian," *Outlook*, June 15, 2015.

48. "How Google Uses Yoga, Meditation to Increase Productivity," Bloomberg Business, March 11, 2015, http://www.bloomberg.com/news/videos/2015-03-10/how-google-uses-yoga-meditation-to-increase-productivity.

49. See, for instance, Melissa Gregg's analysis of the wide range of devices, wellness wearables, and apps designed to promote forms of mindfulness for corporate workers. Digital approaches to work performance rituals blur the boundaries between human body and device. While Gregg traces the genealogy of mindfulness devices to Jon Kabat-Zinn's remediation of Buddhist meditation practices into mindfulness-based stress reduction, genealogies of yoga also contribute to the idea of optimizing the body through the act of appearing to opt out of productivity imperatives. Gregg, *Counterproductive*, 103–26.

50. Department of Homeland Security, "Characteristics of H1B Specialty Occupation Workers: Fiscal Year 2012 Annual Report to Congress: October 1, 2011–September 30, 2012" (Washington, DC, June 26, 2013), 6, http://www.uscis.gov/sites/default/files/USCIS/Resources/Reports%20and%20Studies/H-1B/h1b-fy-12-characteristics.pdf.

51. On informal legal advice discussion boards, yoga instructors seeking the H-1B visa have been encouraged to consider P visas instead. Sunapee, "Is It Better to Apply for H1 as Software Professional or Yoga Instructor?," *Avvo*, October 11, 2012, https://www.avvo.com/legal-answers/is-it-better-to-apply-for-h1-as-software-professio-951850.html.

52. "Yoga Teacher Training," *Data USA*, accessed August 31, 2016, http://datausa.io/profile/cip/513602/#demographics.

53. Ross Bassett, "Aligning India in the Cold War Era: Indian Technical Elites, the Indian Institute of Technology at Kanpur, and Computing in India and the United States," *Technology and Culture* 50, no. 4 (October 2009): 791–98.

54. Andrew B. Kennedy, *The Conflicted Superpower: America's Collaboration with China and India in Global Innovation* (New York: Columbia University Press, 2018),

76–113; Andrew Kennedy, "The Politics of Skilled Immigration: Explaining the Ups and Downs of the US H-1B Visa Program," *International Migration Review* 53, no. 2 (June 2019): 346–70.

55. The program is also used by universities, but most media reporting focuses on corporations.

56. William Branigin, "White-Collar Visas: Back Door for Cheap Labor?," *The Washington Post*, October 21, 1995.

57. Julia Preston, "Pink Slips at Disney. But First, Training Foreign Replacements," *The New York Times*, June 3, 2015, http://www.nytimes.com/2015/06/04/us/last-task -after-layoff-at-disney-train-foreign-replacements.html?_r=0.

58. "Testimony Given by Ronil Hira, Ph.D., P.E. in a Hearing Before the Judiciary Committee, U.S. Senate, on Immigration Reforms Needed to Protect Skilled American Workers," March 17, 2015, http://www.judiciary.senate.gov/imo/media/doc/Hira%20 Testimony.pdf.

59. Matt Smith, Jennifer Gollan, and Adithya Sambamurthy, "Job Brokers Steal Wages, Entrap Indian Tech Workers in US," *Reveal*, October 27, 2014, https://www.revealnews .org/article/job-brokers-steal-wages-entrap-indian-tech-workers-in-us/.

60. Smith, Gollan, and Sambamurthy, "Job Brokers Steal Wages."

61. Vivek Wadhwa and Alex Salkever, *The Immigrant Exodus: Why America Is Losing the Global Race to Capture Entrepreneurial Talent* (Philadelphia: Wharton Digital Press, 2012), Kindle Loc 573.

62. Christian Fuchs, *Digital Labour and Karl Marx* (New York and London: Routledge, 2014), 205.

63. Xiang Biao, *Global "Body Shopping": An Indian Labor System in the Information Technology Industry* (Princeton, NJ: Princeton University Press, 2007), 4–6.

64. Roli Varma argues that Asian immigrants "are permitted to work mainly in those S&E roles that are non-competitive with white males." Roli Varma, "High-Tech Coolies: Asian Immigrants in the US Science and Engineering Workforce," *Science as Culture* 11, no. 3 (2002): 338.

65. Some workers understood themselves through the rhetoric of a laboring body in opposition to a thinking head. Xiang Biao, *Global "Body Shopping,"* 5.

66. ""Testimony Given by Ronil Hira," 7.

67. Edward J.W. Park and John S.W. Park, *Probationary Americans: Contemporary Immigration Policies and the Shaping of Asian American Communities* (New York and London: Routledge, 2005), 103–4; Kaushik Sunder Rajan, *Biocapital: The Constitution of Postgenomic Life* (Durham, NC: Duke University Press, 2006), 228–29.

68. Its 2009 LinkedIn page encouraged its revival. "Immigrants Support Network (ISN)," *LinkedIn*, January 28, 2009, https://www.linkedin.com/groups/Immigrants-Support -Network-ISN-1785609/about.

69. Xiang Biao, *Global "Body Shopping,"* 92.

70. Aziz Haniffa, "'It's Not Brain Drain, It's Brain Circulation,'" *Rediff.com*, August 6, 2009, http://business.rediff.com/report/2009/aug/06/not-brain-drain-but-brain -circulation-says-meera-shankar.htm.

71. "India's Prime Minister Urges Indians to Stay in Their Country," *All Things Considered*, National Public Radio, September 28, 2015, http://www.npr.org/2015/09/28/444236937/indias-prime-minister-urges-indians-to-stay-in-their-country.

72. "153 Congressional Record-Senate S5689-03," *Congressional Record* 153, no. Pt 8 (May 8, 2007): 11589.

73. "Shri Narendra Modi Shares His Vision for Digital India," February 7, 2014, http://www.narendramodi.in/shri-narendra-modi-shares-his-vision-for-digital-india-5944.

74. "Yoga Teacher Training"; Crystal L. Park, Tosca Braun, and Tamar Siegel, "Who Practices Yoga? A Systematic Review of Demographic, Health-Related, and Psychosocial Factors Associated with Yoga Practice," *Journal of Behavioral Medicine* 38, no. 3 (June 2015): 460–71; Holger Cramer, Lesley Ward, Amie Steel, Romy Lauche, Gustav Dobos, and Yan Zhang, "Prevalence, Patterns, and Predictors of Yoga Use," *American Journal of Preventive Medicine* 50, no. 2 (February 2016): 230–35.

75. Pirkko Markula, "Reading Yoga: Changing Discourses of Postural Yoga on the *Yoga Journal* Covers," *Communication and Sport* 2, no. 2 (2015): 143–71, https://doi.org/doi.org/10.1177/2167479513490673; Jennifer B. Webb et al., "Is the 'Yoga Bod' the New Skinny?," *Body Image* 20 (March 2017): 87–98, https://doi.org/10.1016/j.bodyim.2016.11.005; Lina Puustinen and Matti Rautaniemi, "Wellbeing for Sale: Representations of Yoga in Commercial Media," *Temenos* 51, no. 1 (2015): 45–70, https://doi.org/10.33356/temenos.40878; Agi Wittich and Patrick McCartney, "Changing Face of the Yoga Industry, Its Dharmic Roots and Its Message to Women: An Analysis of *Yoga Journal* Magazine Covers, 1975–2020," *Journal of Dharma Studies* 3 (2020): 31–44; Erin Vinoski et al., "Got yoga?: A Longitudinal Analysis of Thematic Content and Models' Appearance-Related Attributes in Advertisements Spanning Four Decades of *Yoga Journal*," *Body Image* 21 (2017): 1–5; Jennifer B. Webb et al., "Downward Dog Becomes Fit Body, Inc.: A Content Analysis of 40 Years of Female Cover Images of Yoga Journal," *Body Image* 22 (2017): 129–35, https://doi.org/10.1016/j.bodyim.2017.07.001.

76. Madan Kataria, *Laugh for No Reason* (Mumbai: Madhuri International, 1999), Kindle Loc 86.

77. "Dr. Kataria's Diary," *Laughter Yoga International*, n.d., https://laughteryoga.org/dr-kataria-diary/.

78. Raffi Khatchadourian, "The Laughing Guru," *The New Yorker*, August 30, 2010.

79. Kataria, *Laugh for No Reason*, Kindle Loc 230.

80. Kataria, *Laugh for No Reason*, Kindle Loc 296.

81. Kataria, *Laugh for No Reason*, Kindle Loc 221.

82. Khatchadourian, "The Laughing Guru."

83. Mira Nair, dir., *The Laughing Club of India* (Filmakers Library, 2002), https://video.alexanderstreet.com/watch/the-laughing-club-of-india.

84. *The Laughing Club of India.*

85. Khatchadourian, "The Laughing Guru."

86. Ulka Anjaria, *Reading India Now: Contemporary Formations in Literature and Popular Culture* (Philadelphia: Temple University Press, 2019), 28.

87. *The Laughing Club of India.*

88. Khatchadourian, "The Laughing Guru."

89. *The Laughing Club of India.*

90. For an analysis of how psychotherapy can personalize political problems, see Dana L. Cloud, *Control and Consolidation in American Culture and Politics: Rhetorics of Therapy* (Thousand Oaks, CA: SAGE, 1998).

91. On the way self-improvement practices for women may reframe political critique into personal growth, see Ujithra Ponniah, "Managing Marriages through 'Self-Improvement': Women and 'New Age' Spiritualities in Delhi," *South Asia: Journal of South Asian Studies* 41, no. 1 (2018): 137–52, https://doi.org/10.1080/00856401.2017 .1366682.

92. Sarah-Kate Lynch, *Heavenly Hirani's School of Laughing Yoga* (New Zealand: Random House New Zealand, 2014), 309.

93. Lynch, *Heavenly Hirani's School of Laughing Yoga*, 310.

94. Shefali Chandra, 'India Will Change You Forever': Hinduism, Islam, and Whiteness in the American Empire," *Signs* 40, no. 2 (Winter 2015): 487–512.

6. FRAMING NEW PARTS

1. Andrea R. Jain, *Peace Love Yoga: The Politics of Global Spirituality* (New York: Oxford University Press, 2020, 6, 8.

2. Suzanne Keen, *Empathy and the Novel* (New York: Oxford University Press, 2007).

3. Keen, *Empathy and the Novel*, 146–47. In this sense, my approach resonates with that of scholars who have investigated yoga as a practice of inquiry through pedagogy and performance. See Jennifer Musial, "Engaged Pedagogy in the Feminist Classroom and Yoga Studio," *Feminist Teacher* 21, no. 3 (2011): 212–28, https://doi.org/10 .5406/femteacher.21.3.0212; Greta Claire Gaard and Bengü Ergüner-Tekinalp, eds., *Contemplative Practices and Anti-Oppressive Pedagogies for Higher Education: Bridging the Disciplines* (New York: Routledge, 2022); Lou Prendergast, *Conscious Theatre Practice: Yoga, Meditation and Performance* (Leiden: Brill, 2022).

4. On the diversity of the Indian diaspora, see, among many others, Ravindra K. Jain, *Nation, Diaspora, Trans-Nation: Reflections from India* (London: Routledge, 2010); Rajesh Rai and Peter Reeves, eds., *The South Asian Diaspora: Transnational Networks and Changing Identities* (New York: Routledge, 2009); Brij V. Lal, Peter Reeves, and Rajesh Rai, eds., *The Encyclopedia of the Indian Diaspora* (Honolulu: University of Hawai'i Press, 2006); Purnima Mankekar, *Unsettling India: Affect, Temporality, Transnationality* (Durham, NC: Duke University Press, 2015); Kama Maclean, *British India, White Australia: Overseas Indians, Intercolonial Relations and the Empire* (Sydney: UNSW Press, 2020); Vivek Bald, *Bengali Harlem and the Lost Histories of South Asian America* (Cambridge, MA: Harvard University Press, 2013); Judith M. Brown, *Global South Asians: Introducing the Modern Diaspora* (Cambridge: Cambridge

University Press, 2006); John C. Hawley, ed., *India in Africa, Africa in India: Indian Ocean Cosmopolitanisms* (Bloomington: Indiana University Press, 2008); Susan Koshy and R. Radhakrishnan, eds., *Transnational South Asians: The Making of a Neo-Diaspora* (New Delhi and New York: Oxford University Press, 2008).

5. See, for example, the labor flexibilities demanded of India's information technology migrants in Xiang Biao, *Global "Body Shopping": An Indian Labor System in the Information Technology Industry* (Princeton, NJ: Princeton University Press, 2007).

6. Chiraag Bhakta, "#WhitePeopleDoingYoga," *Aerogram.com*, 2014, http://theaerogram.com/wp-content/uploads/2014/03/PMH-WPDY-statement.pdf.

7. Bruce Ziff and Pratima V. Rao, eds., *Borrowed Power: Essays on Cultural Appropriation* (New Brunswick, NJ: Rutgers University Press, 1997), 5.

8. Rina Arya, "Debasing the Deity: The Material Culture of Hinduism," *Religion and the Arts* 24, no. 5 (December 16, 2020): 588–603, https://doi.org/10.1163/15685292-02405006.

9. William Crane, "Cultural Formation and Appropriation in the Era of Merchant Capitalism," *Historical Materialism* 26, no. 2 (July 30, 2018): 246, https://doi.org/10.1163/1569206X-00001635.

10. Jain, *Peace Love Yoga*, 74.

11. Dianne Lalonde, "Does Cultural Appropriation Cause Harm?," *Politics, Groups, and Identities*, October 10, 2019, 2–3, https://doi.org/10.1080/21565503.2019.1674160.

12. Véronique Altglas, *From Yoga to Kabbalah: Religious Exoticism and the Logics of Bricolage* (New York: Oxford University Press, 2014), 68.

13. Lalonde, "Does Cultural Appropriation Cause Harm?," 11–12.

14. Liz Bucar, *Stealing My Religion: Not Just Any Cultural Appropriation* (Cambridge, MA: Harvard University Press, 2022), 2–3.

15. While philosophers have described power and profit as "amplifiers" of cultural appropriation, separate from the question of whether a particular act is appropriative, I argue that power and profit are at the heart of the charge. See Patti Tamara Lenard and Peter Balint, "What Is (the Wrong of) Cultural Appropriation?," *Ethnicities* 20, no. 2 (April 2020): 342–46, https://doi.org/10.1177/1468796819866498.

16. J. L. Austin, *How to Do Things With Words* (Cambridge, MA: Harvard University Press, 1962), 4–6. Austin's classic performatives are more literal: for example, "'I give and bequeath my watch to my brother'—as occurring in a will." But what I take is the idea that we can move away from thinking about whether a speech act is true or false, toward the question of what this speech act does.

17. James O. Young, *Cultural Appropriation and the Arts* (Hoboken, NJ: Wiley, 2010).

18. James O. Young and Susan Haley, "'Nothing Comes from Nowhere': Reflections on Cultural Appropriation as the Representation of Other Cultures," in *The Ethics of Cultural Appropriation*, ed. James O. Young and Conrad G. Brunk (Malden, MA: Wiley-Blackwell, 2009), 278.

19. *Pardon My Hindi, #WhitePeopleDoingYoga*, 2014, https://www.chiraagbhakta.com/selectedwork.

20. Chiraag Bhakta, "The Whitewashing of '#WhitePeopleDoingYoga,'" *Mother Jones*, October 17, 2019, https://www.motherjones.com/media/2019/10/white-people-yoga-sf-asian-art-museum/.

21. E-mail to *Mother Jones*, quoted in Bhakta, "The Whitewashing of '#WhitePeople DoingYoga.'"

22. Lovisa Brown et al., "Desegregating Conversations about Race and Identity in Culturally Specific Museums," *Journal of Museum Education* 42, no. 2 (April 3, 2017): 127, https://doi.org/10.1080/10598650.2017.1303602.

23. Matthew Frye Jacobson, *Roots Too: White Ethnic Revival in Post-Civil Rights America* (Cambridge, MA: Harvard University Press, 2006).

24. Shreena Gandhi and Lillie Wolff, "Yoga and the Roots of Cultural Appropriation," *Praxis Center*, December 19, 2017, https://www.kzoo.edu/praxis/yoga/.

25. Amanda J. Lucia, *White Utopias: The Religious Exoticism of Transformational Festivals* (Oakland: University of California Press, 2020); Rumya S. Putcha, "Yoga and White Public Space," *Religions* 11, no. 12 (December 14, 2020): 669, https://doi.org/10.3390/rel11120669.

26. Robin DiAngelo, "White Fragility," *Counterpoints* 497 (2016): 247.

27. Bhakta, "The Whitewashing of '#WhitePeopleDoingYoga.'"

28. See, for example, Priya Swamy, "Neo-Hindutva Affective Economies: Feelings of Pride and Offense among Surinamese Hindus in the Netherlands," *Contemporary South Asia* 26, no. 4 (2018): 439–52, https://doi.org/10.1080/09584935.2018.1545006.

29. Bhakta, "The Whitewashing of '#WhitePeopleDoingYoga.'"

30. On the complex nature of this desire to be seen, see Bakirathi Mani, "Beyond Bollywood: Exhibiting South Asian America," *Journal of Asian American Studies* 18, no. 2 (2015): 193–217, https://doi.org/10.1353/jaas.2015.0013.

31. Nile Green, "Breathing in India, c. 1890," *Modern Asian Studies* 42, no. 2/3 (May 2008): 283–315; Coreen McGuire, Jane Macnaughton, and Havi Carel, "The Color of Breath," *Literature and Medicine* 38, no. 2 (2020): 233–38, https://doi.org/10.1353/lm.2020.0015; Lundy Braun, *Breathing Race into the Machine: The Surprising Career of the Spirometer from Plantation to Genetics* (Minneapolis: University of Minnesota Press, 2014).

32. Howard Norman, "The Healing Powers of the Western Oystercatcher," *Salmagundi*, no. 174/175 (Spring 2012): 33.

33. Jahan Ramazani, "Poetry and Race: An Introduction," *New Literary History* 50, no. 4 (2019): xvii–xviii, https://doi.org/10.1353/nlh.2019.0050.

34. Timothy Yu, "Asian American Poetry in the First Decade of the 2000s," *Contemporary Literature* 52, no. 4 (Winter 2011): 828.

35. Ali Kazim, "The End of Canon," *The Massachusetts Review* 59, no. 4 (2018): 780.

36. Glen Sean Coulthard, *Red Skin, White Masks: Rejecting the Colonial Politics of Recognition* (Minneapolis: University of Minnesota Press, 2014).

37. Reetika Vazirani, "The Art of Breathing," *Prairie Schooner* 75, no. 3 (Fall 2001): 63.

38. Vazirani, "The Art of Breathing," 63.

39. Vazirani, "The Art of Breathing," 72.

40. Luce Irigaray, *Between East and West: From Singularity to Community*, trans. Stephen Pluháček (New York: Columbia University Press, 2002), 44.

41. Vazirani, "The Art of Breathing," 64–65.

42. See, for instance, Mike Lloyd, "Life in the Slow Lane: Rethinking Spectacular Body Modification," *Continuum* 18, no. 4 (December 2004): 555–64, https://doi.org/10.1080/1030431042000297662.

43. Mark Everard, *Breathing Space: The Natural and Unnatural History of Air* (London: Zed Books, 2015); Kenneth E. Harris, "Op-Ed: Breathing While Black," *Michigan Chronicle*, June 17, 2020; Clare Bambra et al., "The COVID-19 Pandemic and Health Inequalities," *Journal of Epidemiology and Community Health*, June 13, 2020, jech-2020-214401, https://doi.org/10.1136/jech-2020-214401; Shermaine M. Jones, " 'I CAN'T BREATHE!:' Affective Asphyxia in Claudia Rankine's *Citizen: An American Lyric*," *South: A Scholarly Journal* 50, no. 1 (Fall 2017): 37–46.

44. Vazirani, "The Art of Breathing," 74.

45. Reetika Vazirani, "From Patanjali," *Prairie Schooner* 75, no. 3 (Fall 2001): 75.

46. Vazirani, "The Art of Breathing," 65.

47. Shameem Black, *Fiction Across Borders: Imagining the Lives of Others in Late Twentieth-Century Novels* (New York: Columbia University Press, 2010), 100–104.

48. Mrinalini Chakravorty, *In Stereotype: South Asia in the Global Literary Imaginary* (New York: Columbia University Press, 2014), 30.

49. Chakravorty, *In Stereotype*, 30.

50. Tracy D. Smith, dir., "Yoga Town Episode 5—TLC, Tandoori Loving Care," *Yoga Town*, 2013, http://watchyogatown.com/watch-the-show/.

51. "Yoga Town Episode 5—TLC, Tandoori Loving Care."

52. Shefali Chandra, " 'India Will Change You Forever': Hinduism, Islam, and Whiteness in the American Empire," *Signs* 40, no. 2 (Winter 2015): 487–512.

53. Chandra, " 'India Will Change You Forever.' "

54. Bucar, *Stealing My Religion: Not Just Any Cultural Appropriation*, 200–201. Artistic form provides strong and complex resources for this inevitably incomplete yet also essential task.

55. Katrina Jaworski, "The Breath of Life and Death," *Cultural Critique*, no. 86 (Winter 2014): 72.

56. Achille Mbembe, "The Universal Right to Breathe," trans. Carolyn Shread, *Critical Inquiry* 47, no. S2 (January 1, 2021): S61, https://doi.org/10.1086/711437.

7. LYING OUT: SPECTRAL YOGA

1. Derek Parfit, *Reasons and Persons* (Oxford: Clarendon Press, 1984), 281.

BIBLIOGRAPHY

Aaron, Cynthia. *Sedlock v. Baird*, No. D064888 (Court of Appeal, Fourth Appellate District, Division One, State of California April 3, 2015).

Acker, Joan. "Gender, Capitalism and Globalization." *Critical Sociology* 30, no. 1 (January 2004): 17–41. https://doi.org/10.1163/156916304322981668.

Agathocleous, Tanya. "'The Coming Clash of East and West': Syncretism, Cosmopolitanism, and Disaffection in the Colonial Public Sphere." *Textual Practice* 31, no. 4 (June 7, 2017): 661–85. https://doi.org/10.1080/0950236X.2016.1189454.

Ali, Tariq. "Karl Marx Led to My Arrest as a Terrorist in Germany." *Independent*, October 30, 2001. https://www.independent.co.uk/voices/commentators/tariq-ali-karl-marx-led-my -arrest-terrorist-germany-9194216.html.

Alter, Joseph S. "Body, Text, Nation: Writing the Physically Fit Body in Post-Colonial India." In *Confronting the Body: The Politics of Physicality in Colonial and Post-Colonial India*, ed. James H. Mills and Satadru Sen, 16–38. Bath, UK: Anthem, 2004.

——. *Gandhi's Body: Sex, Diet, and the Politics of Nationalism*. Philadelphia: University of Pennsylvania Press, 2000.

——. "Pahalwan Baba Ramdev: Wrestling with Yoga and Middle-Class Masculinity in India." *Modern Asian Studies* 55, no. 4 (July 2021): 1359–81.

——. *Yoga in Modern India: The Body Between Science and Philosophy*. Princeton, NJ and Oxford: Princeton University Press, 2004.

Altglas, Véronique. *From Yoga to Kabbalah: Religious Exoticism and the Logics of Bricolage*. New York: Oxford University Press, 2014.

Amish. *The Immortals of Meluha*. Chennai: Westland Publications, 2008.

Anderson, Edward, and Arkotong Longkumer. "'Neo-Hindutva': Evolving Forms, Spaces, and Expressions of Hindu Nationalism." *Contemporary South Asia* 26, no. 4 (2018): 371–77. https://doi.org/10.1080/09584935.2018.1548576.

Anjaria, Ulka, ed. *A History of the Indian Novel in English*. New York: Cambridge University Press, 2015.

——. *Reading India Now: Contemporary Formations in Literature and Popular Culture*. Philadelphia: Temple University Press, 2019.

——. "The Realist Impulse and the Future of Postcoloniality." *Novel* 49, no. 2 (August 2016): 278–94. https://doi.org/10.1215/00295132-3509035.

Annual Report of the Mysore Archaeological Department for the Year 1929 with the Government Review Thereon. Bangalore: Government Press, 1931.

Ansari, Mohd Shoaib. "Evaluation of Role of Traditional Knowledge Digital Library and Traditional Chinese Medicine Database in Preservation of Traditional Medicinal Knowledge." *DESIDOC Journal of Library and Information Technology* 36, no. 2 (March 2016): 73–78.

Antony, Mary Grace. "That's a Stretch: Reconstructing, Rearticulating, and Commodifying Yoga." *Frontiers in Communication* 3, no. 47 (October 23, 2018). https://doi.org/10.3389/fcomm.2018.00047.

Appuhamilage, Udeni M. H. "A Fluid Ambiguity: Individual, Dividual and Personhood." *The Asia Pacific Journal of Anthropology* 18, no. 1 (January 1, 2017): 1–17. https://doi.org/10.1080/14442213.2016.1249020.

Aravamudan, Srinivas. *Guru English: South Asian Religion in a Cosmopolitan Language*. Princeton, NJ: Princeton University Press, 2006.

Arya, Rina. "Debasing the Deity: The Material Culture of Hinduism." *Religion and the Arts* 24, no. 5 (December 16, 2020): 588–603. https://doi.org/10.1163/15685292-02405006.

Ashtakala, Mohan. "The Author." Accessed April 9, 2019. https://www.mohanashtakala.com/the-author/.

——. *The Yoga Zapper*. Calgary: Books We Love, 2015.

Associated Press. "Lawmakers Criticize US Law Enforcement Profiling Guidelines." *The New York Times*, March 11, 2015. http://www.nytimes.com/aponline/2015/03/11/us/ap-us-racial-profiling-guidelines.html.

Associated Press in Washington. "Obama Unveils New Curbs on Racial Profiling in US." *The Guardian*, December 9, 2014. http://www.theguardian.com/world/2014/dec/09/obama-curbs-racial-profiling-us.

Austin, J. L. *How to Do Things with Words*. Cambridge, MA: Harvard University Press, 1962.

Avery, Helen. "The Importance of Holding Space." *Wanderlust*, n.d. https://wanderlust.com/journal/the-importance-of-holding-space/.

Ayres, Alyssa. *Our Time Has Come: How India Is Making Its Place in the World*. New York: Oxford University Press, 2018.

Baier, Karl, Philipp A. Maas, and Karin Preisendanz, eds. *Yoga in Transformation: Historical and Contemporary Perspectives*. Gottingen: V&R Unipress, 2018.

Bailey, K. Alysse, Carla Rice, Melissa Gualtieri, and James Gillett. "Is #YogaForEveryone? The Idealised Flexible Bodymind in Instagram Yoga Posts." *Qualitative Research in Sport, Exercise and Health* 14, no. 5 (2022): 827–42. https://doi.org/10.1080/2159676X.2021.2002394.

Bajoria, Jayshree, and Esther Pan. "The U.S.-India Nuclear Deal." Council on Foreign Relations, November 5, 2010. https://www.cfr.org/backgrounder/us-india-nuclear-deal.

Bald, Vivek. *Bengali Harlem and the Lost Histories of South Asian America*. Cambridge, MA: Harvard University Press, 2013.

Bambra, Clare, Ryan Riordan, John Ford, and Fiona Matthews. "The COVID-19 Pandemic and Health Inequalities." *Journal of Epidemiology and Community Health*, June 13, 2020, jech-2020-214401. https://doi.org/10.1136/jech-2020-214401.

Banerjee, Debesh. "Eat, Pray, Love Promotes Tourism to India." *The Indian Express*, August 16, 2010. http://archive.indianexpress.com/news/eat-pray-love-promotes-tourism -to-india/660833/1.

Barois, Christèle, Suzanne Newcombe, and Dagmar Wujastyk. "Introduction to The Usman Report (1923): Translations of Regional Submissions." *EJournal of Indian Medicine* Supplement 4 (January 26, 2022): ix–xxxi. https://doi.org/10.21827/61e814114457b.

Barry, Ellen. "Prime Minister Modi's Yoga Consultant, H.R. Nagendra." *The New York Times*, June 15, 2015. http://www.nytimes.com/2015/06/16/world/asia/prime-minister-modis -yoga-consultant-hr-nagendra.html?partner=bloomberg.

Bassett, Ross. "Aligning India in the Cold War Era: Indian Technical Elites, the Indian Institute of Technology at Kanpur, and Computing in India and the United States." *Technology and Culture* 50, no. 4 (October 2009): 783–810.

Bauman, Zygmunt. *Liquid Modernity*. Cambridge: Polity Press, 2000.

Beck, Guy L. "Hari Krishna Mahamantra: Gaudiya Vaishnava Practice and the Hindu Tradition of Sacred Sound." In *The Hare Krishna Movement: The Postcharismatic Fate of a Religious Transplant*, ed. Edwin F. Bryant and Maria L. Ekstrand, 35–44. New York: Columbia University Press, 2004.

Berila, Beth, Melanie Klein, and Chelsea Jackson Roberts, eds. *Yoga, the Body, and Embodied Social Change: An Intersectional Feminist Analysis*. Lanham, MD: Lexington Books, 2016.

Bhabha, Homi K. *The Location of Culture*. London: Routledge, 1994.

Bhakta, Chiraag. "The Whitewashing of '#WhitePeopleDoingYoga.'" *Mother Jones*, October 17, 2019. https://www.motherjones.com/media/2019/10/white-people-yoga-sf-asian -art-museum/.

——. "#WhitePeopleDoingYoga." *Aerogram.com*, 2014. http://theaerogram.com/wp-content /uploads/2014/03/PMH-WPDY-statement.pdf.

Bhalla, Nandini, and David Moscowitz. "Yoga and Female Objectification: Commodity and Exclusionary Identity in U.S. Women's Magazines." *Journal of Communication Inquiry* 44, no. 1 (January 2020): 90–108. https://doi.org/10.1177/0196859919830357.

Bhalla, Nandini, Jane O'Boyle, and Leigh Moscowitz. "Selling Yoga 'Off the Mat': A 10-Year Analysis of Lifestyle Advertorials in *Yoga Journal* Magazine." *Journal of Communication Inquiry*, September 15, 2022. https://doi.org/10.1177/01968599221118646.

Bhandari, C. M. "Prime Minister Modi Defies Research Findings." *Devamber Arogya Dham* (blog), August 26, 2015. http://www.bhandariyogayurveda.com/single-post/2015/08/26 /Prime-Minister-Modi-defies-Research-Findings.

Bharatiya Janata Party. *Toward Ram Rajya*. New Delhi: Bharatiya Janata Party, 1991.

Bibi, Asiya. "Abul Fazl's Comparative Study of Hindu Culture: An Analysis." *Journal of Asian Civilizations* 39, no. 1 (2016): 139–62.

"BJP: Those Opposing Yoga Should Drown in Ocean." *The Muslim News*, June 9, 2015. https://muslimnews.co.uk/news/south-asia/india-those-opposing-yoga-surya-namaskar-should-drown-in-ocean/.

"BJP Becomes Largest Political Party in the World." *The Times of India*, March 30, 2015. http://timesofindia.indiatimes.com/india/BJP-becomes-largest-political-party-in-the-world/articleshow/46739025.cms.

Black, Shameem. "Decolonising Yoga." In *Routledge Handbook of Yoga and Meditation Studies*, ed. Suzanne Newcombe and Karen O'Brien-Kop, 13–21. Abingdon, UK: Routledge, 2021.

——. *Fiction Across Borders: Imagining the Lives of Others in Late Twentieth-Century Novels.* New York: Columbia University Press, 2010.

——. "Flexible Indian Labor: Yoga, Information Technology Migration, and U.S. Technoculture." *Race and Yoga* 1, no. 1 (2016): 23–41. https://doi.org/10.5070/R311028974.

——. "State Spectacles of Yoga: Invisible India and India Everywhere." *South Asia: Journal of South Asian Studies* 46, no. 1 (2023): 1–17. https://doi.org/10.1080/00856401.2023.2135847.

——. "Yoga by the Book." *Contemporary South Asia* 28, no. 1 (2020): 15–27. https://doi.org/10.1080/09584935.2019.1666091.

——. "Yoga, Sexual Violation and Discourse: Reconfigured Hegemonies and Feminist Voices." *Australian Feminist Studies* 35, no. 105 (2020): 277–92. https://doi.org/10.1080/08164649.2020.1775067.

——. "Yogic Style in Motion: Experiments in Power and Knowledge." *Textual Practice* 36, no. 4 (2022): 605–25. https://doi.org/10.1080/0950236X.2022.2030515.

Blaine, Diana York. "Mainstream Representations of Yoga: Capitalism, Consumerism, and Control of the Female Body." In *Yoga, the Body, and Embodied Social Change*, ed. Beth Berila, Melanie Klein, and Chelsea Jackson Roberts, 129–40. Lanham, MD: Lexington Books, 2016.

Blinne, Kristen C. *Pop Culture Yoga: A Communication Remix.* Lanham, MD: Lexington Books, 2016.

Blu Wakpa, Tria. "Yoga Brings You Back to Who You Are: A Conversation Featuring Haley Laughter." *Race and Yoga* 3, no. 1 (2018): 1–11.

Bondy, Dianne. "Yoga, Race and Culture." *Yoga International*, n.d. https://yogainternational.com/article/view/yoga-race-and-culture.

Branigin, William. "White-Collar Visas: Back Door for Cheap Labor?" *The Washington Post*, October 21, 1995.

Braun, Lundy. *Breathing Race into the Machine: The Surprising Career of the Spirometer from Plantation to Genetics.* Minneapolis: University of Minnesota Press, 2014.

Brief of Amicus Curiae Yoga Alliance in Support of Respondents and Affirmance, No. 37-2013-00035910-CU-MC-CTL (n.d.). San Diego County Superior Court.

Brosius, Christiane. *India's Middle Class: New Forms of Urban Leisure, Consumption and Prosperity.* Abingdon, UK: Routledge, 2010.

Brown, Candy Gunther. "Christian Yoga: Something New Under the Sun/Son?" *Church History* 87, no. 3 (2018): 659–83. https://doi.org/10.1017/S0009640718001555.

——. *Debating Yoga and Mindfulness in Public Schools: Reforming Secular Education or Reestablishing Religion?* Chapel Hill: University of North Carolina Press, 2019.

Brown, Judith M. *Global South Asians: Introducing the Modern Diaspora.* Cambridge: Cambridge University Press, 2006.

Brown, Lovisa, Caren Gutierrez, Janine Okmin, and Susan McCullough. "Desegregating Conversations about Race and Identity in Culturally Specific Museums." *Journal of Museum Education* 42, no. 2 (April 3, 2017): 120–31. https://doi.org/10.1080/10598650.2017 .1303602.

Brunette-Debassige, Candace. "From Subjugation to Embodied Self-in-Relation: An Indigenous Pedagogy for Decolonization." In *Sharing Breath: Embodied Learning and Decolonization,* ed. Sheila Batacharya and Yuk-Lin Renita Wong, 199–228. Edmonton, AB: Athabasca University Press, 2018.

Bucar, Liz. *Stealing My Religion: Not Just Any Cultural Appropriation.* Cambridge, MA: Harvard University Press, 2022.

Burchett, Patton. "Bhakti Rhetoric in the Hagiography of 'Untouchable' Saints: Discerning Bhakti's Ambivalence on Caste and Brahminhood." *International Journal of Hindu Studies* 13, no. 2 (August 2009): 115–41. https://doi.org/10.1007/s11407-009-9072-5.

Burchett, Patton E. *A Genealogy of Devotion: Bhakti, Tantra, Yoga, and Sufism in North India.* New York: Columbia University Press, 2019.

Burger, Maya. "What Price Salvation? The Exchange of Salvation Goods between India and the West." *Social Compass* 53, no. 1 (March 2006): 81–95. https://doi.org/10.1177/003776 8606061579.

Byrne, Jean. "'Authorized by Sri K. Pattabhi Jois:' The Role of Parampara and Lineage in Ashtanga Vinyasa Yoga." In *Gurus of Modern Yoga,* ed. Mark Singleton and Ellen Goldberg, 107–21. Oxford: Oxford University Press, 2014.

Cady, Kathryn A. "Flexible Labor: A Feminist Response to Late Twentieth-Century Capitalism?" *Feminist Media Studies* 13, no. 3 (July 2013): 395–414. https://doi.org/10.1080 /14680777.2012.678876.

Chacko, Priya. "Marketizing Hindutva: The State, Society, and Markets in Hindu Nationalism." *Modern Asian Studies* 53, no. 2 (March 2019): 377–410. https://doi.org/10.1017 /S0026749X17000051.

Chakrabarty, Dipesh. *Provincializing Europe: Postcolonial Thought and Historical Difference.* Princeton, NJ: Princeton University Press, 2000.

Chakrabarty, Dipesh, and Rochona Majumdar. "Gandhi's Gita and Politics as Such." *Modern Intellectual History* 7, no. 2 (August 2010): 335–53. https://doi.org/10.1017/S1479244 310000107.

Chakraborty, Chandrima. "The Hindu Ascetic as Fitness Instructor: Reviving Faith in Yoga." *The International Journal of the History of Sport* 24, no. 9 (2007): 1172–86.

Chakravorty, Mrinalini. *In Stereotype: South Asia in the Global Literary Imaginary.* New York: Columbia University Press, 2014.

Chandra, Shefali. "'India Will Change You Forever': Hinduism, Islam, and Whiteness in the American Empire." *Signs* 40, no. 2 (Winter 2015): 487–512.

——. "Whiteness on the Margins of Native Patriarchy: Race, Caste, Sexuality, and the Agenda of Transnational Studies." *Feminist Studies* 37, no. 1 (Spring 2011): 127–53.

Chandrasekhar, Charu A. "Flying While Brown: Federal Civil Rights Remedies to Post 9/11 Airline Racial Profiling of South Asians." *Asian Law Journal* 10, no. 2 (2003): 215–52.

Chattopadhyay, Bodhisattva. "Speculative Utopianism in Kalpavigyan: Mythologerm and Women's Science Fiction." *Foundation* 46, no. 127 (2017): 6–19.

Chaturvedi, Amit. "On International Yoga Day, PM Modi to Join 35,000 People at Rajpath." *NDTV*, June 21, 2015. http://www.ndtv.com/cheat-sheet/stage-set-for-international-yoga -day-pm-modi-to-join-35-000-people-at-rajpath-773691.

Chhotray, Vasudha, and Fiona McConnell. "Certifications of Citizenship: The History, Politics and Materiality of Identity Documents in South Asian States and Diasporas." *Contemporary South Asia* 26, no. 2 (2018): 111–26. https://doi.org/10.1080/09584935 .2018.1471042.

Chopra, Ritika. "Panel Picks Patanjali, Ramdev Likely to Head First Vedic Board." *The Indian Express* (blog), February 25, 2019. https://indianexpress.com/article/education/baba -ramdev-likely-to-head-first-vedic-board-patanjali-5599448/.

Ciolkosz, Matylda. "The Quasi-Linguistic Structure of Iyengar Yoga Asana Practice: An Analysis from the Perspective of Cognitive Grammar." *Studia Religiologica* 47, no. 4 (2014): 263–73.

Cloud, Dana L. *Control and Consolidation in American Culture and Politics: Rhetorics of Therapy*. Thousand Oaks, CA: SAGE, 1998.

Conversi, Daniele. "Irresponsible Radicalisation: Diasporas, Globalisation and Long-Distance Nationalism in the Digital Age." *Journal of Ethnic and Migration Studies* 38, no. 9 (2012): 1357–79.

Corliss, Richard. "The Power of Yoga." *Time*, April 15, 2001. http://content.time.com/time /health/article/0,8599,106356,00.html.

Coulthard, Glen Sean. *Red Skin, White Masks: Rejecting the Colonial Politics of Recognition*. Minneapolis: University of Minnesota Press, 2014.

Cramer, Holger, Lesley Ward, Amie Steel, Romy Lauche, Gustav Dobos, and Yan Zhang. "Prevalence, Patterns, and Predictors of Yoga Use." *American Journal of Preventive Medicine* 50, no. 2 (February 2016): 230–35. https://doi.org/10.1016/j.amepre.2015.07.037.

Crane, William. "Cultural Formation and Appropriation in the Era of Merchant Capitalism." *Historical Materialism* 26, no. 2 (July 30, 2018): 242–70. https://doi.org/10.1163 /1569206X-00001635.

Crovetto, Helen. "Ananda Marga and the Use of Force." *Nova Religio* 12, no. 1 (2008): 26–56.

Cvetkovich, Ann. *Depression: A Public Feeling*. Durham, NC: Duke University Press, 2012.

Dabby, Dia, and Amélie Barras. "Bent Out of Shape: Fictions of Yoga and Religion before the Courts." *Religion & Human Rights* 13, no. 3 (2018): 270–96. https://doi.org/10.1163 /18710328-13021142.

Dasgupta, Sayantani. "The Perils of Flying While Brown." *Salon* (blog), July 4, 2014. http:// www.salon.com/2014/07/05/the_perils_of_flying_while_brown_partner/.

De Michelis, Elizabeth. *A History of Modern Yoga: Patanjali and Western Esotericism*. London and New York: Continuum, 2004.

De Vries, Hilary. "Yoga's Great Teacher Draws Crowds on Final U.S. Tour." *The New York Times*, October 13, 2005. http://www.nytimes.com/2005/10/13/arts/yogas-great-teacher -draws-crowds-on-final-us-tour.html?_r=0.

Department of Economic and Social Affairs. "World Social Report 2020: Inequality in a Rapidly Changing World." United Nations, 2020.

Department of Homeland Security. "Characteristics of H1B Specialty Occupation Workers: Fiscal Year 2012 Annual Report to Congress: October 1, 2011–September 30, 2012." Washington, DC, June 26, 2013. http://www.uscis.gov/sites/default/files/USCIS/Resources /Reports%20and%20Studies/H-1B/h1b-fy-12-characteristics.pdf.

Deslippe, Philip. "The Swami Circuit: Mapping the Terrain of Early American Yoga." *Journal of Yoga Studies* 1 (May 1, 2018): 5–44. https://doi.org/10.34000/JoYS.2018.V1.002.

Dey, Sushmi. "Yoga Set to Get WHO Stamp of Approval." *The Times of India*, June 21, 2015. https://timesofindia.indiatimes.com/india/Yoga-set-to-get-WHO-stamp-of-approval /articleshow/47752286.cms.

DiAngelo, Robin. "White Fragility." *Counterpoints* 497 (2016): 245–53.

"Discover True Wellness with Tailor-Made Yoga Tours in India." *Guided Tours India*. Accessed January 2, 2023. http://guidedtoursindia.blogspot.com/2014/12/Discover-True -Wellness-with-Tailor-Made-Yoga-in-India.html.

Dodd, Vikram. "Asian People 42 Times More Likely to Be Held under Terror Law." *The Guardian*, May 24, 2011. http://www.theguardian.com/uk/2011/may/23/counter-terror -stop-search-minorities.

Doniger, Wendy. *The Hindus: An Alternative History*. New York: Penguin, 2009.

Doron, Assa. "Mobile Persons: Cell Phones, Gender and the Self in North India." *The Asia Pacific Journal of Anthropology* 13, no. 5 (2012): 414–33.

Downes, David R. "How Intellectual Property Could Be a Tool to Protect Traditional Knowledge." *Columbia Journal of Environmental Law* 25 (2000): 253–82.

"Dr. Kataria's Diary." *Laughter Yoga International*. N.d. https://laughteryoga.org/dr-kataria -diary/.

"DRDO Ties up with Ramdev to Market Supplements, Food Products." *The Times of India*, August 23, 2015. http://timesofindia.indiatimes.com/india/DRDO-ties-up-with-Ramdev -to-market-supplements-food-products/articleshow/48643649.cms.

Dugger, Celia W. "Religious Riots Loom Over Indian Politics." *The New York Times*, July 27, 2002. http://www.nytimes.com/2002/07/27/international/asia/27INDI.html.

Dworkin, Shari L., and Faye Linda Wachs. *Body Panic: Gender, Health and the Selling of Fitness*. New York: New York University Press, 2009.

Ergas, Oren. "Overcoming the Philosophy/Life, Body/Mind Rift: Demonstrating Yoga as Embodied-Lived-Philosophical-Practice." *Educational Philosophy and Theory* 46, no. 1 (January 2, 2014): 74–86. https://doi.org/10.1111/j.1469-5812.2011.00811.x.

Errington, Frederick, Tatsuro Fujikura, and Deborah Gewertz. *The Noodle Narratives: The Global Rise of an Industrial Food into the Twenty-First Century*. Berkeley: University of California Press, 2013.

Evans, Stephanie Y. *Black Women's Yoga History: Memoirs of Inner Peace*. Albany: State University of New York Press, 2021.

Everard, Mark. *Breathing Space: The Natural and Unnatural History of Air*. London: Zed Books, 2015.

Express Web Desk. "10 Quotes from Narendra Modi's Yoga Day Speech: 'Make Yoga a Part of One's Life.'" *The Indian Express*, June 21, 2016. http://indianexpress.com/article/india /india-news-india/ten-quotes-from-narendra-modis-address-on-international-yoga -day-in-chandigarh-2865991/.

Fish, Allison. "Authorizing Yoga: The Pragmatics of Cultural Stewardship in the Digital Era." *East Asian Science, Technology and Society: An International Journal* 8, no. 4 (2014): 439–60.

——. "The Commodification and Exchange of Knowledge in the Case of Transnational Commercial Yoga." *International Journal of Cultural Property* 13, no. 2 (2006): 189–206.

Flood, Gavin. *The Ascetic Self: Subjectivity, Memory and Tradition*. Cambridge: Cambridge University Press, 2004.

Foucault, Michel. "Technologies of the Self." In *Technologies of the Self: A Seminar with Michel Foucault*, ed. Luther H. Martin, Huck Gutman, and Patrick H. Hutton, 16–49. Amherst: University of Massachusetts Press, 1988.

Foxen, Anya P. *Biography of a Yogi: Paramahansa Yogananda and the Origins of Modern Yoga*. New Delhi: Oxford University Press, 2017.

——. *Inhaling Spirit: Harmonialism, Orientalism, and the Western Roots of Modern Yoga*. New York: Oxford University Press, 2020.

Foxen, Anya, and Christa Kuberry. *Is This Yoga? Concepts, Histories, and the Complexities of Modern Practice*. London: Routledge, 2021.

Friedlander, Peter. "Reassessing Religion and Politics in the Life of Jagjivan Rām." *Religions* 11, no. 5 (May 1, 2020): 224. https://doi.org/10.3390/rel11050224.

Fuchs, Christian. *Digital Labour and Karl Marx*. New York and London: Routledge, 2014.

Gaard, Greta Claire, and Bengü Ergüner-Tekinalp, eds. *Contemplative Practices and Anti-Oppressive Pedagogies for Higher Education: Bridging the Disciplines*. New York: Routledge, 2022.

Gandhi, Shreena, and Lillie Wolff. "Yoga and the Roots of Cultural Appropriation." *Praxis Center*, December 19, 2017. https://www.kzoo.edu/praxis/yoga/.

Ganguly, Debjani. *This Thing Called the World: The Contemporary Novel as Global Form*. Durham, NC: Duke University Press, 2016.

Gaudilliere, Jean-Paul. "An Indian Path to Biocapital? The Traditional Knowledge Digital Library, Drug Patents, and the Reformulation Regime of Contemporary Ayurveda." *East Asian Science, Technology and Society: An International Journal* 8 (2014): 391–415.

Geary, David. "Incredible India in a Global Age: The Cultural Politics of Image Branding in Tourism." *Tourist Studies* 13, no. 1 (2013): 36–61.

Gibbs, Beth. "Holding Space in Yoga Class: What the Yoga Sutras Can Teach Us." *YogaUOnline.com*, October 9, 2017.

Gill, Judith, Julie Mariko Matthews, Lana Zannettino, and Trish Carroll. "Thesis Writing as a Feminist Project: Negotiating Space for Women's Embodied Selves in New

Scholarship." *Australian Feminist Studies* 23, no. 56 (June 2008): 249–61. https://doi.org
/10.1080/08164640802068443.

Godrej, Farah. *Freedom Inside? Yoga and Meditation in the Carceral State*. New York: Oxford
University Press, 2022.

——. "The Neoliberal Yogi and the Politics of Yoga." *Political Theory* 45, no. 6 (2017):
772–800.

Gold, Daniel. "The Hindi Sants' Two Yogic Paths to the Formless Lord." In *Meditation and
Culture: The Interplay of Practice and Context*, ed. Halvor Eifring, 131–46. London:
Bloomsbury, 2015.

Goldberg, Michelle. *The Goddess Pose: The Audacious Life of Indra Devi, the Woman Who
Helped Bring Yoga to the West*. New York: Knopf, 2015.

Goldberg, Philip. *American Veda: From Emerson and the Beatles to Yoga and Meditation—
How Indian Spirituality Changed the West*. New York: Harmony Books, 2010.

Gonzalez, Jr., Juan L. "Asian Indian Immigration Patterns: The Origins of the Sikh Community in California." *International Migration Review* 20, no. 1 (1986): 40–54.

González-Reimann, Luis. "The *Yugas*: Their Importance in India and Their Use by Western Intellectuals and Esoteric and New Age Writers: The Importance of Yugas." *Religion
Compass* 8, no. 12 (December 2014): 357–70. https://doi.org/10.1111/rec3.12139.

Government of India. Income-tax Act, 1961–2016 (2016). http://www.incometaxindia.gov.in
/pages/acts/income-tax-act.aspx.

Government of India, Ministry of AYUSH. "Guidelines for Organizing of Yoga Fest/Utsav
in States/UTs." N.d. http://ayush.gov.in/sites/default/files/Guidelines%20for%20orga-
nizing%20of%20Yoga%20Fest%20and%20utsav_1.pdf.

Gray, Alexandra. *The Yoga Teacher*. New York: Grove/Atlantic, 2008.

Green, Nile. "Breathing in India, c. 1890." *Modern Asian Studies* 42, no. 2/3 (May 2008):
283–315.

Gregg, Melissa. *Counterproductive: Time Management in the Knowledge Economy*. Durham,
NC: Duke University Press, 2018.

Grey Worldwide India. *Ministry of Tourism India—"Yoga 4."* 2006. https://www.adforum
.com/talent/6697276-prathap-suthan/work/6686093.

——. *Yoga*. 2006. https://www.adforum.com/creative-work/ad/player/6686100/yoga/mini
stry-of-tourism-india.

——. *Yoga Microsite*. 2006. https://www.adforum.com/creative-work/ad/player/6686099
/yoga-microsite/ministry-of-tourism-india.

——. *Yoga 2*. 2006. https://www.adforum.com/creative-work/ad/player/6686091/yoga-2
/ministry-of-tourism-india.

Gupta, Akhil. *Red Tape*. Durham, NC: Duke University Press, 2012.

Gupta, Bhuvi, and Jacob Copeman. "Awakening Hindu Nationalism through Yoga: Swami
Ramdev and the Bharat Swabhiman Movement." *Contemporary South Asia* 27, no. 3
(2019): 313–29. https://doi.org/10.1080/09584935.2019.1587386.

Gupta, V. K. "Protecting India's Traditional Knowledge." *WIPO Magazine*, June 2011. http://
www.wipo.int/wipo_magazine/en/2011/03/article_0002.html.

Hagan, Cara, ed. *Practicing Yoga as Resistance: Voices of Color in Search of Freedom*. London: Routledge, 2021.

Hall, Ian. "India's New Public Diplomacy: Soft Power and the Limits of Government Action." *Asian Survey* 52, no. 6 (December 2012): 1089–1110.

Han, Clara. "Precarity, Precariousness, and Vulnerability." *Annual Review of Anthropology* 47 (2018): 331–43.

Haniffa, Aziz. "'It's Not Brain Drain, It's Brain Circulation.'" *Rediff.com*, August 6, 2009. http://business.rediff.com/report/2009/aug/06/not-brain-drain-but-brain-circulation-says-meera-shankar.htm.

Hardt, Michael. "Affective Labor." *boundary 2* 26, no. 2 (Summer 1999): 89–100.

Harpaz, Beth J. "'Eat, Pray, Love' Tourism Courted by Travel Industry." *The Huffington Post* (blog), May 8, 2010. http://www.huffingtonpost.com/2010/08/04/eat-pray-love-tourism-cou_n_671130.html?ir=Australia.

Harris, Craig. "Allauddin Khan | Biography & History." *AllMusic*. Accessed May 10, 2019. https://www.allmusic.com/artist/allauddin-khan-mn0000002677.

Harris, Kenneth E. "Op-Ed: Breathing While Black." *Michigan Chronicle*, June 17, 2020.

Hartman, Saidiya. *Lose Your Mother: A Journey Along the Atlantic Slave Route*. New York: Farrar, Straus and Giroux, 2008.

Harvey, David. *A Brief History of Neoliberalism*. Oxford: Oxford University Press USA, 2005.

Hassan, Narin. "Travelers, Translators, and Spiritual Mothers: Yoga, Gender, and Colonial Histories." *Race and Yoga* 5, no. 1 (2020): 24–41. https://doi.org/10.5070/R351046982.

Hawley, John C., ed. *India in Africa, Africa in India: Indian Ocean Cosmopolitanisms*. Bloomington: Indiana University Press, 2008.

Heidegger, Martin. *The Question Concerning Technology, and Other Essays*. New York: Harper & Row, 1977.

Heifetz, Daniel. "Religion, Science, and the Middle Class in the All World Gayatri Pariwar." *International Journal of Hindu Studies* 23, no. 1 (April 2019): 27–42. https://doi.org/10.1007/s11407-019-09249-0.

Hendrickson, Paul. "Cesar Chavez's Causa." *The Washington Post*, April 22, 1979.

Hines, Alice. "Inside CorePower Yoga Teacher Training." *The New York Times*, April 6, 2019. https://www.nytimes.com/2019/04/06/style/corepower-yoga-teacher-training.html.

Hinz, Angela, Kate Mulgrew, Tamara De Regt, and Geoff Lovell. "Is This What a Female Yogi Looks Like? A Content Analysis of Yoga Images on Instagram." *Body Image* 36 (March 2021): 117–26. https://doi.org/10.1016/j.bodyim.2020.11.003.

——. "Practice or Performance? A Content Analysis of Yoga-Related Videos on Instagram." *Body Image* 39 (December 2021): 175–83. https://doi.org/10.1016/j.bodyim.2021.08.002.

Holdrege, Barbara A. *Bhakti and Embodiment: Fashioning Divine Bodies and Devotional Bodies in Kṛṣṇa Bhakti*. Abingdon, UK: Routledge, 2015.

"How Google Uses Yoga, Meditation to Increase Productivity." Bloomberg Business, March 11, 2015. http://www.bloomberg.com/news/videos/2015-03-10/how-google-uses-yoga-meditation-to-increase-productivity.

Howard, Veena. "Divine Light and Melodies Lead the Way: The Santmat Tradition of Bihar." *Religions* 10, no. 4 (2019): 230. https://doi.org/10.3390/rel10040230.

Hull, Matthew. *Government of Paper: The Materiality of Bureaucracy in Urban Pakistan.* Berkeley: University of California Press, 2012.

Humberstone, Barbara, and Carol Cutler-Riddick. "Older Women, Embodiment and Yoga Practice." *Ageing & Society* 35, no. 6 (July 2015): 1221–41.

Hussain, Mobeen. "Combining Global Expertise with Local Knowledge in Colonial India: Selling Ideals of Beauty and Health in Commodity Advertising (c. 1900–1949)." *South Asia: Journal of South Asian Studies* 44, no. 5 (2021): 926–47. https://doi.org/10.1080/00856401.2021.1968599.

Ichiyo Muto. "Asia, Inter-Asia, and Movement: Decolonization into the Future." *Inter-Asia Cultural Studies* 11, no. 2 (2010): 178–83.

"Immigrants Support Network (ISN)." *LinkedIn,* January 28, 2009. https://www.linkedin.com/groups/Immigrants-Support-Network-ISN-1785609/about.

"India Destroys Stockpile of Chemical Weapons." *India Today,* May 14, 2009. https://www.indiatoday.in/latest-headlines/story/india-destroys-stockpile-of-chemical-weapons-47447-2009-05-14.

"India's Prime Minister Urges Indians to Stay in Their Country." *All Things Considered.* National Public Radio, September 28, 2015. http://www.npr.org/2015/09/28/444236937/indias-prime-minister-urges-indians-to-stay-in-their-country.

"International Day of Yoga." *Wikipedia,* January 9, 2023. https://upload.wikimedia.org/wikipedia/commons/e/e8/The_Prime_Minister%2C_Shri_Narendra_Modi_participates_in_the_mass_yoga_demonstration_at_Rajpath_on_the_occasion_of_International_Yoga_Day%2C_in_New_Delhi_on_June_21%2C_2015_(3).jpg.

Ipsos Public Affairs. "The 2016 Yoga in America Study Conducted by Yoga Journal and Yoga Alliance." January 2016. https://www.yogaalliance.org/2016yogainamericastudy.

Irigaray, Luce. *Between East and West: From Singularity to Community.* Trans. Stephen Pluháček. New York: Columbia University Press, 2002.

Iyengar, B. K. S. *Light on Yoga: Yoga Dipika.* Rev. ed.. New York: Schocken, 1966.

Iyengar, B. K. S., John J. Evans, and Douglas Abrams. *Light on Life: The Yoga Journey to Wholeness, Inner Peace, and Ultimate Freedom.* Emmaus, PA: Rodale, 2005.

Jacobsen, Knut A. *Yoga in Modern Hinduism: Hariharānanda Āraṇya and Sāṃkhyayoga.* Abingdon, UK: Routledge, 2018.

——, ed. *Yoga Powers: Extraordinary Capacities Attained Through Meditation and Concentration.* Leiden: Brill, 2012.

Jacobson, Matthew Frye. *Roots Too: White Ethnic Revival in Post-Civil Rights America.* Cambridge, MA: Harvard University Press, 2006.

Jaffrelot, Christophe. "India's Democracy at 70: Toward a Hindu State?" *Journal of Democracy* 28, no. 3 (July 2017): 52–63.

——. "Narendra Modi between Hindutva and Subnationalism: The Gujarati Asmita of a Hindu Hriday Samrat." *India Review* 15, no. 2 (2016): 196–217.

——. "The Story of Indian Politicians and Tantrics." Carnegie Endowment for International Peace, November 7, 2015. https://carnegieendowment.org/2015/11/07/story-of-indian-politicians-and-tantrics-pub-61928.

Jain, Andrea R. "Branding Yoga: The Cases of Iyengar Yoga, Siddha Yoga and Anusara Yoga." *Approaching Religion* 2, no. 2 (December 2012): 3–17.

———. *Peace Love Yoga: The Politics of Global Spirituality.* New York: Oxford University Press, 2020.

———. *Selling Yoga: From Counterculture to Pop Culture.* New York: Oxford University Press, 2014.

Jain, Ravindra K. *Nation, Diaspora, Trans-Nation: Reflections from India.* London: Routledge, 2010.

Jalote, Pankaj, Bijendra Nath Jain, and Sudhir Sopory. "Classification for Research Universities in India." *Higher Education* 79, no. 2 (February 2020): 225–41. https://doi.org/10.1007/s10734-019-00406-3.

Janmohamed, Zahir. "The Rise of Narendra Modi: The Man Who Doesn't Wear Dark Green." *Boston Review,* June 28, 2013. http://bostonreview.net/world/zahir-janmohamed-narendra-modi-india-gujarat-man-who-refuses-wear-green.

Jaworski, Katrina. "The Breath of Life and Death." *Cultural Critique* 86 (Winter 2014): 65–91.

Jayadeva, Sazana. " 'Below English Line': An Ethnographic Exploration of Class and the English Language in Post-Liberalization India." *Modern Asian Studies* 52, no. 2 (2018): 576–608.

Jia, Susan (Sixue). "Leisure Motivation and Satisfaction: A Text Mining of Yoga Centres, Yoga Consumers, and Their Interactions." *Sustainability* 10, no. 12 (November 27, 2018): 4458. https://doi.org/10.3390/su10124458.

Jones, Sarah. "Yoga Teachers Are Unionizing to Heal the Wellness Industry." *New York Magazine,* September 12, 2019. https://www.thecut.com/2019/09/yogaworks-teachers-first-yoga-teacher-union.html.

Jones, Shermaine M. " 'I CAN'T BREATHE!': Affective Asphyxia in Claudia Rankine's *Citizen: An American Lyric.*" *South: A Scholarly Journal* 50, no. 1 (Fall 2017): 37–46.

Joshi, K. S. "On the Meaning of Yoga." *Philosophy East and West* 15, no. 1 (January 1965): 53–64.

Kablyl, Lubna. "Ramdev Trust Wins I-T War on Tax-Exempt Tag for Yoga." *The Times of India,* February 18, 2017. http://timesofindia.indiatimes.com/business/india-business/ramdev-trust-wins-i-t-war-on-tax-exempt-tag-for-yoga/articleshow/57215759.cms.

Kadetsky, Elizabeth. *First There Is a Mountain.* Westland, MI: Dzanc Books, 2011.

Kale, Sunila S., and Christian Lee Novetske. "Some Reflections on Yoga as Political Theology." *The Wire,* January 28, 2016. https://thewire.in/culture/some-reflections-on-yoga-as-political-theology.

———. "Yoga and the Means and Ends of Secularism." *The Wire,* June 21, 2018. https://thewire.in/government/yoga-means-ends-secularism.

Kang, Bhavdeep. "Indira and the 'Indian Rasputin.'" *The Asian Age,* June 6, 2016. https://www.asianage.com/books/indira-and-indian-rasputin-604.

Karlsson, Bengt G. "The Social Life of Categories." *Focaal: Journal of Global and Historical Anthropology* 65 (2013): 33–41. https://doi.org/10.3167/fcl.2013.650104.

Kataria, Madan. *Laugh for No Reason.* Mumbai: Madhuri International, 1999.

Katz, Max. "Institutional Communalism in North Indian Classical Music." *Ethnomusicology* 56, no. 2 (Spring/Summer 2012): 279–98. https://doi.org/10.5406/ethnomusicology.56.2.0279.

Kaur, Ravinder. *Brand New Nation: Capitalist Dreams and Nationalist Designs in Twenty-First-Century India.* Stanford, CA: Stanford University Press, 2020.

——. "'I Am India Shining': The Investor-Citizen and the Indelible Icon of Good Times." *The Journal of Asian Studies* 75, no. 3 (August 2016): 621–48. https://doi.org/10.1017/S0021911816000619.

——. "Nation's Two Bodies: Rethinking the Idea of 'New' India and Its Other." *Third World Quarterly* 33, no. 4 (2012): 603–21.

Kaushik-Brown, Roopa. "Toward Yoga as Property." In *Yoga, the Body, and Embodied Social Change: An Intersectional Feminist Analysis*, ed. Beth Berila, Melanie Klein, and Chelsea Jackson Roberts, 67–89. Lanham, MD: Lexington Books, 2016.

Kazim, Ali. "The End of Canon." *The Massachusetts Review* 59, no. 4 (2018): 779–82.

Keen, Suzanne. *Empathy and the Novel*. New York: Oxford University Press, 2007.

Kellner, Douglas. "The Media, Democracy, and Spectacle: Some Critical Reflections." *Cultural Politics* 11, no. 1 (2015): 53–69.

Kennedy, Andrew Bingham. *The Conflicted Superpower: America's Collaboration with China and India in Global Innovation*. New York: Columbia University Press, 2018.

——. *The International Ambitions of Mao and Nehru: National Efficacy Beliefs and the Making of Foreign Policy*. New York: Cambridge University Press, 2012.

——. "The Politics of Skilled Immigration: Explaining the Ups and Downs of the US H-1B Visa Program." *International Migration Review* 53, no. 2 (2019): 346–70.

Khalikova, Venera R. "The Ayurveda of Baba Ramdev: Biomoral Consumerism, National Duty and the Biopolitics of 'Homegrown' Medicine in India." *South Asia: Journal of South Asian Studies* 40, no. 1 (2017): 105–22. https://doi.org/10.1080/00856401.2017.1266987.

Khatchadourian, Raffi. "The Laughing Guru." *The New Yorker*, August 30, 2010.

Khilnani, Sunil. *The Idea of India*. New York: Farrar, Straus and Giroux, 1997.

Killian, Diana. *Corpse Pose*. New York: Berkley Prime Crime, 2008.

Killingly, Dermot. "Svādhyāya: An Ancient Way of Using the Veda." *Religions of South Asia* 8, no. 1 (August 22, 2014). https://doi.org/10.1558/rosa.v8i1.109.

Klepinger, Laurah E. *Transnational Yoga at Work: Spiritual Tourism and Its Blind Spots*. Lanham, MD: Lexington Books, 2022.

Koestler, Arthur. "Last of the Saints." *Commentary*, February 1960.

Koshy, Susan, and R. Radhakrishnan, eds. *Transnational South Asians: The Making of a Neo-Diaspora*. New Delhi and New York: Oxford University Press, 2008.

Kumar, Amitava. *Passport Photos*. Berkeley: University of California Press, 2000.

Kumar, V. Ravi. *Yoga: Bharat's Invaluable Gift to the World*. New Delhi: Niyogi Books, 2015.

Lakshmi, Anusha. "Choreographing Tolerance: Narendra Modi, Hindu Nationalism, and International Yoga Day." *Race and Yoga* 5, no. 1 (2020): 42–58.

Lakshmi, Seetha. "Yoga Must Be Proof-Based to Be Popular: PM Narendra Modi's Guru." *The Times of India*, December 20, 2016. http://timesofindia.indiatimes.com/city/bengaluru/yoga-must-be-proof-based-to-be-popular-pm-narendra-modis-guru/articleshow/56072050.cms.

Lal, Brij V., Peter Reeves, and Rajesh Rai, eds. *The Encyclopedia of the Indian Diaspora*. Honolulu: University of Hawai'i Press, 2006.

Lalonde, Dianne. "Does Cultural Appropriation Cause Harm?" *Politics, Groups, and Identities*, October 10, 2019, 1–18. https://doi.org/10.1080/21565503.2019.1674160.

Larios, Borayin. "The Vedamūrti: Embodying the Veda in Contemporary Maharashtra." *International Journal of Hindu Studies* 17, no. 3 (December 2013): 287–312. https://doi.org /10.1007/s11407-014-9141-2.

Lazarus, Susannah Myrtle. "Meet Sarvesh Shashi, India's New Millionaire Yogi." *The Hindu*, May 10, 2019. https://www.thehindu.com/society/meet-27-year-old-sarvesh-shashi-indias -new-millionaire-yogi/article27094190.ece.

Lenard, Patti Tamara, and Peter Balint. "What Is (the Wrong of) Cultural Appropriation?" *Ethnicities* 20, no. 2 (April 2020): 331–52. https://doi.org/10.1177/1468796819866498.

Leonard, Karen. "Historical Constructions of Ethnicity: Research on Punjabi Immigrants in California." *Journal of American Ethnic History* 12, no. 4 (Summer 1993): 3–26.

——. "Punjabi Farmers and California's Alien Land Law." *Agricultural History* 59, no. 4 (October 1985): 549–62.

"Live on the Floor." *The Leader*, August 25, 1921.

Lizzie, Jade. "'Holding Space': What It Means for Yoga Teachers and You." *Yogapedia*, January 29, 2016. https://www.yogapedia.com/holding-space-what-does-it-mean/2 /7018.

Lloyd, Mike. "Life in the Slow Lane: Rethinking Spectacular Body Modification." *Continuum* 18, no. 4 (December 2004): 555–64. https://doi.org/10.1080/1030431042000297662.

Longkumer, Arkotong. "'Nagas Can't Sit Lotus Style': Baba Ramdev, Patanjali, and Neo-Hindutva." *Contemporary South Asia* 26, no. 4 (2018): 400–20. https://doi.org/10.1080 /09584935.2018.1545008.

——. *The Greater India Experiment: Hindutva and the Northeast*. Stanford, CA: Stanford University Press, 2020.

Lorenzen, David N., and Adrian Munoz, eds. *Yogi Heroes and Poets: Histories and Legends of the Naths*. Albany: State University of New York Press, 2011.

Love, Robert. *The Great Oom: The Mysterious Origins of America's First Yogi*. New York: Penguin, 2010.

Lucia, Amanda J. "'Give Me Sevā Overtime': Selfless Service and Humanitarianism in Mata Amritanandamayi's Transnational Guru Movement." *History of Religions* 54, no. 2 (November 2014): 188–207. https://doi.org/10.1086/677812.

——. *White Utopias: The Religious Exoticism of Transformational Festivals*. Oakland: University of California Press, 2020.

Luhr, Eileen. "Seeker, Surfer, Yogi: The Progressive Religious Imagination and the Cultural Politics of Place in Encinitas, California." *American Quarterly* 67, no. 4 (2015): 1169–93. https://doi.org/doi:10.1353/aq.2015.0072.

Lynch, Sarah-Kate. *Heavenly Hirani's School of Laughing Yoga*. New Zealand: Random House New Zealand, 2014.

Maas, Philipp A. "'Sthirasukham Āsanam': Posture and Performance in Classical Yoga and Beyond." In *Yoga in Transformation: Historical and Contemporary Perspectives*, ed. Karl Baier, Philipp A. Maas, and Karin Preisendanz, 49–100. Vienna: Vienna University Press, 2018.

Maclean, Kama. *British India, White Australia: Overseas Indians, Intercolonial Relations and the Empire*. Sydney: UNSW Press, 2020.

Maira, Sunaina. *Missing: Youth, Citizenship, and Empire after 9/11.* Durham, NC: Duke University Press, 2009.

Malabou, Catherine. *The Future of Hegel: Plasticity, Temporality and Dialectic.* Trans. Lisabeth During. Abingdon, UK: Routledge, 2005.

Mallinson, James, and Mark Singleton, trans. *Roots of Yoga.* London: Penguin, 2017.

Malnak v. Yogi. (United States Court of Appeals, Third Circuit 1979).

Mangiarotti, Emanuela. "The Politics of Tending to the Body: Women Doing Yoga in Genoa (Italy)." *European Journal of Women's Studies,* October 27, 2022, 13505068221129o. https://doi.org/10.1177/13505068221129063.

Mani, Bakirathi. "Beyond Bollywood: Exhibiting South Asian America." *Journal of Asian American Studies* 18, no. 2 (2015): 193–217. https://doi.org/10.1353/jaas.2015.0013.

Mankekar, Purnima. *Unsettling India: Affect, Temporality, Transnationality.* Durham, NC: Duke University Press, 2015.

Manuel, Peter. "North Indian Sufi Popular Music in the Age of Hindu and Muslim Fundamentalism." *Ethnomusicology* 52, no. 3 (Fall 2008): 378–400.

March, Stephanie. "International Yoga Day: 35,000-Strong New Delhi Crowd Sets World Record for Largest Yoga Session." *ABC News,* June 22, 2015. http://www.abc.net.au/news/2015-06-22/india-sets-new-world-record-for-international-yoga-day/6562300.

Markula, Pirkko. "Reading Yoga: Changing Discourses of Postural Yoga on the *Yoga Journal* Covers." *Communication and Sport* 2, no. 2 (2015): 143–71. https://doi.org/doi.org/10.1177/2167479513490673.

Martin, Fran, John Nguyet Erni, and Audrey Yue. "(Im)Mobile Precarity in the Asia-Pacific." *Cultural Studies* 33, no. 6 (November 2, 2019): 895–914. https://doi.org/10.1080/09502386.2019.1660690.

Martin, Judith G. "The Pedagogy of Conciliation in the Bhagavata Purana: A 'Sporting' Way of Understanding Jnana-Yoga." MA thesis, McMaster University, 1975.

Martin, Peter. "Yoga Diplomacy: Narendra Modi's Soft Power Strategy." *Foreign Affairs,* January 25, 2015. http://www.foreignaffairs.com/articles/142812/peter-martin/yoga-diplomacy.

Mathur, Swati. "Incredible India 2.0 to Take a Spiritual Bent." *The Times of India,* June 21, 2017. http://timesofindia.indiatimes.com/india/incredible-india-2-0-to-take-a-spiritual-bent/articleshow/59243906.cms.

Mauss, Marcel. *The Gift: Forms and Functions of Exchange in Archaic Societies.* Trans. Ian Cunnison. London: Cohen & West Ltd., 1969.

Mbembe, Achille. "The Universal Right to Breathe." Trans. Carolyn Shread. *Critical Inquiry* 47, no. S2 (January 1, 2021): S58–62. https://doi.org/10.1086/711437.

McCall, Timothy. "Yoga as a Technology for Life Transformation." *Kripalu: Center for Yoga and Health,* Fall 2005. http://kripalu.org/article/179.

McCartney, Patrick. "Jhirī: A 'Sanskrit-Speaking' Village in Madhya Pradesh." *Journal of South Asian Languages and Linguistics* 4, no. 2 (2017): 167–209.

——. "Spiritual Bypass and Entanglement in Yogaland: How Neoliberalism, Soft Hindutva and Banal Nationalism Facilitate Yoga Fundamentalism." *Politics and Religion Journal* 13, no. 1 (2019): 137–75.

———. "Stretching into the Shadows: Unlikely Alliances, Strategic Syncretism, and De-Post-Colonizing Yogaland's 'Yogatopia(s).'" *Asian Ethnology* 78, no. 2 (2019): 373–401.

McGuire, Coreen, Jane Macnaughton, and Havi Carel. "The Color of Breath." *Literature and Medicine* 38, no. 2 (2020): 233–38. https://doi.org/10.1353/lm.2020.0015.

McLean, Bethany. "Whose Yoga Is It, Anyway?" *Vanity Fair*, March 5, 2012. https://www.vanityfair.com/news/business/2012/04/krishna-pattanbhi-trophy-wife-ashtanga-yoga.

Merchant, Atul S. *Taskari*. Mumbai: Atul S. Merchant, 2014.

Miller, Manjari Chatterjee, and Kate Sullivan de Estrada. "Pragmatism in Indian Foreign Policy: How Ideas Constrain Modi." *International Affairs* 93, no. 1 (2017): 27–49.

Miller, Nancy. *But Enough About Me: Why We Read Other People's Lives*. New York: Columbia University Press, 2002.

Mishra, Vijay. *Bollywood Cinema: Temples of Desire*. New York: Routledge, 2002.

Mitchell, Rain. *Tales from the Yoga Studio*. New York: Penguin, 2011.

Mohanty, Satya P. *Literary Theory and the Claims of History: Postmodernism, Objectivity, Multicultural Politics*. Ithaca, NY: Cornell University Press, 1997.

Mookherjee, Nayanika. "Introduction: Self in South Asia." *Journal of Historical Sociology* 26, no. 1 (March 2013): 1–18. https://doi.org/10.1111/johs.12008.

Morey, Peter, and Amina Yaqin. *Framing Muslims: Stereotyping and Representation After 9/11*. Cambridge, MA: Harvard University Press, 2011.

Morning, Ann. "The Racial Self-Identification of South Asians in the United States." *Journal of Ethnic and Migration Studies* 27, no. 1 (January 2001): 61–79. https://doi.org/10.1080/13691830125692.

Morrison, Suzanne. *Yoga Bitch: One Woman's Quest to Conquer Skepticism, Cynicism and Cigarettes on the Path to Enlightenment*. New York: Three Rivers Press, 2011.

Morris-Suzuki, Tessa. "Liquid Area Studies." *positions: asia critique* 27, no. 1 (February 1, 2019): 209–39. https://doi.org/10.1215/10679847-7251897.

"Muhammad Ahmad Writings, Undated." *Archives Unbound*. Accessed June 20, 2019. http://go.galegroups.com/gdsc/i.do?&id=GALE%7CSC5103270679&v=2.1&u=ucberkeley&it=r&p=GDSC&sw=w&viewtype=Manuscript.

Mukerji, Asoke. "Revealed: The Diplomatic Moves That Delivered Modi His Yoga Day." *The Wire* (blog), June 21, 2016. http://thewire.in/44205/revealed-the-diplomatic-moves-that-delivered-modi-his-yoga-day/.

Munshi, Soniya. "Multiplicities of Violence: Responses to September 11 from South Asian Women's Organizations." *Race/Ethnicity: Multidisciplinary Global Contexts* 4, no. 3 (July 2011): 419–36. https://doi.org/10.2979/racethmulglocon.4.3.419.

Musial, Jennifer. "Engaged Pedagogy in the Feminist Classroom and Yoga Studio." *Feminist Teacher* 21, no. 3 (2011): 212–28. https://doi.org/10.5406/femteacher.21.3.0212.

Nanda, Meera. *The God Market: How Globalization Is Making India More Hindu*. New York: Monthly Review Press, 2009.

Nandy, Ashis. "Obituary of a Culture." *Seminar*, May 2002. http://www.india-seminar.com/2002/513/513%20ashis%20onandy.htm.

Narayan, Kirin. *Everyday Creativity: Singing Goddesses in the Himalayan Foothills*. Chicago: University of Chicago Press, 2016.

———. *My Family and Other Saints.* Chicago: University of Chicago Press, 2007.

———. "Refractions of the Field at Home: American Representations of Hindu Holy Men in the 19th and 20th Centuries." *Cultural Anthropology* 8, no. 4 (November 1993): 476–509.

———. "Statement." In *Living in America: Poetry and Fiction by South Asian American Writers*, ed. Roshni Rustomji-Kerns, 155–66. New York: Routledge, 1995.

Nawaz, MS. "Almost Half the Yoga Centres in Rishikesh, Regarded as the Yoga Capital of the Country, Forced to Shut as Many Can't Afford Rent." *The Times of India*, August 10, 2020.

Newcombe, Suzanne. "Stretching for Health and Well-Being: Yoga and Women in Britain, 1960–1980." *Asian Medicine* 3, no. 1 (October 16, 2007): 37–63. https://doi.org/10.1163/157342107X207209.

———. "Yoga and Meditation as a Health Intervention." In *Routledge Handbook of Yoga and Meditation Studies*, ed. Suzanne Newcombe and Karen O'Brien-Kop, 156–68. Abingdon, UK: Routledge, 2021.

———. *Yoga in Britain: Stretching Spirituality and Educating Yogis.* Sheffield, UK: Equinox, 2019.

Newcombe, Suzanne, and Philip Deslippe. "Anglophone Yoga and Meditation Outside of India." In *Routledge Handbook of Yoga and Meditation Studies*, 350–65. Abingdon, UK: Routledge, 2021.

Newcombe, Suzanne, and Karen O'Brien-Kop, eds. *Routledge Handbook of Yoga and Meditation Studies.* Abingdon, UK: Routledge, 2021.

Ng, Yuk-hang, and Natalie Ornelland Lana Lam. "Seventh Yoga Centre Goes Bust." *South China Morning Post*, June 27, 2011.

Nicholson, Andrew J. *Unifying Hinduism: Philosophy and Identity in Indian Intellectual History.* New York: Columbia University Press, 2010.

Noble, Freya. "That's A LOT of Downward Dogs!" *Daily Mail Australia*, June 21, 2015. http://www.dailymail.co.uk/news/article-3133167/That-s-LOT-downward-dogs-Incredible-photos-millions-people-world-taking-International-Day-Yoga-army-prime-minister-involved.html.

Norman, Howard. "The Healing Powers of the Western Oystercatcher." *Salmagundi* 174/175 (Spring 2012): 21–56.

O'Brien, Tom. "Episode 2: 'Something Great.'" *Om City: The Series*, n.d. http://omcityseries.com/episodes.

———. "Episode 5: 'Think Of Others.'" *Om City: The Series*, 2014. http://omcityseries.com/episodes.

O'Brien-Kop, Karen. *Rethinking "Classical Yoga" and Buddhism: Meditation, Metaphors and Materiality.* London: Bloomsbury, 2022.

"153 Congressional Record-Senate S5689-03." *Congressional Record* 153, no. Pt 8 (May 8, 2007).

Ong, Aihwa. *Flexible Citizenship: The Cultural Logics of Transnationality.* Durham, NC: Duke University Press, 1999.

———. "(Re)Articulations of Citizenship." *PS: Political Science and Politics* 38, no. 4 (October 2005): 697–99.

Osho. "Sanskrit Is a Divine Language." *Speaking Tree*, n.d. https://www.speakingtree.in/article
/sanskrit-is-a-divine-language#:~:text=The%20Sanskrit%20language%20is%20called%20
Devavani%20%E2%80%94%20the,certain%20music%20and%20aroma.%20How%20did%20
this%20happen?

"Our Five National Movement." Bharat Swabhiman, n.d. http://bharatswabhimantrust.org
/ReadMore.aspx?ContentType=Bharat%20Swabhiman%20details&ContentID=28.

Outlook Web Desk. "PM Modi Gets Clean Chit From SC In 2002 Gujarat Riots Case: A
Timeline Of Events." *Outlook*, June 24, 2022. https://www.outlookindia.com/national
/pm-modi-gets-clean-chit-in-2002-gujarat-riots-case-a-timeline-of-events-news
-204382.

——. "'The Modi Question': India Slams BBC Documentary On PM Modi And 2002 Gujarat
Riots, Calls It 'Propaganda Piece.'" *Outlook*, January 19, 2023. https://www.outlookindia
.com/national/-a-propaganda-piece-india-slams-bbc-documentary-on-pm-modi-and
-2002-gujarat-riots-youtube-takes-down-video-news-255000.

Padmanabhan, Satish. "If Yoga Is Hindu, Then Gravity Is Christian." *Outlook*, June 15, 2015.

Page, Enoch H. "The Gender, Race, and Class Barriers: Enclosing Yoga as White Public
Space." In *Yoga, the Body, and Embodied Social Change: An Intersectional Feminist Anal-
ysis*, ed. Beth Berila, Melanie Klein, and Chelsea Jackson Roberts, 41–65. Lanham, MD:
Lexington Books, 2016.

Palkhivala, Rashmi. *A Life of Light: The Biography of B. K. S. Iyengar*. Noida, Uttar Pradesh:
Harper Element, 2017.

Palshikar, Suhas. "The BJP and Hindu Nationalism: Centrist Politics and Majoritarian
Impulses." *South Asia: Journal of South Asian Studies* 38, no. 4 (2015): 719–35. https://doi
.org/10.1080/00856401.2015.1089460.

Pande, Manisha. "BJP Does Shirshasana over Ramdev Remark: Yoga Guru's Distasteful
Anti-Dalit Remarks May Harm Party's Cause." *DNA: Daily News and Analysis*. May 3,
2014.

Pandey, Neelam. "CBSE Students Will Earn Grades in Class 10 by Doing Yoga, Showing Patriotism." *Hindustan Times*, February 1, 2017. https://www.hindustantimes.com/education
/cbse-students-will-earn-grades-in-class-10-by-practising-yoga-showing-patriotism
/story-990rKCgmqP6X1rtLOx6RQJ.html.

Pant, Ketaki. "A Poet's Ocean: Merchants and Imagination across Indian Ocean Gujarat."
South Asia: Journal of South Asian Studies 44, no. 4 (2021): 684–702. https://doi.org/10
.1080/00856401.2021.1939104.

Panton, Rachel, and Stephanie Evans, eds. "Sassin' Through Sadhana." *Race and Yoga* 2, no. 1
(2017).

Pardon My Hindi. #WhitePeopleDoingYoga. 2014. https://www.chiraagbhakta.com
/selectedwork.

Parfit, Derek. *Reasons and Persons*. Oxford: Clarenden Press, 1984.

Park, Crystal L., Tosca Braun, and Tamar Siegel. "Who Practices Yoga? A Systematic Review
of Demographic, Health-Related, and Psychosocial Factors Associated with Yoga Practice." *Journal of Behavioral Medicine* 38, no. 3 (June 2015): 460–71.

Park, Edward J.W., and John S.W. Park. *Probationary Americans: Contemporary Immigration Policies and the Shaping of Asian American Communities*. New York and London: Routledge, 2005.

Patankar, Prachi. "Ghosts of Yogas Past and Present." *Jadaliyya*, February 26, 2014. http://www.jadaliyya.com/Details/30281/Ghosts-of-Yogas-Past-and-Present.

Patel, Kajal Nisha. "White Womanhood, Hindutva and Spiritual Bypass: Museum Yoga and the Mass-Participation Spectacle." *The Jugaad Project* 5, no. 1 (2023). www.thejugaad project.pub/museum-yoga.

Patil, Vrushali. "Reproducing-Resisting Race and Gender Difference: Examining India's Online Tourism Campaign from a Transnational Feminist Perspective." *Signs: Journal of Women in Culture and Society* 37, no. 1 (September 2011): 185–210.

Pedersen, Julia, ed. *Guruji BKS Iyengar and His Institute in the '70s*. London: YogaWords, 2020.

Pednekar, Puja. "Patanjali to Hold Monthly Yoga Sessions in Schools." *Hindustan Times*, August 19, 2016. https://www.hindustantimes.com/cities/patanjali-to-hold-monthly-yoga -sessions-in-schools/story-XQk2gHzWRhKBepB4CNzd2I.html.

Pethiyagoda, Kadira. "India's Soft Power Advantage." *Australia India Institute* (blog), November 4, 2014. http://www.aii.unimelb.edu.au/news/blog/india%E2%80%99s-soft-power -advantage.

Pinch, William R. *Warrior Ascetics and Indian Empires*. Cambridge: Cambridge University Press, 2006.

"PM Narendra Modi Launches 'Fit India Movement.'" *Money Control*, August 29, 2019. https://www.moneycontrol.com/news/india/pm-narendra-modi-to-launch-fit-india -movement-at-10-am-where-to-watch-live-4383891.html.

Pollack, Neal. *Downward-Facing Death*. Las Vegas: Thomas & Mercer, 2013.

——. *Open Your Heart*. Las Vegas: Thomas & Mercer, 2013.

——. *Stretch: The Unlikely Making of a Yoga Dude*. New York: HarperCollins, 2010.

Ponniah, Ujithra. "Managing Marriages through 'Self-Improvement': Women and 'New Age' Spiritualities in Delhi." *South Asia: Journal of South Asian Studies* 41, no. 1 (2018): 137–52. https://doi.org/10.1080/00856401.2017.1366682.

Prashad, Vijay. "The Day Our Probation Ended." *Race/Ethnicity: Multidisciplinary Global Contexts* 4, no. 3 (July 2011): 361–71. https://doi.org/10.2979/racethmulglocon.4.3.361.

——. *The Karma of Brown Folk*. Minneapolis: University of Minnesota Press, 2000.

——. *Uncle Swami: South Asians in America Today*. Noida, Uttar Pradesh: HarperCollins India, 2013.

"Prathap Suthan, NCD, Cheil India." *Desi Creative*, September 7, 2010. http://www .desicreative.com/prathap-suthan-ncd-cheil-india/.

Prendergast, Lou. *Conscious Theatre Practice: Yoga, Meditation and Performance*. Leiden: Brill, 2022.

Press Information Bureau, Government of India. "Ministry of AYUSH and WHO Working Group Meeting on Benchmarks for Training in Yoga from Today." February 26, 2019. http://pib.nic.in/newsite/PrintRelease.aspx?relid=188950.

Preston, Carrie J. *Learning to Kneel: Noh, Modernism, and Journeys in Teaching.* New York: Columbia University Press, 2016.

Preston, Julia. "Pink Slips at Disney. But First, Training Foreign Replacements." *The New York Times,* June 3, 2015. http://www.nytimes.com/2015/06/04/us/last-task-after-layoff-at -disney-train-foreign-replacements.html?_r=0.

Putcha, Rumya S. "Yoga and White Public Space." *Religions* 11, no. 12 (December 14, 2020): 669. https://doi.org/10.3390/rel11120669.

Putcha, Rumya Sree. "After Eat, Pray, Love: Tourism, Orientalism, and Cartographies of Salvation." *Tourist Studies* 20, no. 4 (2020): 450–66. https://doi.org/10.1177/1468797620946808.

Puustinen, Lina, and Matti Rautaniemi. "Wellbeing for Sale: Representations of Yoga in Commercial Media." *Temenos* 51, no. 1 (2015): 45–70. https://doi.org/10.33356/temenos .40878.

Radjou, Navi, Jaideep Prabhu, Simone Ahuja, and Kevin Roberts. *Jugaad Innovation: Think Frugal, Be Flexible, Generate Breakthrough Growth.* Hoboken, NJ: Wiley, 2012.

Rahman, Maseeh. "Indian Prime Minister Claims Genetic Science Existed in Ancient Times." *The Guardian,* October 29, 2014. https://www.theguardian.com/world/2014/oct/28/indian -prime-minister-genetic-science-existed-ancient-times.

Rai, Amit S. *Jugaad Time: Ecologies of Everyday Hacking in India.* Durham, NC: Duke University Press, 2019.

Rai, Rajesh and Peter Reeves, eds. *The South Asian Diaspora: Transnational Networks and Changing Identities.* New York: Routledge, 2009.

Rai, Saritha. "India's Tourism Banks on 'Eat, Pray, Love.'" *Globalpost* (blog), August 22, 2010. http://www.globalpost.com/dispatch/india/100804/tourism-international-travel-eat -pray-love.

Raj, Dhooleka Sarhadi. "The Overseas Citizen of India and Emigrant Infrastructure: Tracing the Deterritorializations of Diaspora Strategies." *Geoforum* 59 (February 2015): 159–68. https://doi.org/10.1016/j.geoforum.2014.11.015.

Rajan, Kaushik Sunder. *Biocapital: The Constitution of Postgenomic Life.* Durham, NC: Duke University Press, 2006.

Rajaram, Sowmya. "'Indian Readers Largely Read Realism Fiction.'" *Bangalore Mirror,* July 8, 2018.

Ramanathan, Suguna. "Ordeal by Fire." *Seminar,* May 2002. http://www.india-seminar.com /2002/513/513%20suguna%20ramanathan.htm.

Ramazani, Jahan. "Poetry and Race: An Introduction." *New Literary History* 50, no. 4 (2019): vii–xxxvii. https://doi.org/10.1353/nlh.2019.0050.

Rawal, Priyanka. "Indian Monk Who Wants a Billion-Dollar Company: A Yogic Business Revolution." *International Journal of Management Research and Review* 6, no. 9 (September 2016): 1169–81.

Reddy, Vanita. "The Nationalization of the Global Indian Woman: Geographies of Beauty in *Femina*." *South Asian Popular Culture* 4, no. 1 (April 2006): 61–85. https://doi.org/10 .1080/14746680600555691.

"Religious Landscape Study." Pew Research Center. Accessed February 9, 2021. https://www .pewforum.org/religious-landscape-study/.

Remski, Matthew. "Modern Yoga Will Not Form a Real Culture Until Every Studio Can Also Double as Soup Kitchen, and Other Observations from the Threshold between Yoga and Activism." In *21st Century Yoga: Culture, Politics and Practice*, ed. Carol Horton and Roseanne Harvey, 104–27. Chicago: Kleio Books, 2012.

"Review: Memoir of the Late Major Antony Bumble, of the Bengal Army. By John William Braye. London: 1867." *The Pioneer*, May 10, 1867.

Richards, Michael. "B. K. S. Iyengar." *Time*, April 26, 2004. http://content.time.com/time/specials/packages/article/0,28804,1970858_1970910_1972051,00.html.

Rohatynskyj, Marta. "Empowering the Dividual." *Anthropological Theory* 15, no. 3 (September 2015): 317–37. https://doi.org/10.1177/1463499615570919.

Sadana, Rashmi. *English Heart, Hindi Heartland: The Political Life of Literature in India.* Berkeley and Los Angeles: University of California Press, 2012.

Samuel, Geoffrey. *The Origins of Yoga and Tantra: Indic Religions to the Thirteenth Century.* Cambridge: Cambridge University Press, 2008.

Sarkar, Radha, and Amar Sarkar. "Sacred Slaughter: An Analysis of Historical, Communal, and Constitutional Aspects of Beef Bans in India." *Politics, Religion & Ideology* 17, no. 4 (October 2016): 329–51. https://doi.org/10.1080/21567689.2016.1259108.

Scarimbolo, Justin. "Brahmans Beyond Nationalism, Muslims Beyond Dominance: A Hidden History of North Indian Classical Music's Hinduization." PhD diss., University of California, Santa Barbara, 2014.

Schmidt, Michael S., and Eric Lichtblau. "Racial Profiling Rife at Airport, U.S. Officers Say." *The New York Times*, August 11, 2012. http://www.nytimes.com/2012/08/12/us/racial-profiling-at-boston-airport-officials-say.html?paewanted=all&_r=1.

Schnäbele, Verena. *Yoga in Modern Society.* Hamburg: Verlag Dr Kovac, 2010.

Sedlock v. Baird, No. 37-2013-00035910-CU-MC-CTL (Superior Court of San Diego County 2013).

Sen, Sharmila. *Not Quite Not White: Losing and Finding Race in America.* Gurgaon, Haryana: Penguin Viking, 2018.

Sharma, Pragati Ratti. "Yoga: A Multi-Billion Dollar Opportunity Market Poised to Grow." *Wellness India.com*, November 21, 2016. http://www.franchiseindia.com/wellness/Yoga-A-multi-billion-dollar-opportunity-market-poised-to-grow.8983.

Sharma, Sarah. *In the Meantime: Temporality and Cultural Politics.* Durham, NC: Duke University Press, 2014.

Sharma, Swati. "Here's What Narendra Modi's Fashion Says about His Politics." *The Washington Post*, January 26, 2015. https://www.washingtonpost.com/news/worldviews/wp/2014/06/06/heres-what-narendra-modis-fashion-says-about-his-politics/?utm_term=.5a9b8d699e80.

Shastry, Gauri Kartini. "Human Capital Response to Globalization: Education and Information Technology in India." *Journal of Human Resources* 47, no. 2 (2012): 287–330.

Shaw, Alison, and Esra S. Kaytaz. "Yoga Bodies, Yoga Minds: Contextualising the Health Discourses and Practices of Modern Postural Yoga." *Anthropology & Medicine* 28, no. 3 (2021): 279–96. https://doi.org/10.1080/13648470.2021.1949943.

"Shri Narendra Modi Shares His Vision for Digital India." February 7, 2014. http://www
.narendramodi.in/shri-narendra-modi-shares-his-vision-for-digital-india-5944.

"Siddha at a Glance." *Traditional Knowledge Digital Library.* Accessed January 31, 2023. http://
www.tkdl.res.in/tkdl/langdefault/Siddha/Sid_Siddha-Glance.asp?GL=Eng.

Siegel, Lee. *Trance-Migrations: Stories of India, Tales of Hypnosis.* Chicago: University of Chicago Press, 2014.

Siganporia, Harmony. "Who Dreams This Dreaming? Patanjali's Symbolic Usurpation of the Trope of the 'Enslaved' Indian Economy." *Continuum* 32, no. 6 (November 2, 2018): 758–69. https://doi.org/10.1080/10304312.2018.1525926.

Singh, IP, and Siddhartha Sarma. "'Ravana's Airports,' 'Modi Waves' Leave Science Congress Stunned." *The Times of India,* January 6, 2019. https://timesofindia.indiatimes .com/india/ravanas-airports-modi-waves-leave-science-congress-stunned/articleshow /67402208.cms.

Singh, Karan. "Nets of Maya: Gorakhnath as a Trickster Saint in the Folktale of Raja Bharthari and Gopi Chand." *Marvels & Tales* 32, no. 1 (2018). https://doi.org/10.13110/marvelstales .32.1.0013.

Singh, Manmohan. "PM's Remarks at Presentation of Kabir Puraskar and National Communal Harmony Awards." May 1, 2006. https://archivepmo.nic.in/drmanmohansingh /speech-details.php?nodeid=318.

Singh, Satya Prakash, ed. *History of Yoga.* New Delhi: Munshiram Manoharlal Publishers, 2010.

Singleton, Mark. *Yoga Body: The Origins of Modern Posture Practice.* New York: Oxford University Press, 2010.

Singleton, Mark, and Jean Byrne, eds. *Yoga in the Modern World: Contemporary Perspectives.* London and New York: Routledge, 2008.

Singleton, Mark, and Borayin Larios. "The Scholar-Practitioner of Yoga in the Western Academy." In *Routledge Handbook of Yoga and Meditation Studies,* ed. Suzanne Newcombe and Karen O'Brien-Kop, 37–50. Abingdon, UK: Routledge, 2021.

Smith, Benjamin Richard. "Body, Mind and Spirit? Towards an Analysis of the Practice of Yoga." *Body & Society* 13, no. 2 (June 2007): 25–46. https://doi.org/10.1177/1357034X07077771.

Smith, Matt, Jennifer Gollan, and Adithya Sambamurthy. "Job Brokers Steal Wages, Entrap Indian Tech Workers in US." *Reveal,* October 27, 2014. https://www.revealnews.org/article /job-brokers-steal-wages-entrap-indian-tech-workers-in-us/.

Smith, Sabrina, and Matthew Atencio. "'Yoga Is Yoga. Yoga Is Everywhere. You Either Practice or You Don't': A Qualitative Examination of Yoga Social Dynamics." *Sport in Society* 20, no. 9 (2017): 1167–84. https://doi-org.virtual.anu.edu.au/10.1080/17430437.2016 .1269082.

Spadola, Christine E., Rebecca Rottapel, Neha Khandpur, Emily Kontos, Suzanne M. Bertisch, Dayna A. Johnson, Mirja Quante, Sat Bir S. Khalsa, Robert B. Saper, and Susan Redline. "Enhancing Yoga Participation: A Qualitative Investigation of Barriers and Facilitators to Yoga among Predominantly Racial/Ethnic Minority, Low-Income Adults." *Complementary Therapies in Clinical Practice* 29 (November 2017): 97–104. https://doi.org /10.1016/j.ctcp.2017.09.001.

Stanley, Jessamyn. *Yoke: My Yoga of Self-Acceptance.* New York: Workman, 2021.

"State of California Hopes to Boost Trade Ties with India." *The Economic Times,* January 16, 2020. https://economictimes.indiatimes.com/news/economy/foreign-trade/state-of -california-hopes-to-boost-trade-ties-with-india/articleshow/73276995.cms.

Strauss, Sarah. *Positioning Yoga: Balancing Acts Across Cultures.* Oxford: Berg, 2005.

Strube, Julian. *Global Tantra: Religion, Science, and Nationalism in Colonial Modernity.* New York: Oxford University Press, 2022.

Suleri, Sara. *Meatless Days.* Chicago: University of Chicago Press, 1989.

Sunapee. "Is It Better to Apply for H1 as Software Professional or Yoga Instructor?" *Avvo,* October 11, 2012. https://www.avvo.com/legal-answers/is-it-better-to-apply-for-h1-as -software-professio-951850.html.

Surti, Aalif. "Annapurna Devi: The Tragedy And Triumph Of Ravi Shankar's First Wife." *Man's World India,* May 2000. https://www.mansworldindia.com/people/annapurna -devi-the-tragedy-and-triumph-of-ravi-shankars-first-wife/.

S-VYASA Swami Vivekandanda Yoga Anusandhana Samsthana. "Swami Vivekananda Yoga Anusandhana Samsthana—S-VYASA." Accessed May 16, 2019. https://svyasa.edu.in/#.

Swamy, Priya. "Neo-Hindutva Affective Economies: Feelings of Pride and Offense among Surinamese Hindus in the Netherlands." *Contemporary South Asia* 26, no. 4 (2018): 439– 52. https://doi.org/10.1080/09584935.2018.1545006.

Swarup, Vikas, ed. *International Day of Yoga.* New Delhi: MaXposture Media Group (1) Pvt Ltd., 2015.

Syman, Stefanie. *The Subtle Body: The Story of Yoga in America.* New York: Farrar, Straus and Giroux, 2010.

"Tamar Indien." *The Pioneer,* November 12, 1877.

Taneja, Shweta. *The Rakta Queen.* Noida, Uttar Pradesh: HarperCollins India, 2018.

Taylor, McComas. *Seven Days of Nectar: Contemporary Oral Performance of the Bhāgavatapurāṇa.* New York: Oxford University Press, 2016.

——. "'Stories of God': Contemporary Oral Performance of Bhāgavatakathā." *International Journal of Hindu Studies* 17, no. 3 (December 2013): 261–86. https://doi.org/10.1007/s11407 -014-9145-y.

Tenfelde, Sandi M., Lena Hatchett, and Karen L. Saban. "'Maybe Black Girls Do Yoga': A Focus Group Study with Predominantly Low-Income African-American Women." *Complementary Therapies in Medicine* 40 (October 2018): 230–35. https://doi.org/10.1016/j .ctim.2017.11.017.

"Testimony Given by Ronil Hira, Ph.D., P.E. in a Hearing Before the Judiciary Committee, U.S. Senate, on "Immigration Reforms Needed to Protect Skilled American Workers," March 17, 2015. http://www.judiciary.senate.gov/imo/media/doc/Hira%20Testimony.pdf.

"The Best Yoga Sequence to Do After Work." *Shape,* July 12, 2003. http://www.shape.com /blogs/working-it-out/best-yoga-sequence-do-after-work.

The Laughing Club of India. Dir. Mira Nair. Filmakers Library, 2002. https://video .alexanderstreet.com/watch/the-laughing-club-of-india.

The Uncommon Yogi: A History of Blacks and Yoga in the U.S. Dir. Jana Long, 2016. https:// www.youtube.com/watch?v=xQqSdB9PD38.

Thomas, Pradip N. "Traditional Knowledge and the Traditional Knowledge Digital Library: Digital Quandries and Other Concerns." *The International Communication Gazette* 72, no. 8 (2010): 659–73.

Timalsina, Sthaneshwar. "Songs of Transformation: Vernacular Josmanī Literature and the Yoga of Cosmic Awareness." *International Journal of Hindu Studies* 14, no. 2–3 (December 2010): 201–28. https://doi.org/10.1007/s11407-011-9091-x.

"Traditional Knowledge and Traditional Medicine." World Trade Organization. N.d. https://www.wto.org/english/tratop_e/trips_e/trilatweb_e/ch2d_trilat_web_13_e.htm.

Tribble, Evelyn B., and John Sutton. "Minds in and out of Time: Memory, Embodied Skill, Anachronism, and Performance." *Textual Practice* 26, no. 4 (August 2012): 587–607. https://doi.org/10.1080/0950236X.2012.696485.

Tripathy, Jyotirmaya. "Consuming Indigeneity: Baba Ramdev, Patanjali Ayurveda and the Swadeshi Project of Development." *Journal of Developing Societies* 35, no. 3 (September 2019): 412–30. https://doi.org/10.1177/0169796X19873213.

Truschke, Audrey. *Culture of Encounters: Sanskrit at the Mughal Court.* New York: Columbia University Press, 2016.

Tsioulcas, Anastasia. "She Was Poised To Be A Star—Instead, She Spent 60 Years In Her Apartment." *National Public Radio*, October 23, 2018. https://www.npr.org/2018/10/23/659786993/annapurna-devi-poised-star-surbahar-spent-60-years-her-apartment.

United Nations. Convention on Biological Diversity (1992). https://treaties.un.org/doc/Treaties/1992/06/19920605%2008-44%20 p.m./Ch_XXVII_08p.pdf.

United Nations A/Res/69/131 (2014). http://undocs.org/A/RES/69/131.

United States v. Bhagat Singh Thind. 261 U.S. 204, No. 204 (U.S. Supreme Court 1923).

Urban, Hugh B. *Tantra: Sex, Secrecy, Politics and Power in the Study of Religions.* Berkeley: University of California Press, 2003.

——. *Zorba the Buddha: Sex, Spirituality and Capitalism in the Global Osho Movement.* Oakland: University of California Press, 2015.

van der Veer, Peter. "Global Breathing: Religious Utopias in India and China." *Anthropological Theory* 7, no. 3 (September 2007): 315–28. https://doi.org/10.1177/1463499607080193.

Varma, Roli. "High-Tech Coolies: Asian Immigrants in the US Science and Engineering Workforce." *Science as Culture* 11, no. 3 (2002): 337–61.

Varughese, E. Dawson. "Celebrate at Home: Post-Millennial Indian Fiction in English and the Reception of 'Bharati Fantasy' in Global and Domestic Literary Markets." *Contemporary South Asia* 22, no. 4 (2014): 350–61. https://doi.org/10.1080/09584935.2014.963513.

Vazirani, Reetika. "From Patanjali." *Prairie Schooner* 75, no. 3 (Fall 2001): 75.

——. "The Art of Breathing." *Prairie Schooner* 75, no. 3 (Fall 2001): 63–74.

Vikram, Shringi Diva. "Mystery, Mythology and Masala." *The Hindu*, June 14, 2017. https://www.thehindu.com/books/books-authors/mystery-mythology-and-masala/article19047862.ece.

Vinoski, Erin, Jennifer B. Webb, Jan Warren-Findlow, Kirstyn A. Brewer, and Katheryn A. Kiffmeyer. "Got Yoga?: A Longitudinal Analysis of Thematic Content and Models' Appearance-Related Attributes in Advertisements Spanning Four Decades of *Yoga Journal.*" *Body Image* 21 (2017): 1–5.

Voix, Raphaël. "Denied Violence, Glorified Fighting: Spiritual Discipline and Contro-versy in Ananda Marga." *Nova Religio* 12, no. 1 (2008): 3–25. https://doi.org/10.1525/nr.2008.12.1.3.

——. "Hindu Ascetics and the Political in Contemporary India." In *Routledge Handbook of Yoga and Meditation Studies*, ed. Suzanne Newcombe and Karen O'Brien-Kop, 146–55. Abingdon, UK: Routledge, 2021.

"W+K's Incredible India! Campaign Puts Spotlight on Die-Hard Indophiles." *Campaign India*, January 22, 2009. https://www.campaignindia.in/article/wks-incredible-india-campaign-puts-spotlight-on-die-hard-indophiles/409566.

Wadhwa, Vivek, and Alex Salkever. *The Immigrant Exodus: Why America Is Losing the Global Race to Capture Entrepreneurial Talent*. Philadelphia: Wharton Digital Press, 2012.

Wagner, Shannon. "Workers Say They Were Manipulated into Free Labor For National Yoga Brand." *Vice*, October 30, 2020.

Warikoo, Niraj. "Ohio Woman Sues FBI, Airline for Racial Profiling." *USA Today*, January 22, 2013. http://www.usatoday.com/story/news/nation/2013/01/22/racial-profiling-lawsuit/1856619/.

Warth, Gary. "Yoga Funders Offer New Grant to EUSD." *The San Diego Union-Tribune*, July 31, 2013. http://www.sandiegouniontribune.com/news/2013/Jul/31/tp-yoga-funders-offer-new-grant-to-eusd/2/#article-copy.

Webb, Jennifer B., Erin R. Vinoski, Jan Warren-Findlow, Marlene I. Burrell, and Davina Y. Putz. "Downward Dog Becomes Fit Body, Inc.: A Content Analysis of 40 Years of Female Cover Images of *Yoga Journal*." *Body Image* 22 (2017): 129–35. https://doi.org/10.1016/j.bodyim.2017.07.001.

Webb, Jennifer B., Erin R. Vinoski, Jan Warren-Findlow, Meagan P. Padro, Elizabeth N. Bur-ris, and Elizabeth M. Suddreth. "Is the 'Yoga Bod' the New Skinny?" *Body Image* 20 (March 2017): 87–98. https://doi.org/10.1016/j.bodyim.2016.11.005.

Weber, Tracy. *Murder Strikes a Pose*. Woodbury, MN: Midnight Ink, 2013.

Weiss, Richard S. *Recipes for Immortality: Healing, Religion, and Community in South India*. New York: Oxford University Press, 2009.

White, David Gordon. *Sinister Yogis*. Chicago: University of Chicago Press, 2009.

——. *The Alchemical Body: Siddha Traditions in Medieval India*. Chicago: University of Chicago Press, 1996.

——. *The Yoga Sutra of Patanjali: A Biography*. Princeton, NJ and Oxford: Princeton University Press, 2014.

——, ed. *Yoga in Practice*. Princeton, NJ: Princeton University Press, 2011.

"Whose Yoga Is It Anyway?" *Tehelka*, June 21, 2016.

Wildcroft, Theodora. *Post-Lineage Yoga: From Guru to #MeToo*. Sheffield, UK: Equinox Ebooks Publishing, 2020.

Williams, R. John. *The Buddha in the Machine: Art, Technology, and the Meeting of East and West*. New Haven, CT: Yale University Press, 2014.

Wittich, Agi. "Iyengar Yoga for Women: A Practising Tradition in the Making." *Religions of South Asia* 11, no. 2–3 (August 1, 2018): 231–53. https://doi.org/10.1558/rosa.37025.

Wittich, Agi, and Patrick McCartney. "Changing Face of the Yoga Industry, Its Dharmic Roots and Its Message to Women: An Analysis of *Yoga Journal* Magazine Covers, 1975–2020." *Journal of Dharma Studies* 3 (2020): 31–44. https://doi.org/10.1007/s42240-020-00071-1.

Wong, Karen-Anne. "Inclusive Identities: The Lens of Critical Theory." In *Routledge Handbook of Yoga and Meditation Studies*, ed. Suzanne Newcombe and Karen O'Brien-Kop, 473–89. Abingdon, UK: Routledge, 2021.

Wouters, Jelle J.P., and Tanka B. Subba. "The 'Indian Face,' India's Northeast, and 'The Idea of India.'" *Asian Anthropology* 12, no. 2 (December 2013): 126–40. https://doi.org/10.1080/1683478X.2013.849484.

Xiang Biao. *Global "Body Shopping": An Indian Labor System in the Information Technology Industry*. Princeton, NJ: Princeton University Press, 2007.

"Yoga Industry Growth, Market Trends & Analysis 2021." Wellness Creative Co., January 21, 2021. https://www.wellnesscreatives.com/yoga-industry-trends/.

"Yoga Teacher Training." *Data USA*. Accessed August 31, 2016. http://datausa.io/profile/cip/513602/#demographics.

"Yoga to Be Made Compulsory in Schools." *DNA: Daily News and Analysis*, May 6, 2016. http://www.dnaindia.com/india/report-yoga-to-be-made-compulsory-in-schools-govt-2209866.

"Yoga Town Episode 5—TLC, Tandoori Loving Care." Dir. Tracy D. Smith. *Yoga Town*, 2013. http://watchyogatown.com/watch-the-show/.

Yogananda, Paramahansa. *Autobiography of a Yogi*. Los Angeles: Self-Realization Fellowship, 1946.

Young, James O. *Cultural Appropriation and the Arts*. Hoboken, NJ: Wiley, 2010.

Young, James O., and Susan Haley. "'Nothing Comes from Nowhere': Reflections on Cultural Appropriation as the Representation of Other Cultures." In *The Ethics of Cultural Appropriation*, ed. James O. Young and Conrad G. Brunk, 268–89. Malden, MA: Wiley-Blackwell, 2009.

Yu, Timothy. "Asian American Poetry in the First Decade of the 2000s." *Contemporary Literature* 52, no. 4 (Winter 2011): 818–51.

Ziff, Bruce, and Pratima V. Rao, eds. *Borrowed Power: Essays on Cultural Appropriation*. New Brunswick, NJ: Rutgers University Press, 1997.

INDEX

body (*continued*)
137–38; sedentary, 151; spread of yoga, 5,
14; subtle, 45; superhuman, 44;
svādhyāya, 31–34, 46, 196, 200;
technologized, 158–59, 247n49; thin
white, 172; United States, 116
body image, 45
body shops, 161–62
Bollywood, 12, 44, 76, 234n105, 234n1
bookstores, 69, 83–86, 104, 109
border management, 102, 104, 109, 117
borders, 11, 88; cross-cultural
representation, 16, 85, 139; fiction, 102;
India, 44, 68, 87, 102, 109; selfhood, 215
breathing, 33, 46, 111–12, 125, 192–97,
199–200, 205–6; Incredible India, 61–62;
India Brand Equity Foundation, 6; race,
193, 196
breathing practices, 67, 252n31, 263
Britain, 73, 244n68
Buddhism, 93, 109, 127, 129–30, 247n49

capitalism, global, 14–15, 21, 37, 62–63, 151,
159, 164
Chavez, Cesar, 116
China, 41, 43, 58, 63, 67, 102, 115, 124, 172,
203; tourism videos, 8; yoga studios, 57
Christian perspectives, 41, 81, 124–25,
135
Corpse Pose, 119
courts, 37, 73, 116, 125–29
crowds, 43, 64, 75–77, 81
cultural appropriation, 139, 179;
#WhitePeopleDoingYoga, 190; as
cross-cultural exchange, 181; emotional
energy, 184–85; as injury, 182; as inquiry,
185, 205; museum controversy, 187; as
norms of cultural correctness, 181; as
performative, 184; in philosophy, 184,
251n15; as uneven spread of benefits, 183

Devanagari script, 2, 63, 158
Downward-Facing Death, 121–22

economic liberalization, 12, 24, 163
empathy, 178
empire, 27, 115
Encinitas, CA, 124–26, 128, 130; school
district, 126, 139
enclosing, of nations, 19–20
English, 7–8, 50, 60, 235n1, 256, 266; B. K. S.
Iyengar, 30, 225n95; border zone, 3;
colonialism and capitalism, 9;
contradictions in ideas of India, 6;
creative visions of yoga, 3, 5, 10–11, 30, 35;
discourse of International Day of Yoga,
70; Encinitas, CA, 124; flexibility, 22;
flexible India, 11; Guru English, 9; in
India, 9, 49–50, 84–85, 87, 160, 220n24,
234n1; Incredible India, 60; Indianness,
9–11, 50; market advantage, 50; modern
yoga, 9; *svādhyāya*, 25, 30; Traditional
Knowledge Digital Library, 67;
transformations of colonial modernity,
4; and yoga, 9; yoga studios, 158

fiction, 4, 17, 35, 37, 86, 89–90, 97–98, 108–9,
132, 145, 151
Fit India Movement, 24
fitness, 4, 22, 24, 131; capitalism, 23; media,
134; pandemic, 24; physical, 52, 57;
flexibility, 17, 43, 206; capitalism, 23, 38,
142–43, 145, 169; concealed
contradictions, 20, 35, 37, 48, 87, 91, 103,
110, 146, 179; in English, 22; flexible
citizenship, 18–19; gender, 23, 94, 144,
150; health and fitness, 22; Indian
diaspora, 16, 19–21, 140, 179–80, 195, 200,
205; Indianness, 88, 97, 109, 191, 201–3;
jugaad, 21; national enclosure, 19;
personhood, 22; plasticity, 18; precarity,
144, 150, 171; folklore, 50, 53, 82, 92, 119,
226n6; freedom, 8, 14, 38–39, 142, 144, 193

Gandhi, Indira, 53
Gandhi, Mohandas K., 51–52, 62, 72, 101, 125
Google, 159